UCB

D1343897

NAILS

Level 2

Lindsey Anderson
Alice Avenell
Lisa Kniveton

www.pearsonschoolsandfecolleges.co.uk

✓ Free online support
✓ Useful weblinks
✓ 24 hour online ordering

0845 630 44 44

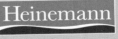

Heinemann

Part of Pearson

Heinemann is an imprint of Pearson Education Limited, Edinburgh Gate, Harlow, Essex, CM20 2JE.

www.pearsonschoolsandfecolleges.co.uk

Heinemann is a registered trademark of Pearson Education Limited

Text © Pearson Education Ltd, 2011
Edited by Susan Ross and Helen Atkinson
Designed by Pearson Education
Original illustrations © Pearson Education, 2011
Illustrated by nb illustrations/Ben Hasler
Cover design by Woodenark Studio
Picture research by Sally Cole
Cover photo/illustration © Pearson Education Ltd/Stuart Cox

The rights of Lisa Kniveton, Lindsey Anderson and Alice Avenell to be identified as authors of this work have been asserted by them in accordance with the Copyright, Designs and Patents Act 1988.

First published 2011

14 13 12 11
10 9 8 7 6 5 4 3 2 1

British Library Cataloguing in Publication Data
A catalogue record for this book is available from the British Library

ISBN 978 0 435 04755 9

Copyright notice
All rights reserved. No part of this publication may be reproduced in any form or by any means (including photocopying or storing it in any medium by electronic means and whether or not transiently or incidentally to some other use of this publication) without the written permission of the copyright owner, except in accordance with the provisions of the Copyright, Designs and Patents Act 1988 or under the terms of a licence issued by the Copyright Licensing Agency, Saffron House, 6–10 Kirby Street, London EC1N 8TS (www.cla.co.uk). Applications for the copyright owner's written permission should be addressed to the publisher.

Typeset by Phoenix Photosetting, Chatham, Kent
Printed in the UK by Scotprint

Websites
The websites used in this book were correct and up to date at the time of publication. It is essential for tutors to preview each website before using it in class so as to ensure that the URL is still accurate, relevant and appropriate. We suggest that tutors bookmark useful websites and consider enabling students to access them through the school/college intranet.

Acknowledgements
The authors and publisher would like to thank the following individuals and organisations for permission to reproduce photographs:
(Key: b-bottom; c-centre; l-left; r-right; t-top)

Alamy Images: Dmitry Goygel-Sokol 28, Foodfolio 21, Jack Sullivan 148, 151b, 157c, Jeffery Blacker 46b; **Camera Press Ltd:** Kruell laif 112; **Ciate:** 72, 72c, 72b; **Corbis:** Bridge 163, Herry Choi 100, Sonja Pacho 223; **cut2white:** 21t, 93, 169t; **Denise Wright:** 270, 276r; **Getty Images:** Ariel Skelley 47c, Jonathan Storey 147, Martin Barraud / Stone 47t; **Image courtesy of The Advertising Archives:** 267; **John Grace:** 196tl; **Masterfile UK Ltd:** 1; **Mediscan:** 150b; **Minx Inc:** Brandon Wiggins 85, 119; **Pearson Education Ltd:** Stuart Cox 9, 9bc, 19, 23/5, 37, 40, 45t, 55, 65, 113, 121, 186c, 186b, 195, 196b, 198, 198t, 199, 200, 200b, 201, 202, 204, 204t, 205t, 205c, 205b, 206, 207, 210t, 210l, 210r, 210bc, 212l, 212c, 212r, 212b, 213t, 213r, 214t, 214b, 215t, 215b, 216t, 216b, 217t, 228, 233t, 233b, 234, 235, 239, 240/1, 240/2, 240/3, 240/4, 240/5, 240/6, 243/1, 243/2, 243/3, 243/4, 245/1, 245/2, 245/3, 245/4, 245/5, 245/6, 246, 247, 248, 249, 249/2, 249/3, 249/5, 249/6, 250/1, 250/3, 250/4, 250/5, 250/6, 251/1, 251/2, 251/3, 251/4, 251/7, 251/8, 252/1, 252/2, 252/3, 252/4, 253/5, 253/6, 261; Gareth Boden 23, 24, 31, 171, 176tr, 176cl, 176cr, 176bl, 176br; Mindstudio 7tl, 7tr, 7bl, 7br, 18, 36, 39tl, 39tr, 39b, 45, 45bl, 46t, 50, 51, 68, 81, 84, 91, 165tr, 175, 175b, 176tl, 177t, 177b, 179, 179bl, 180/3, 180/4, 180/5, 180/6, 180/7, 180/8, 181/9, 181/10, 181/11, 181/12, 181/13, 181/14, 182/15, 182/16, 182/17, 182/19, 182/20, 183/1, 183/2, 183/3, 183/4, 184/7, 184/8, 184/9, 184/10, 185/11, 185/12, 186, 187, 197, 209tl, 209tr, 209r, 278/18; **Photolibrary.com:** Adam Gault 66, Datacraft Co Ltd 165br, Jay Baker 75, Mendil 160c, Trinette Reed / BlendImages 47b; **Science Photo Library Ltd:** 152, 156cl, BSIP, Jolyot 160, Cordelia Molloy 9t, Custom Medical Stock photo 151c, Dr H.C.Robinson 156c, Dr P. Marazzi 150, 151, 152c, 153, 153t, 154, 155tl, 155c, 155cl, 155b, 156b, 157, 157t, 158t, 159c, 159cl, 160b, 208b, 255; Francoise Sauze 159b, JANE SHEMILT 151cl, 152b; MEDICAL PHOTO NHS LOTHIAN 159, Mike Devlin 158b, 208, Science Photo Library 152cl, 154c, 156, 156tl; ST BARTHOLOMEW'S HOSPITAL 155t, Steve Gschmeissner 122, 127cr, Susumu Nishinaga 127t; **Shutterstock.com:** Anton Albert 231, Blend Images 118, Brian Chase 265, Dima Kalinin 42, grublee 67, iofoto 48, 167, Karoline Cullen 274, Konstantin Stepanenko 276, l i g h t p o e t 32, PashOK 80, RamonaS 217b, Ruslan Kudrin 174, Sakala 60, Sheftsoff 83; **Sweet Squared:** 172; **The Carlton Group:** 25; **www.imagesource.com:** 35.
All other images © Pearson Education

Every effort has been made to contact copyright holders of material reproduced in this book. Any omissions will be rectified in subsequent printings if notice is given to the publishers.

The authors and publisher would also like to thank the following organisations for their assistance with the cover shoot: Nailtopia (Nail art items and Toma nail varnish were provided by Nailtopia Ltd, www.nailtopia.co.uk, 020 8674 8824, info@nailtopia.co.uk); NSI (NSI (UK) Ltd, James Nasmyth Way, Eccles, Manchester M30 0SF; Website: www.nsinails.co.uk; Tel: 0161 788 2860).

Grateful thanks go to Keeley Dennyschene for her assistance at the cover shoot, her help with photo selection and for resolving authoring queries in the Nail extensions unit. Her expertise and professional approach were greatly appreciated.

Our thanks also go to Angie Walker for her assistance with authoring of the Nail Art unit.

Contents

The answers to *Check your knowledge* have been provided on the Pearson Education website.
Visit the following link: www.pearsonfe.co.uk/Level2Nailsanswers

Introduction

Why choose a career in the nail industry?

The nail industry is one of the most creative fields and having a career in nails can take you to some of the most interesting places both globally and professionally. A career as a nail technician can suit all different types of lifestyles, career interests and aspirations. It will allow you to create a fulfilling and rewarding career pathway. Being a nail technician can be versatile — it can be a full-time or part-time profession. Freelance technicians can fit their clients around other commitments. You can also aspire to work in a range of environments, including:

- specialised nail studios or bars
- spas
- hotels
- health farms or health clubs
- cruise liners
- hair and beauty salons
- fashion and modelling companies.

This profession focuses on specific areas including the hands, arms, legs and feet. They are possibly the most intensively used areas of the body and they require the most maintenance to stay healthy and attractive.

VRQs and Diplomas

What are VRQs and Diplomas (NVQ)s?

Diplomas (formerly NVQs — National Vocational Qualifications) are related to the National Occupational Standards. They are competence-based qualifications and identify that a person is work-ready. To complete a Diploma, you must perform treatments and demonstrate skills on real, paying clients, in a realistic working environment under commercial pressures and within commercially acceptable service times.

VRQs (Vocationally Related Qualifications) are also based on the National Occupational Standards. They combine the academic and practical skills necessary to prepare a person for work or further studies. VRQs are not competence-based qualifications, so anyone completing a VRQ will require further training from their employer once they are working in industry. You will not be required to work on real, paying clients, in a realistic working environment under commercial pressures and within commercially acceptable service times. However, you will still develop employability skills.

How do I gain a VRQ or Diploma (NVQ) in Level 2 Nail Services?

You must complete the mandatory units and selected optional units that your place of study will discuss with you. The qualification you choose will determine the units you will study — see the example below.

VRQs – Level 2 Certificate in Nail Technology	Level 2 Diploma (NVQ) in Beauty Therapy (Nail Services)
Core mandatory units:	**Core mandatory units:**
• Working in beauty-related industries • Follow health and safety practice in the salon • Client care and communication in beauty-related industries • Promote products and services to clients in a salon • Provide and maintain nail enhancement	• Fulfil salon reception duties • Develop and maintain your effectiveness at work • Promote additional services or products to clients • Ensure responsibility for actions to reduce risks to health and safety • Provide manicure services • Provide pedicure services • Carry out nail art services • Apply and maintain nail enhancements to create a natural finish

How will I be assessed ?

Both Diplomas (NVQs) and VRQs consist of observed practical assessments and tasks to test your knowledge and understanding, such as multiple-choice questions. Your place of study will explain the assessment methods for your chosen qualification.

What progression opportunities do I have?

After achieving a Level 2 Nail Services qualification, you can progress onto Level 3 Nail Services. Alternatively, you could take short courses in specific skills at Level 2, such as acrylic nails.

How do I use this book?

This book maps the units from both the Diploma (NVQ) and VRQ qualifications and focuses on the theory and practical-based knowledge you need to know. It also covers the underpinning knowledge of anatomy and physiology, skin and nail analysis that you will need to support the practical units. The learning features of the book will help to reinforce the knowledge and understanding you must utilise to assist you in the application of your practical skills and theory.

Learning features

- **Salon life** (my story):
  - Personal experiences of people from the nail industry sharing problems they have had at work. These also reflect upon how the individual overcame their problems and the valuable lessons they learned. You will be encouraged to assess what you might have done in their place or reflect on a problem that you might have already experienced.
  - Benefits of offering particular services, from both the client's and nail technician's view point. These will help you to understand why you offer these services and their importance to your career and the business as a whole.
  - Ask the experts. These include commonly asked questions with expert answers.
- **Think about it:** short activities to help you remember valuable information from that unit.
- **Check it out:** short tasks or activities to help you apply the theory you have learned and to generate evidence for your assessments.
- **Frequently asked questions:** commonly asked questions with expert answers.
- **Key terms:** tricky or unfamiliar words with an explanation of their meanings. These usually involve nail terminology that it is important you understand fully.
- **Top tips:** expert tips or suggestions to make you aware of important information to promote good practice.
- **Check your knowledge:** questions at the end of each unit to test your knowledge. They will be either multiple-choice or short-answer questions.
- **Getting ready for assessment:** guidance notes on the unit to help prepare you for assessments in either the Diploma (NVQ) or VRQ qualification.

The mapping grid on the next page demonstrates how this book supports a range of qualifications. GLH stands for guided learning hours.

UCB
179799

	Level 2 (NVQ) Diploma Nail Services GLH 329 40 credits	VTCT L2 Certificate in Nail Treatments GLH 183 20 credits	VTCT Level 2 Certificate in Nail Technologies GLH 162 20 credits	City & Guilds Level 2 Certificate in Nail Technology GLH 149 19 credits	City & Guilds Level 2 Diploma in Nail Technology Enhancement GLH 460 55 credits	City & Guilds Level 2 Diploma in Nail Technology Services GLH 320 37 credits	City & Guilds Level 2 Certificate in Nail Art GLH 151 18 credits	City & Guilds Level 2 Certificate in Manicure GLH 151 17 credits	City & Guilds Level 2 Certificate in Pedicure GLH 151 17 credits
Follow health and safety practice in the salon (G20)	Mandatory	Mandatory	Mandatory	Mandatory	Mandatory	Mandatory	Mandatory	Mandatory	Mandatory
Client care and communication in beauty-related industries (G7 L2 Hairdressing)		Mandatory	Mandatory	Mandatory	Mandatory	Mandatory	Mandatory	Mandatory	Mandatory
Display stock to promote sales in a salon (G18)*	Optional								
Promote products and services to clients in a salon (G18)	Mandatory			Mandatory	Mandatory		Mandatory	Mandatory	Mandatory
Salon reception duties (G4)	Mandatory				Mandatory	Mandatory	Mandatory		
Create an image based on a theme within the hair and beauty sector					Mandatory	Mandatory			
Working in beauty-related industries				Mandatory	Mandatory	Mandatory	Mandatory	Mandatory	Mandatory
Provide manicure treatments (N2)	Mandatory	Mandatory	Mandatory	Mandatory	Mandatory	Mandatory		Mandatory	
Provide pedicure treatments (N3)	Mandatory	Mandatory	Optional		Mandatory	Mandatory			Mandatory
Provide and maintain nail enhancement (N5)	Optional	Optional	Mandatory	Mandatory	Mandatory	Mandatory			
Provide nail art (N4)	Mandatory	Optional	Optional				Mandatory		

Follow health and safety practice in the salon

What you will learn

- Maintain health, safety and security practices
- Follow emergency procedures

Introduction

A successful nail studio will always appear to be working efficiently and professionally to clients and the public. Behind the scenes, it is very important that health and safety is maintained. A client may only notice if the salon appears to be clean and tidy on the surface, but it is also the responsibility of the employees to sanitise and sterilise the working areas, tools and equipment. This will prevent cross-infection and harm to others. This unit will explore the health and safety legislation and workplace policies that help to protect employees and clients from harm, including what to do in the event of an emergency.

Maintain health, safety and security practices

As a successful nail technician, one of the most important aspects of your career will be health and safety. The way you work will have an impact on your clients, colleagues, the business and yourself. You will be expected to understand, follow and enforce all relevant health and safety laws and to comply with the **health and safety policies** of your employer or place of study. You will need to be able to identify potential **hazards** and **risks** so that you help to prevent accidents or incidents from occurring in the salon. Clients will not necessarily be aware that health and safety procedures are being followed, so often potential dangers will not be spotted by them — it is your responsibility, as the nail technician, to be vigilant at all times. You will need to create a professional, safe, hygienic and relaxing work environment so that your client feels safe, confident and relaxed. You should have regular health and safety meetings with your team to ensure you always have the most up-to-date information.

The difference between legislation, codes of practice and workplace policies

Legislation

Legislation is the set of laws made by government and passed as Acts of Parliament. Acts are the law of the land and must be followed by both businesses and individuals. Health and safety laws are designed to create a safe environment for everyone in the salon. If, by not following the law, a business or technician causes injury to a client, this is a criminal offence, which could lead to prosecution and may result in fines, the business closing or even imprisonment.

In addition to legislation, there are local government by-laws set by local authorities and **European Union (EU) laws**, which relate to health, safety, hygiene and treatments that use a needle or piercings.

Codes of practice

Industry codes of practice set out professional guidelines on all aspects of being a nail technician. They offer information on how to achieve high standards and

Key terms

Health and safety policies – health and safety rules that employees must follow to ensure everyone's personal health and safety.

Hazard – something that has the potential to cause an accident or harm (injury).

Risk – the likelihood of a hazard causing an accident or harm.

Legislation – laws passed by Parliament.

European Union (EU) laws – laws passed by the European Union (27 countries including the UK) that must be followed by all EU countries.

describe what is acceptable. Habia, the body that sets the standards for the UK nail industry, publishes a Code of Practice for Nail Services, which covers:

- client consultation and aftercare advice
- dress code
- infection control and hygiene
- electric nail files
- operating procedures
- ventilation
- salon safety
- insurance
- training, education, **CPD** and qualifications
- mobile technicians.

Workplace policies

Workplace policies are designed to maintain a safe environment for all and provide a detailed explanation of how to achieve this. By referring to health and safety legislation and codes of practice, nail services businesses are able to create workplace policies specific to the industry. These policies specify the things that must be provided by the employer or manager. They include:

- creating a health and safety policy that must be adhered to
- completing **risk assessments** for all activities that occur in the workplace, for example performing fibreglass nails or refilling bottles of enamel remover
- providing first aid facilities and a designated and trained first aider(s)
- creating emergency procedures, including fire evacuation
- appointing a health and safety officer to whom staff would report any accidents, hazards or risks and who would be responsible for taking appropriate action such as staff training in using the autoclave correctly or what to do in the event of a spillage.

The employer or manager is responsible for ensuring that employees understand health and safety laws and workplace policies and for enforcing safe working practices, including:

- washing and sterilising tools
- sterilisation and sensitisation of working area
- dress code and salon hygiene rules
- storing tools, products and equipment correctly
- what to do in the event of an accident or incident
- what to do in the event of a spillage or breakage
- how to dispose of waste correctly
- which personal protective equipment to use and to ensure it is used.

Check it out

The Health and Safety Executive (HSE) publishes guidance on all areas of health and safety. Search the HSE website for current publications.

Key term

CPD – continual professional development. Technicians attend training sessions to stay abreast of new developments in the nail industry. To learn more about CPD, see Working in beauty-related industries, page 116.

Check it out

Look at the Code of Practice for Nail Services on the Habia website.

Key term

Risk assessments – the identification of possible health and safety risks, creating a safer environment for all.

Course:		Course Code:		Day:	Time:
Hazard – likelihood	Tick if applies	Tick if info leaflet given	Tick if specific advice given	Tick if formal assessment made (Head of Curriculum only)	Controls in place
Slips, trips and falls					
Electrical equipment in use					
Blockage of fire escape					
Use of furniture as a hazard					
Hazardous substances					
Trailing wires					
Increased fire risk					
Fumes					
Physical exercise					
Manual handling					
Lone working					
Tools being used					
Sharp objects being used					
Ergonomics (IT)					
Food and drink (IT)					
Electrical equipment owned by tutor/learner must have a valid Portable Appliance Test (PAT)					
At-risk learner(s) (Give name and nature of risk – Please use separate sheet if more room is required)					
Signature:				Date:	
Job role:					

An example of a risk assessment used in training

Everyone who works in a nail bar, salon or spa must comply with health and safety legislation, codes of practice and workplace policies, but there should always be a key person who ensures that everyone complies.

The main provisions of health and safety legislation

There are many health and safety laws that nail technicians must adhere to. The Health and Safety at Work Act 1974 is the main legislation covering health and safety in the UK. It provides the rules that must be followed by employers, employees and the self-employed and also enables other health and safety regulations to be made.

Top tip

When starting your own business, you will need to contact the HSE who will inspect your workplace. Inspection requirements vary depending upon your location, so check out the HSE website and contact your local authority for specific information for your area.

As a nail technician, the legislation that you will need to be aware of is covered below.

Health and Safety at Work Act (HASAW) 1974

The act aims to provide a safe working environment for employers, employees and clients. Employees and employers are expected to care for the health and safety of others and cooperate with each other to ensure this happens.

The employer has a duty to:

- keep all doorways and walkways clear to prevent an accident and to ensure access to fire exits

- ensure staff are adequately trained

- provide storage for equipment and products.

Employees need to be constantly aware of potential hazards and dangers in the workplace. They must:

- comply with **PPE** regulations, for example by wearing gloves, an apron, mask and protective goggles

- report accidents to the health and safety officer or the manager and ensure an accident report form has been completed

- report faulty equipment and label it 'faulty'.

The Workplace (Health, Safety and Welfare) Regulations 1992

These regulations are designed to ensure a healthy and safe working environment. They require the employer to provide:

- regular, scheduled maintenance and daily checks of the salon and equipment

- correct **environmental conditions** — including adequate ventilation with extractor fans or air filtration at the nail desk/station, reasonable room temperature (minimum 16°C), good natural lighting and client comfort

- correct disposal of waste

- a clean and hygienic salon

- workstations and stools of the correct size and height

- a safe walkway with no obstructions or damaged/uneven floors

- amenities — including toilet facilities, washing facilities, drinking water, kitchen facilities, changing room facilities with storage for personal effects and a break-time seating area

- safety glass and locks on all doors and windows.

RISK ASSESSMENT FORM:

NAME OF EQUIPMENT:

Paraffin wax heater

STEP 1 WHAT ARE THE HAZARDS?

Accident:
- heater on unstable surface
- trailing wires
- faulty plug casing
- equipment not serviced regularly
- faulty equipment
- testing the temperature of the wax on technician and/or client before use

STEP 2 WHO MIGHT BE HARMED?

Client
General public
Nail technician
All staff

WHAT IS ALREADY IN PLACE?

Equipment regularly serviced
PAT tested
Regular and updated risk assessments
Follow manufacturer's instructions
Staff training of equipment
Heater securely positioned on a stable work surface
Wires are not trailing

WHAT FURTHER ACTION COULD BE TAKEN?

Training new staff in safe use of the heater
Regular visual safety check of treatment areas and the equipment
Continual regular servicing, PAT and updated risk assessments

| The **risk rating** is: 10 | The **probability rating** is: 2 | The **severity rating** is: 2-5 |

Example of workplace risk assessment

PPE – personal protective equipment. These are items such as gloves, towels and gowns that protect the technician, client and working area from damage.

Environmental conditions – the environment within a workplace in terms of temperature, lighting, ventilation and so on.

Follow health and safety practice in the salon

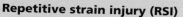

Top tip

Ensure your working area has enough space, especially around your trolley and equipment. This will enable you to perform an effective treatment safely.

Check it out

After reading about the Workplace (Health, Safety and Welfare) Regulations 1992, evaluate your workplace. Does it meet the law's requirements?

Key term

Repetitive strain injury (RSI) – injury that occurs from performing a treatment using bad posture and over-stretching, throughout each working day. Over time it will cause posture problems, including muscular and skeletal damage and pain.

Suitable environmental conditions in the workplace are essential to produce outstanding results:

- Good lighting enables technicians to prevent the incorrect application of products.

- Correct working temperatures ensure good product results – some products will not work effectively if conditions are too hot or too cold.

- Adequate ventilation ensures that the salon is a pleasant place to work – extraction units remove dusty, unclean air and strong odours and replace them with clean air.

- Comfortable working conditions prevent technicians suffering from **repetitive strain injury (RSI)** or muscular and skeletal pain.

The Provision and Use of Work Equipment Regulations 1998

The regulations cover the maintenance of equipment, its use and training.

- Equipment must be fit for purpose with regular, scheduled maintenance by a competent person, preferably a qualified electrician, every six months.

- Technicians must be trained by the manufacturer before using any piece of equipment.

- It is the employer's responsibility to organise regular training for all technicians.

- Technicians must only use the equipment for its intended purpose.

- Always follow the manufacturer's instructions to prevent injury or damage to the equipment.

The Manual Handling Operations Regulations 1992

The employer must carry out a risk assessment on employees for manual lifting and handling at work. Employees need training on how to handle and lift heavier items, to prevent muscular or skeletal damage and repetitive strain injury (RSI).

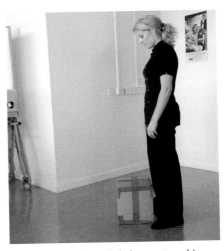

Position your feet slightly apart and in line with your shoulders.

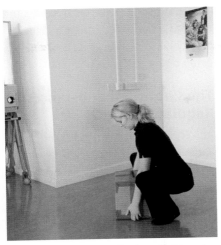

Bend down with your back straight and hold the box securely in your hands.

Top tip

If you are placing a box on a shelf, ask for help and use a safe ladder, never a chair. Never lift a box that is too heavy or too wide. Always ask for help or, if appropriate, use a trolley.

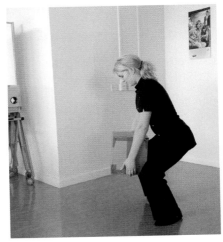

Lift up the box and push up with your feet and legs, keeping your back straight – do not use your back to pull up the weight of the box.

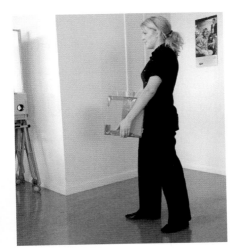

Carry the box close to your body.

The Personal Protective Equipment at Work Regulations 1992 and Personal Protective Equipment Regulations 2002

Personal protective equipment (PPE) is designed to protect employees and clients from injuries, damage to clothing or the working area during a treatment. The employer must supply PPE, train staff how to use it and ensure that they use it.

PPE consists of:

- for the technician – gloves, apron, safety glasses and mask
- for the client – towel, paper or plastic covers, a gown
- for the working area – towels and plastic or paper covers.

Top tip

Chemical products can be **toxic** and flammable, and may be absorbed via the skin, eyes, nose or mouth, causing damage. Ensure you always follow PPE guidelines.

Key terms

Chemical products – for example enamel remover, fibreglass resin.

Toxic – poisonous, harmful

Check it out

Find three products in your workplace and read the manufacturer's instructions. Does the client need a skin test before use? How should you use, handle, store and dispose of them (COSHH)? Have you been using these products correctly?

Top tip

When dealing with damaged or leaking chemical containers, always wear PPE to protect you from harmful exposure.

The employer is expected to carry out risk assessments to decide what PPE is required for each treatment or activity. Employees are responsible for maintaining the condition of PPE and must report any damage or low stock levels to the salon manager.

The Control of Substances Hazardous to Health (COSHH) Regulations 2002

All employees must understand the health and safety implications of how **chemical products** are used, handled, stored and disposed of and their potential harm if procedures are not followed. Employers are responsible for ensuring employees comply with these regulations and that they are trained correctly to control exposure to substances hazardous to health in the workplace.

Exposure to harmful products can be reduced or prevented by:

- following the correct procedures for use, handling, storage and disposal
- reading the manufacturer's instructions before use — especially if you change to another company's product
- performing risk assessments on all products and training staff before use.

The employer is responsible for carrying out risk assessments covering the following areas, as shown on the product's COSHH leaflet.

- Use — for example, does a skin test need to be performed?
- Handling — for example, are protective gloves, a mask, glasses and an apron required?
- Storage — for example, does it need to be stored in a dry, dark, cool, locked cupboard or storeroom?
- Disposal — for example, what are the manufacturer's instructions and local by-laws concerning disposal? Is the product toxic? If so, do not dispose of it down the sink or it will contaminate the water supply.

Chemicals should be clearly labelled to state if they are hazardous and harmful. The labels to look out for are shown below.

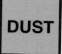
Dust

Toxic   Flammable

Irritant   Corrosive

Oxidising agent

COSHH labels that are used to warn about hazardous chemicals

8

The Electricity at Work Regulations 1989

These regulations cover the use of electrical equipment in the salon.

- All electrical equipment must be checked by a competent person, preferably a qualified electrician, every six months.

- Employees must be trained to use electrical equipment by the manufacturer.

- Always follow manufacturer's instructions regarding use and storage of equipment to prevent injury.

- Employees must check electrical equipment before using it on a client (visual check first — check the wires, the plug and the machine, before switching on to check if it is working). They should report faulty equipment and label it 'faulty'. These electrical safety checks are known as portable appliance testing (PAT) and must meet the Institution of Electrical Engineers (IEE) code of practice for in-service inspection and testing of electrical equipment. Only a qualified PAT tester can perform a PAT test, as they will need to have obtained a level of competency.

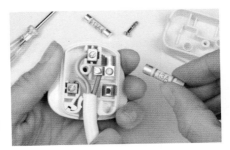

Have you been trained to change a fuse in a plug?

The Health and Safety (Display Screen Equipment) Regulations 1992 (amended 2002)

These regulations aim to provide a safe working environment for staff working on computers. The employer must provide information and training for employees to enable them to use computers safely and also undertake a risk assessment to check that:

- computer desks or workstations are at the correct height, with adequate space to work

- computer chairs have a back support and are at the correct height (a foot stool must be provided if your feet do not touch the ground)

- work is planned to ensure regular breaks

- employees have eyesight tests on request and special spectacles if required.

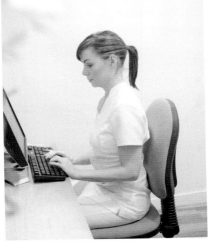

Correct posture will prevent muscular or skeletal injury

Check it out

Practise performing electrical checks when you are not busy. Find a piece of equipment:

- Is there a label on it stating when it had a professional service (should be every six months)?

- Check for faulty wires, plugs, loose cables, safety lights (on/off/ heating and so on).

- Does it perform well?

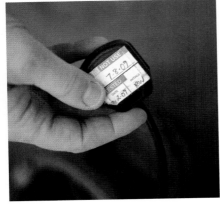

After portable appliance testing, the electrical professional will place a sticker on your equipment stating the date it passed

Top tips

- Turn all equipment off or to zero before switching off at the electric socket, so that it does not create a hazard when it is next used.

- When working at the computer, make sure you sit correctly and have adequate working space. Take regular breaks to avoid eye strain, mental stress, repetitive strain injury and muscular and skeletal pains.

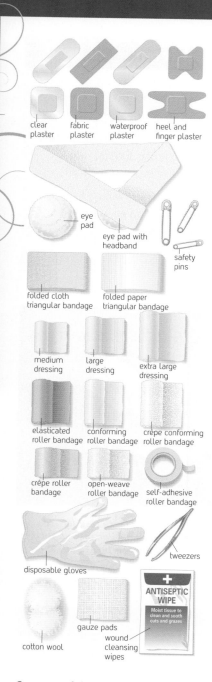

clear plaster

fabric plaster

waterproof plaster

heel and finger plaster

eye pad

eye pad with headband

safety pins

folded cloth triangular bandage

folded paper triangular bandage

medium dressing

large dressing

extra large dressing

elasticated roller bandage

conforming roller bandage

crêpe conforming roller bandage

crêpe roller bandage

open-weave roller bandage

self-adhesive roller bandage

disposable gloves

tweezers

cotton wool

gauze pads

wound cleansing wipes

Contents of the first aid box

Key term

Reportable disease – a work-related disease such as occupational dermatitis, infections like hepatitis or tetanus, or certain poisonings. See the HSE website for a full list.

The Health and Safety (First-Aid) Regulations 1981

To comply with the regulations, the employer should provide first aid facilities on the premises with a first aid box that is fully stocked. There should be a designated first aider who is fully trained and first aid procedures in place in case of an accident or illness.

An example of a first aid box:

- a leaflet giving guidance on first aid
- individually wrapped sterile adhesive dressings (assorted sizes)
- individually wrapped sterile triangular bandages
- individually wrapped medium-sized wound dressings
- individually wrapped large-sized wound dressings
- medical gauze
- antiseptic wipes
- eye-wash bottle
- sterile eye pads
- cotton wool
- safety pins
- scissors and tweezers
- disposable aprons and gloves
- antiseptic cream or liquid
- one litre of sterile water or sterile normal saline (0.9 per cent) in sealed, disposable container.

The Reporting of Injuries, Diseases and Dangerous Occurrences (RIDDOR) Regulations 1995

RIDDOR covers the recording and reporting of serious accidents. If an accident occurs in the salon, it must be reported to the HSE who will investigate serious cases (this is a legal requirement).

Accidents must be reported:

- if an injury or death occurs and the victim is taken to hospital
- if an injury to an employee occurs that results in their not being able to work for three days or more
- if someone other than an employee injures themselves while on the premises and cannot work for three days or more
- if a doctor informs the employer that an employee has a **reportable disease**.

Follow health and safety practice in the salon

The Fire Precautions (Workplace) Regulations 1999

Employers have several responsibilities under these regulations, including:

- conducting fire risk assessments
- training staff to know what to do in the event of a fire
- displaying fire notices, such as fire exit signs, route and a floor plan
- providing firefighting equipment, for example extinguishers, fire blankets.

Data Protection Act 1998

All employees must comply with this act when handling clients' personal information that is stored on the premises, such as record cards, computer files and accident report forms, and maintaining its confidentiality. To learn more about the act, see Client care and communication in beauty-related industries, page 44. If you disclose a client's personal data to an unauthorised person, you will be in breach of the Data Protection Act and you may be prosecuted.

Employers' Liability (Compulsory Insurance) Act 1969

It is a legal requirement for all businesses to have public liability insurance, which protects employers and employees if they are sued by a third party (such as an employee, a client, trades person, or visitor) who injures themselves on the premises or, in extreme cases, where an accident has resulted in death or if they contract a disease from their employment. Insurance must comply with the following:

- The level of cover must be at least the minimum amount required by law, which is currently £5 million.
- It must cover the whole company, and should identify who is covered. Where a salon is part of a group, it must be covered by the main company's insurance.
- The certificate must show the name of the insurer and must be signed by the authorised insurer. Names of authorised insurers can be found on a register held by the Financial Services Authority (FSA).

To protect against fire or damage to the building, the salon owner must take out buildings insurance. They must also have contents insurance to cover damage to such items as tools, products, equipment, fixtures and fittings.

Local Government (Miscellaneous Provisions) Act 1982

Section 8 of the act refers to registration of professionals who pierce the skin, including treatments such as epilation, ear and body piercing, acupuncture and tattooing, in either a salon or mobile environment. Local authorities are responsible for validating practitioners' qualifications and control hygiene levels for these treatments.

Top tip

Employers and/or employees must have professional indemnity insurance to protect themselves against being sued by a client if injury to the client or damage to their property occurs through negligence.

Top tip

Visit the Health and Safety Executive's (HSE) website for further information on the Employers' Liability (Compulsory Insurance) Act 1969 and download its free guide.

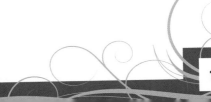

Occupiers Liability Act 1957 and 1984

These acts protect visitors and trespassers when on the occupier's property. The occupier is the person who occupies either a fixed structure such as a building, land or a moveable structure such as a vehicle and may be held liable for injury to another person.

Under the 1957 act, the occupier could be the owner, a person with exclusive possession, a person with the right to enter/use the property, a manager, local authorities, companies, individuals or partnerships, which means more than one person could be the occupier. This act covers the following:

- There is a duty of care towards visitors, who are individuals that have been invited onto the premises by the occupier. Also covered are those enforcing the law, such as the police. This duty of care is to ensure that the visitor is safe, not that the premises are safe.

- Visitors could include children, and the occupier must take a higher duty of care, as children will probably be less careful than adults.

- Workmen do not require a higher duty of care, as they will already be aware of potential hazards and risks associated with their trade and will not require supervision.

- Work completed by contractors that causes injury to a visitor will not subject the occupier to a higher duty of care if the occupier has warned the visitor about possible hazards.

The 1984 act deals with trespassers and the occupier's duty of care, if they are aware of the following:

- a current danger

- that an individual is near a known danger

- they already knew that protection was required from the danger.

There is no duty of care if a trespasser accepts a risk, and they can only claim for injury or death but not for damage to personal property.

Management of Health and Safety at Work Regulations 1999

These regulations protect individuals who work in conjunction with employees, contractors, clients or customers. Under the regulations, employers must assess potential risks at work or if employees work elsewhere, for example from home, have action plans in place to deal with emergencies. Employers must:

- update risk assessments, especially when new equipment or procedures are introduced

- improve safety procedures where or when appropriate

- be aware of potential hazards and risks

- have in place salon policies and procedures on health and safety which employees must adhere to

- ensure employees have regular health and safety training

- identify hazards and make changes to working practices to minimise the risk.

Top tip

Health and safety legislation is vast and difficult to remember, so you need to revise this unit well, ask lots of questions and apply your theory in practice to retain the knowledge necessary to make you an outstanding nail technician.

The employer's and employee's health and safety responsibilities

Employer	Employee
Identify health and safety risks and hazards	Be aware of risks and hazards and do not endanger others
Provide information and training for employees on services and equipment	Participate in regular training sessions, follow manufacturer's instructions and use, handle, store and dispose of products correctly
Provide storage for products and equipment	Store products and equipment correctly
Provide and maintain PPE	Comply with PPE regulations
Organise regular scheduled maintenance and checks of the salon and equipment by a competent person	Report faulty equipment and perform checks before use
Provide the correct environmental conditions	Maintain the correct environmental conditions
Observe and remove any obstructions	Do not obstruct walkways or doorways
Provide the correct waste and recycling bins	Correctly dispose of waste
Ensure scheduled/regular breaks occur	Take regular breaks
Provide eyesight tests when requested	Inform your employer if you require a sight test
Provide workstations, stool and desks at correct height and size	Use equipment for intended purpose
Provide staff training on how to correctly lift and carry objects	Lift and carry objects correctly
Provide a designated first aider and first aid box	Identify the first aider and location of the first aid box
Report injuries, diseases and dangerous occurrences to the HSE	Inform your manager of any injuries, diseases and dangerous occurrences
Display safety signs	Observe and follow safety signs
Provide firefighting equipment and fire evacuation training	Participate in firefighting equipment/evacuation training and only use in an emergency
Carry out risk assessments and ensure accident report forms are completed	Ensure risk assessments and accident report forms are completed
Provide amenities	Use amenities
Provide safety glass and locks on windows and doors	Ensure windows and doors are locked at the end of the day
Hold valid and current liability insurance	
Have salon policies and procedures in place and have regular meetings	Attend training and follow salon policies and procedures
Keep accurate records	Keep accurate records and follow Data Protection Act
Consult experts and implement knowledge within all aspects of the business	Participate in training sessions and implement any updates

The difference between a hazard and a risk

When working in any business you must always be aware of the hazards and risks. If you understand what might happen when using a piece of equipment, products or even performing a simple cleaning activity, you should be able to prevent an accident or damage occurring.

Businesses use risk assessment forms to identify hazards and potential outcomes. Using the results of the risk assessment, they can then put procedures in place to make employees aware of potential dangers in order to reduce the likelihood of them happening.

Key terms

Cross-infection – transferring an infection or disease from one person to another.

Erythema – reddening of the skin from an increase of the blood circulation.

Hazards that may occur in a salon

The table below lists some examples of hazards in the salon and their potential risks.

Hazard	Potential risks
Boxes left in doorways, passageways or corridors	Person trips or falls
Wet, slippery floor – spillage not noticed or cleaned up	Person slips, trips or falls
Trailing wires across the working area	Person trips or falls Damage to equipment
Equipment not stored away correctly	Person trips or falls Damage to equipment
Visual and manual checks not performed on electrical equipment before use on a client	Damage to equipment Electrical burns, electrical shock and, in severe cases, death
Skin test not performed before a treatment	Client has allergic reaction
Consultation not performed – failure to diagnose disease or disorder	**Cross-infection** of disease Causes client discomfort Makes condition worse
Incorrect use of equipment or tools when performing a treatment	Client's skin or cuticle cut or damaged Causes client discomfort Causes skin or nail infection
Water too hot in manicure or pedicure bowl when performing a treatment	Causes deep **erythema**, burns, blister, infection, scarring, discomfort

Hazards in the salon and their potential risks

Hazards which need to be referred

If any hazards result in damage or infection to the client's skin, cuticles or nails, you should refer the client to their GP or the hospital. If you become aware of any serious hazards, you will need to report them to your employer or manager so that they can take action to remove them. In the case of faulty equipment, contact the manufacturer. If the hazard is not of a serious nature and you are able to deal with it safely, then take prompt action.

Dealing with hazards within your own area of responsibility

Employers or managers must be vigilant at all times, performing spot checks to identify any hazards that might cause an accident. Nail technicians must be alert too – if you identify any of the hazards shown below, you should deal with them promptly. Any employee who fails to follow health and safety procedures must be reported to the employer or manager immediately to prevent an accident from occurring. The table below summarises hazards or risks in the workplace that could result in damage, injury or death.

Key term

Contra-indication – a disease or disorder that could restrict or prevent a treatment (see Skin analysis, page 150).

Fire evacuation procedures and equipment	Working procedures	Maintenance of building	COSHH	General health and safety
• Obstructions in walkways or door-ways (fire exits) • Faulty equipment or equipment that has not been serviced, either by an electrical or Gas Safe registered professional • No electrical checks on equipment before use • Employees not trained in fire evacuation procedures • Locked fire exits • Fabrics that are not fire resistant • Locked windows and doors, especially where there are no keys	• Equipment not stored away • Using unsafe trolleys to place equipment on • Using equipment without being aware of others, e.g. trailing wires • Workstations, chairs or stools not used at the correct height or position • Brakes not working on workstations or couches • Portable trolleys not provided to move heavy items around premises • Technicians not reading manufacturer's instructions or having training before using products and equipment on clients • Not checking for **contra-indications** during the consultation • Not following PPE procedures	• Poor condition of passageways, e.g. uneven floors • No safety glass in doors or windows • Unsecure signage on the exterior of building • Asbestos present in older buildings • Subsidence and unsafe foundations in older buildings • No first aid facilities or designated first aider	• Storing chemicals in daylight or a warm environment • Leaving lids off products • Not locking away products in a dark, dry, cool store cupboard • Products not clearly labelled • Refilling chemicals using unclear or unlabelled bottles and/or bottles made of the wrong material • Not performing a skin test when required or not recording a skin test • Not wearing PPE when cleaning up or dealing with leaking chemical containers • Not storing chemicals correctly, causing damage to the containers	• Not following the salon dress code • Not completing a treatment plan or record card • No facilities for storage of valuables • Not cleaning up spillages or over-polishing floors • Unsecured carpets and floor covering • Poor ventilation or extractor fans not working • Unsecured fixtures and fittings • Unsterilised equipment, tools or workstations • Waste disposal bins not provided • Bins not emptied regularly • Using a chair, instead of a ladder, when reaching for something • Lifting heavy objects incorrectly • No procedures in the event of an intruder

Hazards in the salon

To get ready for your health and safety assessment, look around your workplace and use the headings in the table above to begin listing potential hazards and risks and identifying the action that you will need to take. The first one has been filled in for you.

Health and safety hazards and risks in my workplace		
Hazards	**Risks**	**Action**
Electrical Faulty equipment that has not been checked before use, has not been PAT tested or has not had regular maintenance by a competent person.	This could result in the client or technician receiving an electric shock; there could be an electrical fire or permanent damage to the equipment.	Electric shock – dial 999 for an ambulance and contact first aider. Electrical fires – follow your salon fire procedures. Report damaged equipment to the manager.
Obstructions		
Spillages		
Breakages		
Cross-infection		
Lifting and carrying		
Storage, safe usage, handling and disposal of chemicals		

Check it out

As part of your practical or written assessment for this unit, you will need to follow your salon's health and safety procedures to reduce the health and safety risks in your workplace. Start to think about categorising potential hazards and risks such as electrical, obstructions and so on – re-read the above section to help you.

Key term

Respiratory system – our breathing system, which includes the lungs and airways.

The purpose of personal protective equipment (PPE) used in a salon during different services

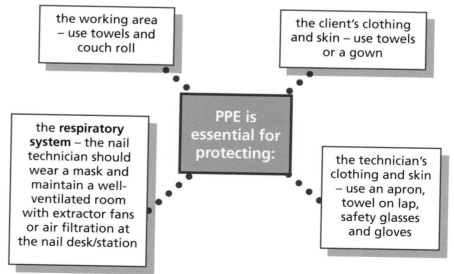

the working area – use towels and couch roll

the client's clothing and skin – use towels or a gown

PPE is essential for protecting:

the **respiratory system** – the nail technician should wear a mask and maintain a well-ventilated room with extractor fans or air filtration at the nail desk/station

the technician's clothing and skin – use an apron, towel on lap, safety glasses and gloves

Follow health and safety practice in the salon

Top tips

- Wear safety goggles when dispensing chemicals or if there is a chance of flying debris when clipping toenails.
- Use non-latex (synthetic) or nitrile, powder-free gloves in case either you or the client is allergic to latex.
- Wear a dust mask to avoid inhaling dust particles when filing nails. Some manufacturers recommend you apply an oil or solution to make the dust particles heavier during filing, to minimise dust in the air.
- There is a 60 cm area around the head – the breathing zone – where we inhale air from. The use of an extraction unit should minimise an employee's and client's exposure to toxic chemicals and dust.

The importance of personal presentation, hygiene and conduct in maintaining health and safety

As a nail technician, you must be professional at all times and ensure that you comply with the salon policy on **conduct** in the workplace, not only to create a good relationship with clients but also to maintain high standards of health, hygiene and safety in the workplace. The way you interact with colleagues and clients is important as you need to behave appropriately in order to create a positive image. It is important that you cooperate with your colleagues to ensure harmony within the salon and that the business runs smoothly and effectively. It is important that you remain professional and **unbiased**, as you must be **non-judgemental**, **non-discriminatory** and not argumentative, as you should respect the beliefs of others, as they should respect yours. When working with colleagues or communicating with clients, as a professional you must show understanding (empathy) towards others rather than sympathy, which will enable you to create **professional boundaries**. This can be accomplished by excellent **verbal** and **non-verbal communication** skills. (To learn more about communication skills, see Client care and communication in beauty-related industries, page 35.)

Your personal presentation, hygiene and conduct must be maintained throughout the day – how you conduct yourself as a technician will reflect upon your colleagues, the business and you, so always follow the salon guidelines for appropriate behaviour and conduct. A nail technician must:

- comply with all health and safety laws
- follow the salon's policies
- adhere to the salon's dress code
- wash and sterilise all tools and equipment after every client
- dispose of waste correctly
- wear personal protective equipment (PPE).

Key terms

Conduct – the way you behave in the workplace, for example professionally.

Unbiased – neutral position, impartial.

Non-judgemental – do not judge others' beliefs or ideas

Non-discriminatory – fair, not judging or discriminating against others.

Professional boundaries – limits on overly friendly behaviour

Verbal communication – communicating by speaking

Non-verbal communication – communicating using other forms of communication such as body language, smiling, nodding, posture, hand gesture.

Top tips

- Professional conduct is vital in the role of a successful nail technician and taking recreational drugs and drinking is prohibited.
- Eating and drinking should only occur during scheduled breaks and in designated areas, as it looks unprofessional and is unhygienic to others.

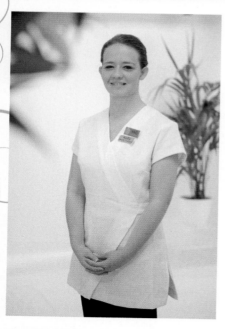

A professional image will give your clients confidence in your ability

Top tip

When training to become a nail technician, your awarding body will provide guidelines for acceptable dress code, which you must adhere to. Failure to follow these guidelines could mean an **unsuccessful assessment**.

Key term

Unsuccessful assessment – when you are being assessed and have not yet fully met the assessment criteria set by the awarding body.

Personal presentation requirements

You will need to be aware of your personal presentation throughout the day, making sure you maintain a fresh and professional appearance. Pay particular attention to your uniform, hair, make-up (if applicable) and nails, as a professional image will help you to gain your clients' confidence.

Uniform

Your employer, college or training provider will determine what the dress code will be and you will be expected to abide by this. Uniforms should be laundered daily and ironed, to prevent a build-up of body odour and stains. Having a spare uniform to change into in case there is a spillage or stain is advisable, or you could wear a nail technician apron.

Make-up

A light, subtle, day make-up can give a fresh appearance and could be suggested by employers. Avoid heavy make-up, especially if you wear a high-collar tunic that can form a build-up of make-up. Heavy make-up can also give a false impression of a bold and unapproachable person – a fresh look is more appealing to clients and it creates a professional appearance. Wear colours and tones that suit your complexion and touch up when required.

Hair

Hair styles can vary in style and length. Long hair must be tied back away from the face and any short wisps should be clipped back. If your hair is shorter but will fall forward when performing a treatment, tie or clip it back appropriately. It is not hygienic to touch your hair during a treatment, so be prepared – style your hair neatly, look professional and make sure your hair is always clean.

Nails

Your nails are an advertisement for you and your place of work, so it is essential to maintain the condition and presentation of your nails. Nails should be short, clean, with healthy cuticles and no enamel or nail extensions when performing manicure or pedicure treatments (the client might be allergic to the enamel or nail extensions).

Shoes

Clean, odour-free and polished shoes will complete the uniform look and comply with the required dress code. Shoes should feel comfortable, so a closed-in shoe with a low heel is required to fulfil health and safety aspects and protect your feet.

Jewellery

Jewellery must never come in contact with a client as it is unhygienic, a distraction and may scratch or catch the client during the treatment. In some instances, facial jewellery may be considered unprofessional and could discourage the client from returning. When working on a client, it is best to wear minimal jewellery, such as a wedding band, small earrings and a fob watch.

Personal hygiene

In the area of personal hygiene it is important to understand the difference between a deodorising antiperspirant and a body spray. Body sprays are intended to give you a pleasant fragrance but they do not prevent body odour — a light body spray or fragrance is acceptable as long as it is not overpowering. You can purchase sprays that have both a deodorant (to remove unpleasant odours) and an antiperspirant (to control the amount of sweat released). Refresh yourself by reapplying during the day.

You will also need to shower daily to stay fresh, as bacteria on the skin's surface feed on sweat and excrete a strong, unpleasant odour. Also, hands must be washed before, during and after each treatment to maintain levels of hygiene — the client should be able to observe you doing this.

Safely positioning the nail technician and the client

When carrying out a treatment, it is essential that you are positioned correctly to prevent aches, pains and repetitive strain injury (RSI). If you are uncomfortable, the client is also likely to feel uncomfortable and this will affect your performance and result in a poor-quality treatment. If you cannot safely reach the client or they are not supported correctly, you could cause damage when working, for example by accidently cutting the cuticles too short or nicking the skin. To prevent bad posture, assess your work area before and during the treatment:

- Ensure your stool or chair is positioned at the correct height. It should have a back support with a height adjuster.

- The client should be in a static chair with a back, or in a pedicure spa chair.

- Ensure you are facing the client head-on and not at a slight angle.

- The workstation should not be too wide — this will prevent overstretching. For example, never perform a manicure over a couch as it is likely to be too wide; instead opt for a manicure station.

- Both you and the client should have elbow or wrist pad support when working on the hands.

- If you cannot place your feet directly on the floor, use a footrest.

- Position the workstation away from sunlight, as it can affect certain products.

Techniques to prevent repetitive strain injury

- Perform hand, finger and wrist exercises regularly.

- Hold tools correctly — avoid holding them tightly.

- When working long hours, take sufficient breaks.

- Rotate the treatments you perform.

- Position yourself and your client correctly during the treatment.

- Do not overstretch during the treatment.

- Maintain good posture — do not slouch.

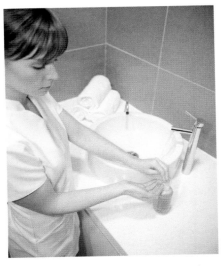

Use an antibacterial hand soap to wash your hands

Top tips

- Ensure you follow your salon's dress code, wear a clean uniform, use deodorising antiperspirant and shower daily. Remember, you might not be able to smell your unpleasant body odour, but your client will and it is offensive.

- Some salons provide antibacterial gel for employees and clients to use to minimise cross-infection – door handles, for example, harbour **micro-organisms**.

Key term

Micro-organisms – very small organisms that enter the body through the ears, mouth, nose, genitals, cuts in the skin and blood (if the skin is pierced). They can be bacterial, viral or fungal organisms, and are contra-indicated to treatments.

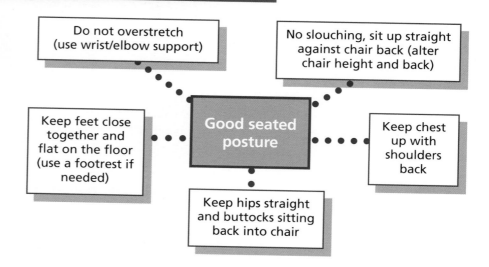

Do not overstretch (use wrist/elbow support)

No slouching, sit up straight against chair back (alter chair height and back)

Keep feet close together and flat on the floor (use a footrest if needed)

Good seated posture

Keep chest up with shoulders back

Keep hips straight and buttocks sitting back into chair

Handle, use and store products, materials, tools and equipment safely

During your training to become a nail technician, you will be shown how to correctly handle, use, dispose and store all products, materials, tools and equipment, but you must also read the manufacturer's guidelines before using anything new. Throughout your career you will need to stay abreast of the latest developments in the industry, including products, treatments and equipment. Before using anything new you will need to receive full training – often companies or education institutes will hold training sessions after which you will receive a certificate. If it is something new, for example a nail varnish remover or cuticle oil, you will need to read the manufacturer's guidelines and ingredients to prepare you for any eventuality, such as skin test requirements or a change in treatment timing or procedures.

Safe storage of products, materials, tools and equipment

Equipment that is not being used should be stored in a cupboard or storeroom to keep the salon tidy, prevent damage to the equipment and create a safe, accident-free environment. Products should be kept in a dark, dry, cool, locked cupboard or storeroom, especially chemical products that could react to heat or sunlight. Storing them in a locked area will also deter thieves and comply with legislation. Working areas should be left clean and tidy at the end of the day to present a professional business and to enable treatments to begin on time the following day.

To learn more about the guidelines that refer to the use, handling, storage and disposal of products, see the COSHH regulations on page 8.

Maintaining the security of belongings

The owner or manager of the salon should include security procedures in their workplace policy in order to protect employees, clients, stock, cash, valuables and the premises. For insurance purposes, businesses will need to have adequate security measures and procedures in place. Unfortunately, anyone

Top tip

At the end of the day, dry metal tools thoroughly to prevent them from rusting and store them safely.

20

can be suspected of being a thief or of vandalism, and that includes clients and employees. Necessary steps must be put in place to deter and prevent opportunities for crime.

Vandalism

Security cameras installed at the front and rear of the premises should discourage vandals. This also means that their actions will be recorded, which can be used later as evidence.

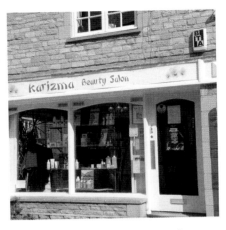

Alarm on the exterior wall of a salon

Theft when the premises are closed

A range of measures can be used to act as a deterrent against theft when there is no one on the premises. They include:

- a security alarm, or at least a fake box on the wall so it appears as if there is an alarm

- lights left on in the premises to illuminate the workplace, making intruders more visible to passersby or the police

- double-glazed windows and doors — more difficult to break than single-glazed glass

- locks on windows and deadlocks on doors

- metal shutters installed over doors and windows at the front and/or rear of the property

- additional locks on internal doors and stock cupboards that contain valuable items.

Theft during the working day

- The salon should provide a safe, secure place for clients to leave their valuables, such as handbags, wallets, mobile phones, car keys or coats, during a treatment if they cannot be left close by.

- Employees should have a designated place or lockers to store their handbags or valuables to keep them safe and also to deter people from stealing.

- Money should be kept in a till with the till key removed when there is no one on reception. If there are large amounts of cash on the premises, it should be stored in a locked safe until it can be taken to the bank.

- When taking money to the bank for depositing, always go with a colleague and do not go at the same time each day. Avoid carrying a bag that looks as if it contains cash.

- Stock on reception or in the treatment rooms should be kept in a locked cupboard, with the key kept in a safe place. Perform regular stock checks to identify missing stock — if an employee is stealing, this could help to identify them. Display bottles can be purchased to promote products instead.

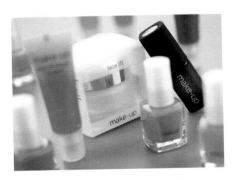

Small, expensive items are attractive to thieves

Protecting clients

Generally, during the day, the biggest risk for a client is theft, so a safe place must be provided for the client's coat, which is usually close to reception or

Top tip

Never wear expensive jewellery at work and never perform treatments with it on. First, it is against dress code, and second, it could be stolen or damaged.

within a treatment room. The client's handbag or personal effects, such as a wallet or car keys, must be kept close at all times to protect not only the client but also the nail technician — to avoid the client claiming that the technician has stolen from them. When a client removes their jewellery they need to be responsible for it, so they need to put it in a safe place such as their handbag or a pocket.

If the client has an evening appointment, it is important that they get home safely, so the technician could call a taxi or wait with the client while someone comes to collect them.

Protecting the employee

Employees should never work alone, especially during the winter months when it is dark. Lock the front door to the salon in the evening, as long as there is someone to remain on reception to greet clients.

Employees should understand the salon's workplace policy on security procedures so that they know where to store valuables and what action to take in cases of theft. At the end of the working day, more than one person should be responsible for locking up the premises.

The principles of hygiene and infection control

Tools, equipment and materials must meet the salon's hygiene standards and comply with health and safety legislation. Manufacturers' instructions will also give you guidance, as some items have specific considerations. All tools and equipment must be sterilised after each client to prevent cross-infection and maintain hygiene standards. Where disposable items such as wooden spatulas are used, it is recommended that you dispose of them after each client. Towels and gowns must be placed in a covered laundry bin and then laundered after each client on a 60°C wash cycle.

Cross-infection

There are two ways that cross-infection can occur from a contra-indication during a treatment:

Top tip
When you are training, you will not always be able to name all possible skin and nail diseases, so if the treatment area is tender, looks red and swollen and there is pus present, ask your tutor for guidance, as the client is contra-indicated to the treatment.

Direct cross-infection: a client with an undiagnosed, contagious condition, e.g. a nail or skin disease, touches the nail technician and infects them with micro-organisms

• • • • • **Cross-infection** • • • • •

Indirect cross-infection: a client with an undiagnosed, contagious condition, e.g. a nail or skin disease, has a treatment which contaminates the tools. These tools are not washed and sterilised and are then used on another client. The tools infect the second client with micro-organisms.

Methods used in the salon to ensure hygiene and their effectiveness and limitations

The table below lists the health and safety terminology that you will need to know to ensure that that you maintain a high standard of hygiene in the salon.

Term	Definition
Sterilisation	the total destruction of all living organisms
Sanitisation	removal of dirt and germs
Disinfection	the destruction of most micro-organisms
Bactericide	a chemical that will destroy bacteria but not always the bacterial spores, which can begin reproduction again
Antiseptic	a chemical that destroys or inhibits the growth of micro-organisms
Asepsis	free from disease
Sepsis	infected with either a bacterial, fungal, parasitic or viral infection

Health and safety terminology

Top tip

Use antiseptic on the client's skin and disinfectant on your working area.

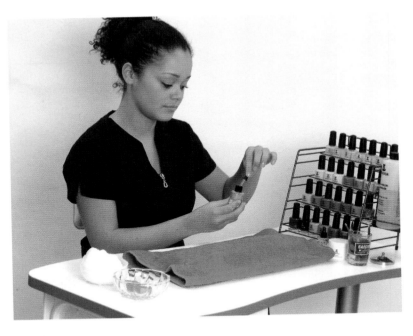

Working at a nail station

Sterilisation equipment

Autoclave

An autoclave is the most effective form of sterilisation, but it can only be used on metal tools such as knives or nippers. The autoclave runs on electricity and resembles a pressure cooker. It produces high-pressurised steam that maintains a temperature of 121–34°C, which destroys micro-organisms.

Procedure for using an autoclave:

1 Wash metal tools in hot, soapy water and remove any debris such as dead skin cells.

2 Fill the autoclave with water to the measure line – do not overfill.

3 Place the metal tools in the basket.

4 Place the top on the basket – this provides an area for smaller tools, creating a stacking option with larger tools inside the basket.

5 Put on the autoclave lid – line up the arrows and twist to lock.

6 Make sure the steam release valve is set at 0, so no steam can escape.

7 Switch on the machine. Most modern autoclaves have indicator lights to show that the equipment is heating up, that it has reached the correct temperature and that the cycle has finished.

8 Once the cycle is finished, turn the steam release valve to the steam icon to release the pressurised steam, which will be quite loud and visible (but will not happen if the autoclave has cooled).

9 Place metal tools in a jar of Barbicide® to keep them sterile until use. Never leave metal tools in a damp or wet environment, such as Barbicide® or the autoclave, as they will rust.

Top tips

- Always follow the manufacturer's instructions – the procedure may vary with different autoclaves.

- Never remove the autoclave lid without releasing the steam – it could cause serious burns.

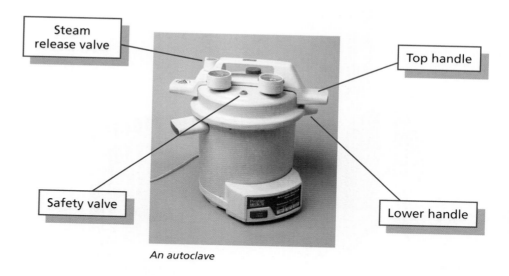

Steam release valve

Top handle

Safety valve

Lower handle

An autoclave

UV cabinet

The UV (ultraviolet) cabinet is more versatile than the autoclave, as it can be used on almost anything from metal, plastic, foam or wooden tools, including emery boards and brushes. It sterilises at a low rate of penetration and will only sterilise areas of the tools where the light reflects upon them, so if scissors are placed in the cabinet with the blades closed, the inside of the blades will not be sterilised. UV cabinets have a **quartz mercury vapour lamp**, similar to a sunbed lamp, which will eventually need to be replaced.

Key term

Quartz mercury vapour lamp – produces an artificial UV light that mimics the sun's UV light

24

Procedure for using a UV cabinet:

1 Wash tools in hot, soapy water to remove any debris such as dead skin cells and dry, or spray with specialised cleanser (emery boards).

2 Place the tools on the shelf inside the UV cabinet and close the lid.

3 Switch on the UV cabinet and leave for 15 minutes, then turn over the tools — remember to switch off the cabinet before opening it.

4 Leave for a further 15 minutes. Switch off the cabinet.

5 Place tools in a jar of Barbicide® to keep sterile until use and place on your workstation.

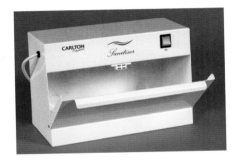
An ultraviolet cabinet

Glass bead sterilisation

The sterilising unit consists of small glass beads that can heat up to temperatures in excess of 300°C. Small metal instruments are placed in the glass beads. They will be sterilised in 10–60 seconds, but will require 30–60 seconds to cool. This sterilising unit will kill most types of fungal, bacterial and viral infections. The glass beads will last approximately one month before needing to be replaced.

Disinfectants

Disinfectants are concentrated, liquid chemicals that can be used either on the skin or with tools and equipment. The chemicals are sometimes diluted with water, depending upon their purpose, so always follow manufacturer's instructions. Disinfectants destroy micro-organisms but not always the bacterial spores, which can begin reproducing again. The following table describes the main disinfectants used in the salon.

Disinfectant	Usage
Gluteraldehyde	A 2% chemical solution that is used within a chemical bath, which disinfects metal tools. The tools are placed in a basket that is lowered into the chemical bath and left to soak. The chemical will remain active for approximately two weeks, and then it must be changed. However, if too many tools are in the bath at once the chemical will stop working.
Surgical spirit	A 70% alcohol-based disinfectant product that cannot be reused. It may be used to clean equipment or the skin. However, it can be extremely drying to the skin, so alternatives such as antiseptic lotion are recommended.
Barbicide®	Concentrated Barbicide® is poured into a Barbicide® jar and mixed with water, according to manufacturer's instructions. It is a well-known disinfectant solution that is used to store pre-sterilised tools, such as knives, nippers, clippers and scissors, to keep them sterilised during treatment.

Disinfectants

Top tips

- UV cabinets do not usually have timers, so make sure that you time the process accurately or the tools will not be sterilised effectively.

- UV light is dangerous to the eyes, so never look directly at it. Switch off the UV cabinet before opening the lid.

Check it out

Before carrying out a treatment, check your tools work properly, wash them in hot soapy water (if applicable) or use a spray sanitiser (in the case of an emery board, for example), sterilise them in either the autoclave or UV cabinet (the two most effective types), store tools correctly on the workstation (Barbicide® for metal or plastic tools). Follow this procedure every time, as you will be assessed on preparation.

Top tip

Always rinse off Barbicide® solution before using tools, as it will be harmful to the client's skin.

Disinfectants are also used for general cleaning purposes on a range of surfaces, including floors, walls, drains, sanitary ware, glass, workstations and equipment (for example trolleys). Examples include hypochlorous acid or sodium/calcium hypochlorites (for example bleach). They are usually cheap to buy. However, they should not be used as a chemical bath to soak metal tools in, as they are corrosive. Quats (quaternary ammonium compounds) are cleaning agents that prevent bacteria from spreading, but as certain organisms are resistant to them it is better to use an alternative such as disinfectant.

Detergents

There are different formulations of detergent, for example soap, washing-up liquid, laundry, dishwasher and surface detergents. They are synthetic products that act as an emulsifier, which allows water and oil to mix to remove grease and grime from the area. Laundry detergents also contain small quantities of bleach to de-colour stains.

Antiseptics

Antiseptic is a chemical-based product that destroys or inhibits the growth of micro-organisms. It can be applied to the skin with cotton wool or you can purchase pre-soaked antiseptic wipes, often known as medi-wipes. Antiseptic can be used at the beginning of a treatment to sanitise the hands or feet or on an open cut or wound to prevent infection.

Ventilation

Good ventilation in the salon is essential, as nail treatments and the products and chemicals used create a dusty, warm and dry environment with strong odours. This is especially important in smaller salons, where the air can become very unpleasant and stuffy. Ventilation may come from a natural source such as open windows and doors, which allow external air to enter the workplace and the salon air to exit. There are also artificial sources, including extractor fans or air filtration at the nail desk/station or free-standing units that will improve the air considerably. The table below looks at the disadvantages.

Type of ventilation	Disadvantage
Natural (open doors and windows)	Lets noise in from the outside Affects room temperature Can create a cold draft
Extractor fans or air filtration	Can be costly to purchase and run
Free-standing unit	Potential risk that it could be knocked over

Disadvantages of different types of ventilation

> **Top tip**
>
> To maintain high standards of hygiene and prevent cross-infection, after each client:
>
> - wash, sterilise and store tools correctly
> - launder towels and gowns
> - disinfect your working area.

> **Top tip**
>
> Some chemical products will not work effectively if the salon is too hot or too cold.

How to dispose of different types of salon waste

Every day salons create waste — a mixture of general, broken glass, chemical and recycled waste — which must be handled and disposed of correctly (see the following table). All businesses should try to recycle wherever possible, especially where recycling bins are provided.

Type of waste	How to dispose of/recycle
Disposable items, e.g. wooden spatulas/orange sticks, cotton wool, tissues	Treat as general waste. In the salon, place in an ordinary lined pedal bin. When full dispose of outside in the general black wheelie bin.
Broken glass	Collect in a cardboard box (not a plastic bin bag, as it will rip and tear). Dispose of outside in the recycling wheelie bin, if one has been provided by your local authority; alternatively, you could use a local recycling centre.
Chemicals, solvents and cleaning products, e.g. nail varnish remover, acetone	Do not dispose of down the sink, as it will contaminate water supplies. Soak up excess in a bowl with tissues and put into a lined pedal bin.
Massage oil	Soak up with tissues then dispose of like chemicals, as pouring down the sink will block your water pipes.
Paraffin wax	Do not pour down the sink, especially if it is still a liquid – it will solidify and block the water pipes. Dispose of in lined pedal bin.
Masks	Treat as general waste.
Recyclable waste, e.g. paper, cardboard, plastic bottles, glass	Depending on where you live, your local council will supply you with recycling wheelie bins and often bags for paper. Follow the council's guidelines on coloured bins for glass, plastics and tins. Remember, there are many recycling bins provided at supermarkets, shopping centres and local car parks that take other items such as old mobile phones, clothing and so on.

How to dispose of/recycle salon waste

Access the following websites to learn more about waste disposal: Habia, Directgov, your local council, the Health and Safety Executive (HSE), Greenpeace, Allergy UK and the NHS.

Recycled waste facts

Recycling packaging is very important in our attempts to reduce the amount of raw materials that we use. It also helps us to reduce the amount of rubbish we send to landfill sites and cuts air and water pollution. It is the responsibility of manufacturers to be aware of environmental issues when creating new

Think about it

As a nail technician, you need to be aware of advancements in the nail industry, as there is a worldwide focus on recycling and environmental sustainability. Often these advancements are linked to the production of products containing less harmful irritants, possibly for the use of clients who have allergies or dermatitis. They may also affect guidelines for the disposal of harmful toxins that all nail technicians must adhere to.

Top tips

If you are studying at college, there might be an environmental campaign that your tutors will make you aware of, known as sustainability. This looks at ways to sustain our environment to reduce our 'carbon footprint' – the impact our daily activities have on the environment and climate change. These daily activities include the burning of fossil fuels for electricity, heating and transport, which results in the production of greenhouse gases such as carbon dioxide. You will look at recycling, reducing the amount of electricity, water, gas, petrol and food packaging you use. Think about what you can do.

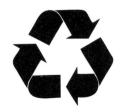

An object with the Möbius loop can be recycled, but it does not mean it has been made of recycled materials

Follow health and safety practice in the salon

Check it out

As well as the Möbius loop symbol, you might see the green dot symbol or the PET plastics symbol. Can you find these symbols online or on your products? Find out what they mean.

products and packaging. Many nail treatment containers, such as plastic tubs of hand cream, are recyclable, but remember when you are having lunch, plastic sandwich boxes, plastic yogurt pots and tins of tuna can all be recycled too.

Follow emergency procedures

As a nail technician, the types of emergencies that you will need to be aware of could include a fire, thief, vandal, intruder, water/gas leak, bomb alert, an allergic reaction, an accident or serious illness. Employers must complete risk assessments to understand every eventuality of any possible situation, and employees must be trained to deal with any emergency and understand what procedures to follow to minimise risk, hazards and severity of what could happen. An evacuation drill must be performed regularly to prepare employees in case of a real evacuation.

Procedures for dealing with emergencies

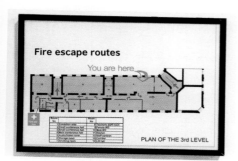

Example of fire escape routes

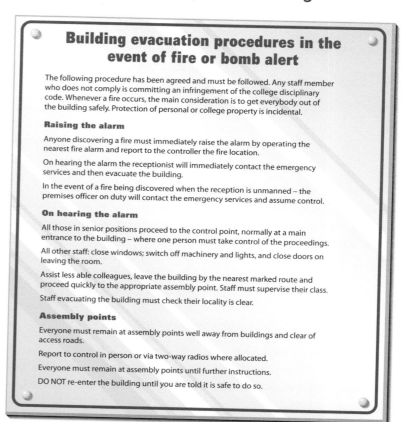

Building evacuation procedures in the event of fire or bomb alert

The following procedure has been agreed and must be followed. Any staff member who does not comply is committing an infringement of the college disciplinary code. Whenever a fire occurs, the main consideration is to get everybody out of the building safely. Protection of personal or college property is incidental.

Raising the alarm

Anyone discovering a fire must immediately raise the alarm by operating the nearest fire alarm and report to the controller the fire location.

On hearing the alarm the receptionist will immediately contact the emergency services and then evacuate the building.

In the event of a fire being discovered when the reception is unmanned – the premises officer on duty will contact the emergency services and assume control.

On hearing the alarm

All those in senior positions proceed to the control point, normally at a main entrance to the building – where one person must take control of the proceedings.

All other staff: close windows; switch off machinery and lights, and close doors on leaving the room.

Assist less able colleagues, leave the building by the nearest marked route and proceed quickly to the appropriate assembly point. Staff must supervise their class.

Staff evacuating the building must check their locality is clear.

Assembly points

Everyone must remain at assembly points well away from buildings and clear of access roads.

Report to control in person or via two-way radios where allocated.

Everyone must remain at assembly points until further instructions.

DO NOT re-enter the building until you are told it is safe to do so.

Example of a poster for evacuation procedures

Top tips

- It is advisable to have a list of contact numbers for all types of emergencies, for example if you need a first aider, emergency services (dial 999), electrician, plumber and so on.

- How to recognise a gas leak – there will be a distinctive smell and you might feel sick, tired and have a headache.

- Local fire stations will offer training sessions for staff as well as provide guidance on firefighting equipment and alarms.

Fire evacuation procedures

In the event of a fire, carry out the following procedures.

- Activate the nearest fire alarm to inform others.

- Everyone must leave the building by the designated fire evacuation route. Use the closest exit – do not panic, walk calmly and do not use the lift. Leave your belongings behind.

- Lead your client to safety – they can put on their shoes to prevent any accidents from happening (if applicable).

- Assemble at the fire assembly point and do not re-enter the building.

- Perform a head count to check that everyone has evacuated the building.

- Ring the emergency services to report the fire.

A thief, vandal or intruder in the workplace

If the thief, vandal or intruder is an unknown person, do not confront them. Remember, a thief could become hostile when confronted and safety is more important. If necessary, evacuate everyone from the salon and call the police to deal with the situation. If you have internal or external cameras, they will record what has happened and could help identify the person.

If you identify that a client or employee has stolen from the premises, it will be the responsibility of the employer to decide if they wish to call the police.

Water or gas leak

Turn off the water or gas supply at the **stopcock** and telephone for a professional to fix the pipe. You should know the location of stopcocks in your workplace in case of emergency. If it is a gas leak, evacuate the building. Do not switch off lights as it could ignite the gas, causing an explosion. If the gas has been leaking overnight and you are concerned about a potential gas explosion, telephone the emergency services and do not enter the building.

In case of a water leak, do not touch sockets or light switches, as the water could have soaked into them and you could get an electric shock.

Client with an allergic reaction

If a client has an allergic reaction during a treatment, remove the products immediately and apply a cold compress. If irritation persists, refer the client to their GP.

Accident or serious illness in the workplace

If a client or colleague has an accident such as a serious fall, or has a heart attack, ask someone to locate the first aider and telephone for an ambulance. Remember to complete an accident report form and inform the employer.

A bomb alert

During a bomb alert, evacuate the building, do not re-enter, perform a head count and follow the workplace procedures. Remember never inspect bags, parcels or look for a bomb – it could be concealed in anything and you might trigger the detonator.

Think about it

Do you know your workplace fire evacuation emergency procedure and assembly point? You will need to perform an evacuation or describe this as part of the health and safety assessments.

Key term

Stopcock – a valve or tap used to regulate the flow of water or gas.

Think about it

Have a look at the products you have in your workplace or place of study. Which products do you supply to clients who have known allergies or skin sensitivities? If there are none, research suitable alternatives and make some recommendations. This will expand your product knowledge and provide an opportunity for these types of client to have a wider range of products and services, which will help to increase the salon's profits.

Think about it

Who is your first aider or health and safety officer? Find out before you need them.

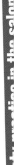

Top tips

- Every workplace needs a fire warden to supervise evacuation and to ensure everyone is safe while waiting for the emergency services.

- A smoke alarm is an essential requirement and can detect a fire in the early stages, so everyone can be evacuated safely. Remember to test alarms frequently and display fire exit signs and floor plans.

The correct use of firefighting equipment for different types of fire and the dangers of incorrect use

In case a fire occurs in the salon, firefighting equipment must be located throughout the premises and it should be appropriate to the room in which the fire may occur, for example the kitchen or treatment room.

Fire extinguishers and other types of firefighting equipment

Only trained employees may use fire extinguishers as long as they are not in danger – it is more important to leave the building safely. Extinguishers must be specific to the business and its needs. A risk assessment will identify what is required. The following table shows the different types of fire extinguisher, which fires they may be used on and the dangers of incorrect use.

Fire extinguisher	Colour of panel on extinguisher	Type of fire (class)	Do not use – dangers of incorrect use
Water with additives	Red	Class A: fires involving solid materials, e.g. paper, wood, textiles, fabric	Electrical fires – spreads the fire and possibility of electric shock Burning liquid and flammable metal fires – spreads fire
Foam	Cream/yellow	Class A: fires involving solid materials, e.g. paper, wood, textiles, fabric Class B: fires involving flammable liquids	Electrical fires – spreads the fire and possibility of electric shock Flammable metal fires – spreads fire
Dry powder	Blue	Classes A–F: all types of fires (including fires relating to kitchen appliances with oil)	Flammable metal fires – spreads fire
CO_2	Black	Class B: fires involving flammable liquids Class C: fires involving flammable gases Class E: fires involving electrical hazards	Flammable metal fires – spreads fire

Types of fire extinguisher

Water with additives

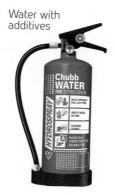

Foam

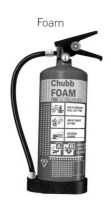

Powder

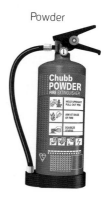

CO_2 gas

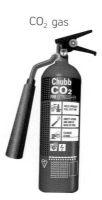

Fire extinguishers

Other types of firefighting equipment are shown below.

Equipment	How it works	How to use it
Fire blanket	Made of fire-resistant material that will cover a fire and extinguish the flames	If clothing is on fire, wrap the blanket tightly around the victim Use at home in case of a kitchen fire and may be placed over the top of cooking oil flames
Bucket of sand	Extinguishes the flames Soaks up any oils or liquids from a fire	Pour over the top of a small fire
Fire hose	Water extinguishes fire	Like a garden hose, turn on the tap and use the water to extinguish the flames

Firefighting equipment

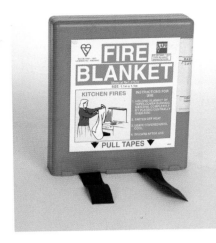

Fire blanket

Reporting and recording accidents

Once an illness or accident has occurred and first aid has been given, the first aider must complete an accident report form regardless of the severity, as what appears to be a minor accident could develop, with the person needing medical attention later. The report could also be used in legal proceedings if the person who has had the accident wishes to sue the business for negligence (carelessness). Store the accident report form in a locked, secure place and adhere to the Data Protection Act.

Types of accidents:

- Cuts to the skin (caused by incorrect use of tools, etc)

- Physical injury to client (caused by falling equipment, unstable or unsafe workstation, etc)

- Slips, trips and falls (caused by uneven or damaged floor covering, spillages, obstruction, trailing wires, cluttered walkway, etc)

- Electrocution (caused by faulty equipment; failure to perform checks or regular services, etc)

- Burns, deep erythema or blisters (caused by very hot water, equipment that is too hot, etc)

- Allergic reaction (caused by failure to perform a skin test, unidentified allergy, etc)

Think about it

Look around your workplace to see what firefighting equipment is available. Always be aware of your surroundings – it may be important on the day that you really need it.

ACCIDENT / ILLNESS REPORT FORM

Beautiful Nails

This form is to be completed by the injured party. If this is not possible, the form should be completed by the person making the report. If more than one person was injured, please complete a **separate form for each person**.

Completing and signing this form does not constitute an admission of liability of any kind, either by the person making the report or any other person.

This form should be completed immediately and forwarded to the Health and Safety Officer and Salon Manager.

If it is possible that an accident has been caused by a defect in machinery, equipment or a process, isolate / fence off the area and contact the Health and Safety Officer or Manager immediately.

SECTION 1 PERSONAL DETAILS

Surname: Lung   (Mr/(Mrs)/Ms/Miss) Forename(s): Jenny
Date of birth: 29/01/57   Address: 89, New Street, Glasgow
STAFF ☐   CONTRACTOR ☐   VISITOR ☐   GENERAL PUBLIC ☑

SECTION 2 ACCIDENT / INCIDENT / ILLNESS DETAILS

Accident (Injury) ☑ Illness ☐ Date: 19/04/11 Time: 13:07 (24-hour clock)
Location: Nail studio
Nature of injury or condition and the part of the body affected:
Slipped on floor, twisted ankle

Account
Describe what happened and how. In the case of an accident state clearly what the injured person was doing.
Small patch of water on the floor – client got up from nail station and slipped on it.
Name and address of adult witness(es): Jo Benfield, Beautiful Nails

Details of action taken
Ambulance summoned ☐   Taken to hospital ☐   Sent to hospital ☑
First aid given ☐   Taken home ☐   Sent home ☐   Returned to work ☐

SECTION 3 PREVENTATIVE ACTION
Recommended: to ensure that all spillages are mopped up straight away
Implemented: (Yes)/ No   Date: 19/04/11

Report raised by
Name: Catrina Waldron
Position: Nail technician
Signature: C Waldron   Date: 19/04/11

FOR OFFICE USE ONLY	
Copy sent to: Nail Studio Manager	☐
Health and Safety Officer	☐

Example of an accident/illness report form

Salon life

My story

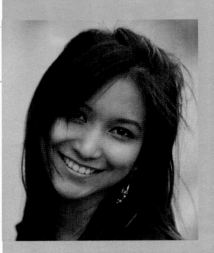

My name is Priya and I am studying to become a nail technician. During a summer holiday work placement I suffered from repetitive strain injury (RSI). My placement was in a small hairdressing salon that had one nail technician who performed manicures, pedicures, nail art and applied artificial nails. The treatments were performed at the front of the hair salon and there was one manicure station provided. I had already completed Level 2 Nail Services and after the summer I was enrolled to study Level 3 Nail Services. As I was already qualified to perform manicure, pedicure, nail art and fibreglass nail extensions, I began to work on real clients. However, the nail technician always used the workstation and I had to perform my treatment either across a table or on my lap, as the clients had their hair done. Over time I started to have pains in my back and neck; with working such long days, the pain gradually worsened.

When I went to see my GP she said I was suffering from RSI and my working conditions needed to be evaluated. My employer should have provided the correct working environment for me and if he had performed a risk assessment then this would have been identified. Even though I was only working for him during the summer holidays, my employer still had a duty of care to his employees. This has been a real life lesson for me, as I did not realise how important my working conditions are on my health and now I understand what I am entitled to as an employee under the health and safety legislation.

Ask the experts

Q1. What should I do if my employer has not provided me with the correct working area or personal protective equipment (PPE)?

A. Under current health and safety legislation, it is your employer's responsibility to provide you with a safe and comfortable working environment. Discuss your needs with your employer and explain the impact it will have on your health and the treatments you perform.

Q2. What type of working area should my employer provide?

A. If you are performing hand and nail treatments they should be done over a manicure/nail work station. A pedicure can be performed with a client sitting on a couch or a pedicure chair, with you seated at the correct height.

Top Tip

This unit provides detailed information about how to perform a safe treatment. Remember — never overstretch, use good posture, take regular breaks, alternate treatments and reposition yourself if you are uncomfortable during a treatment.

Check your knowledge

1. What is the distance of breathing zone area around the head when performing a nail treatment?
   a) 40 cm
   b) 60 cm
   c) 60 inch
   d) 40 m

2. What are the environmental conditions a nail technician must maintain throughout the working day?

3. How can cross-infection be prevented when performing a treatment on the skin and nails?

4. What fire extinguisher would you use if a pair of electrical bootees caught fire?
   a) Water (red label)
   b) Foam (cream label)
   c) Dry powder (blue label)
   d) CO_2 (black label)

5. Under the Personal Protective Equipment (PPE) at Work Regulations 2002, what PPE must an employer provide a nail technician with?

6. What does the term 'sterilisation' mean to a nail technician?
   a) The total destruction of all living organisms
   b) Removal of dirt and germs
   c) The destruction of most micro-organisms

7. What equipment should an employer provide in a dusty and strong-smelling environment that a nail technician works within?

8. What is the title of the main health and safety law that all other laws derive from?

9. How is RSI caused?
   a) Bad posture and working conditions
   b) PPE not provided
   c) No skin test performed
   d) Not following manufacturer's instructions

10. What is the most efficient method of sterilisation for metal tools?
    a) UV cabinet
    b) Autoclave
    c) Barbicide®
    d) Chemical baths

Getting ready for assessment

Health and safety is differently assessed in VRQs and NVQs, using a combination of assessment methods, as specified below. You cannot simulate any practical assessment but you must be aware of the criteria and be proactive during practical sessions to cluster assessments for more than one unit at a time.

City & Guilds		VTCT	
NVQ	**VRQ**	**NVQ**	**VRQ**
Service times: Not applicable to this unit	Service times: Not applicable to this unit	Service times: There are no maximum service times that apply to this unit	Service times: There are no maximum service times that apply to this unit
Evidence : • Should be gathered in a realistic working environment, and simulation avoided • You must demonstrate that you have met the required standard for all the outcomes, assessment criteria/skills and ranges	Evidence: • You can take either the online test or complete knowledge tasks in the assignments • There is no particular time limit set for the completion of an assignment (tasks) • Assignment is pass or fail only	Evidence: • It is strongly recommended that the evidence for this unit be gathered in a realistic working environment • Simulation should be avoided where possible • You must practically demonstrate that you have met the required standard for this unit • All outcomes, assessment criteria and range statements must be achieved • Your performance will be observed on at least three occasions for each assessment criteria	Evidence: • It is strongly recommended that the evidence for this unit be gathered in a realistic working environment • Simulation should be avoided where possible • You must practically demonstrate that you have met the required standard for this unit • All outcomes, assessment criteria and range statements must be achieved • Your performance will be observed on at least three occasions for each assessment criteria
Knowledge and understanding will be assessed by: • Oral assessment: oral questions are assessed through either verbal questioning, or paper-based or GOLA online tests to cover all the essential knowledge and understanding • Practical assessment: on at least two occasions – for these two practical observations there is no range to cover but the outcomes specify what points you must cover when performing a service: i. Identify the hazards and risks in your workplace; ii. Reduce the risks to health and safety in your salon	Knowledge and understanding will be assessed by: Knowledge tasks or an online GOLA test	Knowledge and understanding will be assessed by: internally-assessed workplace performance using a variety of methods	Knowledge and understanding will be assessed by: • mandatory written question paper • oral questioning • portfolio of evidence

Client care and communication in beauty-related industries

What you will learn

- Communicate with clients
- Provide client care

Client care and communication in beauty-related industries

Top tip

To encourage clients to return to the salon, offer **incentives** such as money-off vouchers and monthly promotions.

Think about it

Access the **Habia** website for the Code of Practice for Nail Services and read about client care and aftercare advice to learn more.

Key terms

Incentives – something to entice clients to return, for example discounted treatments or 3-for-2 offers.

Habia – is the standard-setting body and creates the industry codes of practice for the hair, beauty, nails and spa industries.

Introduction

Excellent client care and communication skills are essential in the nail industry. Clients expect more than just fantastic results — they are also paying for outstanding client care and want to have a good relationship with the nail technician. There are two types of clients:

- those who have treatments occasionally and go to a nail studio as a treat — perhaps they have received a gift voucher
- regular clients who enjoy being pampered and want their nails maintained.

Whichever type of client, treatments can be costly, so it is important to pamper clients as well as ensuring perfect nails. You can do this by performing the treatments correctly and demonstrating good communication skills. With so many nail studios, salons and spas providing nail treatments, there is a lot of competition and clients can afford to be selective. Having outstanding client care and communication skills can give you the edge your business needs.

Communicate with clients

Different forms of communication used to deal with clients

You will need to communicate effectively with everyone you come in contact with, develop specific relationships and adapt how you communicate, depending upon the situation and the person you are with, as shown in the diagram below.

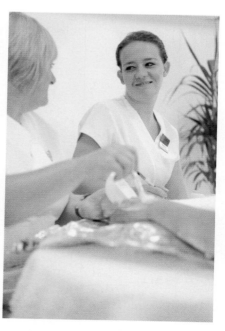

Working well together as a team creates a harmonious environment

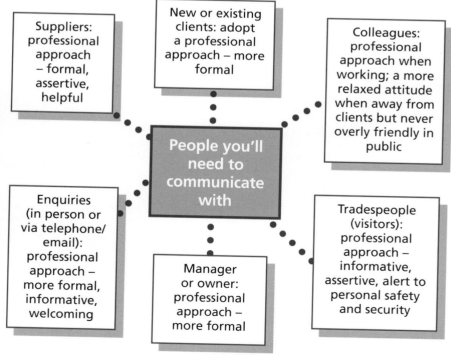

Suppliers: professional approach – formal, assertive, helpful

New or existing clients: adopt a professional approach – more formal

Colleagues: professional approach when working; a more relaxed attitude when away from clients but never overly friendly in public

Enquiries (in person or via telephone/email): professional approach – more formal, informative, welcoming

People you'll need to communicate with

Manager or owner: professional approach – more formal

Tradespeople (visitors): professional approach – informative, assertive, alert to personal safety and security

The table below identifies the personality **traits** required to be a high-performing nail technician and how to avoid being a poorly performing one.

High-performing nail technician	Poor-performing nail technician
• Good communication skills – an **active listener**, speaks at appropriate times, good questioning skills, good body language, can communicate with all, without discrimination • Skilled and motivated – has the qualifications, experience and drive to succeed • Efficient and **proactive** – has excellent time management skills and can allocate tasks and activities themselves • Discreet – demonstrates high level of professionalism and maintains client confidentiality in line with the **Data Protection Act 1998** (see page 44) • Pleasant and friendly approach – evidenced by the way they deal with clients, making them feel special, and demonstrating a passion for the nail industry. You need to be approachable so that clients feel confident in you • Good manners – demonstrates a level of respect for others by always being polite or generally being helpful to others • Following **dress code and personal hygiene** – helps clients to feel confident in their abilities and will not create barriers.	• Not following dress code or personal hygiene – creates barriers, as clients will lack confidence in their abilities and poor personal hygiene will be offensive to all • Poor communication skills – clients, employees and employers will lack confidence in their abilities and this will not generate repeat bookings or retail sales • Not following salon policies – creates risks and hazards that could result in injury, damage to a client's personal effects or salon equipment and, in serious cases, death

Personality traits of a good and poor nail technician

Key terms

Traits – personality qualities, behaviour, character.

Active listener – someone who listens carefully to what the other person is saying.

Proactive – being able to self-manage, i.e. not requiring someone to tell you what you need to do.

Data Protection Act 1998 – the law that protects clients' personal information.

Dress code and personal hygiene – rules from the salon's workplace policy on what you must wear and do (see also Follow health and safety practice in the salon, page 17).

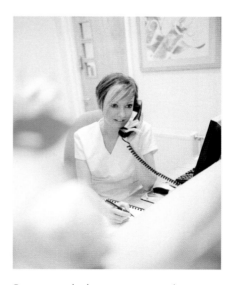

Be prepared when you communicate over the telephone

Think about it

Look at the personality traits of a good and poor technician, then write a list of your own personality traits. Are there any areas you can improve on?

Client care and communication in beauty-related industries

Top tips

- Always make eye contact and smile when a client walks into the salon, as it makes them feel important. Imagine how you would feel if you were a client and the receptionist ignored you when you entered the salon. Never treat clients in this way.

- When the telephone rings, answer it quickly, demonstrate good verbal skills and have the information you might need, which could include business opening times, appointment availability, treatments offered and prices. An example of a telephone greeting might be: 'Good morning, The Nail Studio, Samuel speaking. How may I help you?'

Types of communication

As soon as a client walks through the door, you will naturally start to communicate with them, first by making eye contact and smiling. This initial greeting acknowledges the client's importance and makes them feel welcome.

The diagram below summarises the main types of communication.

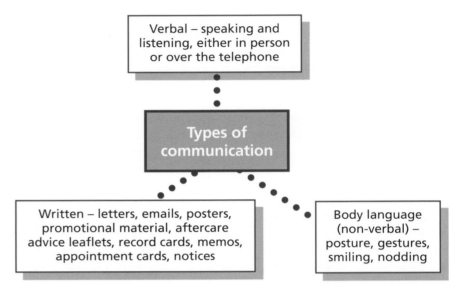

Using verbal communication

- Speak clearly.
- Avoid jargon; use plain English.
- Actively listen and do not interrupt.
- Be polite and attentive.
- Use good questioning techniques.
- Some hearing-impaired clients can lip read, so demonstrate good communication skills by keeping still when you speak and they are trying to lip read.
- Clients who are visually impaired will need you to be very descriptive, as often they cannot see the treatment results fully, or at all.
- Never use over-familiar or overly friendly words, such as 'Love' or 'Babe', as this is not professional and some clients may find it offensive.

Using non-verbal communication (body language)

- Nod when you are actively listening to a client to acknowledge them.
- Make eye contact and smile.
- Never fold your arms, keep them relaxed.
- Do not point with your fingers.

- Give clients 'personal space' – never get too close, as it may cause them to feel very uncomfortable.

- Stand up when a client approaches you.

Using written communication

- Check presentation is clear.

- Use ICT skills when appropriate, for example when creating a poster or writing an email.

- Avoid jargon; use plain English.

- Use correct spelling, good grammar and punctuation.

- Provide correct information, for example when filling in an appointment card or taking a message.

- Clients who are dyslexic will have special requirements. For example, they might need promotion letters to be on yellow paper. Ask them what you can do to help, as this will demonstrate good client care.

Understanding a client's body language

When recommending a treatment or retail product to a client, you need to learn how to recognise whether they are interested or not. Their body language will give you clues, for example they:

- may look uninterested

- do not ask any questions

- provide little or no eye contact

- fiddle or play with their hair or jewellery

- look nervous or confused

- frown.

How to use consultation techniques to identify treatment objectives

The main purpose of completing a **consultation** is to:

- build a good **rapport** with the client

- gain the client's confidence

- discuss the treatment plan and the client's requirements

- establish any **contra-indications**

- discuss future treatments and retail recommendations

- complete the record card and obtain the client's signature.

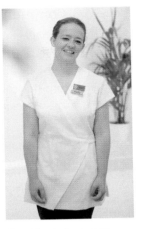
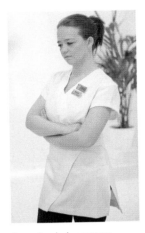

Good body language   *Poor body language*

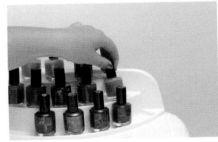

During the consultation and when you give the client aftercare advice, remember to recommend retail products that they would benefit from

Top tips

- When you give important information to a client who speaks English as a second language, check that they have understood by asking them to repeat back what you have said or reinforce their understanding by providing a written copy.

- Clients who are visually impaired will often have guide dog. Ensure the client is positioned safely so the dog is not obstructing walkways or doorways.

Key terms

Consultation – a discussion before a treatment begins.

Rapport – relationship between people.

Contra-indications – skin and nail diseases or disorders that would prevent or restrict a treatment.

Top tip

Avoid the 'hard-sell' approach, as it never really works. Even if the client buys a product, you could intimidate them so much that they do not return.

Client care and communication in beauty-related industries

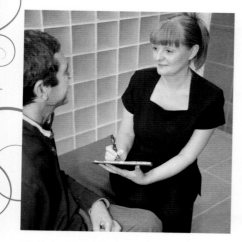

Sit facing your client during a consultation and use positive body language

Key terms

Open questioning techniques – questions asked in a way to get a detailed answer.

Closed questions – questions that only obtain a yes or no answer.

Technical jargon – words used by nail industry professionals, for example 'epidermis'; when talking to clients, refer to the skin instead.

Contra-action – a bad or adverse reaction of a client to a treatment, for example redness or blistering of the skin.

Check it out

Look at the communication techniques shown in the table.

In pairs, use role play to practise your communication techniques, taking it in turns to be the technician and the client. Perform a consultation and discuss aftercare advice, then evaluate your performance. What areas do you need to perfect before you are assessed on this unit for your qualification?

Communication techniques in practice

Gathering all the information required may be difficult if the client is shy or nervous and perhaps does not feel comfortable discussing either themselves or the treatment. This is where you will need to demonstrate excellent communication and questioning skills. The following table shows the techniques you will need to be an effective communicator.

Communication technique	What is involved
Active listening	Listen carefully to what the client is saying. Do not be distracted when performing the consultation – sit down in front of the client at the same level and focus on what they are saying. Never interrupt or finish a client's sentence to avoid any misunderstandings.
Questioning techniques	Use **open questioning techniques** to obtain as much information as possible from the client; e.g. 'How do you care for your feet at home?' will give you a detailed response. Avoid **closed questions**, such as 'Do you have a routine at home to look after your feet?', which will give you a yes or no answer.
Understanding	Ask the client questions to check they have understood what you have said. You might need to rephrase and repeat a question or information. Never use **technical jargon** – use plain English so clients will understand.
Location of the consultation	Only the nail technician performing the treatment should complete the consultation, which should be carried out at the workstation, in a discreet manner.
Body language	Use open, friendly gestures, e.g. smile, nod and maintain a good posture.
Written communication	The nail technician must complete the record card and ask the client to check and sign it before the consultation process is complete. The client must sign the record card to document what has been discussed and for insurance purposes to protect the technician and business. Any retail products purchased by the client, aftercare or homecare advice can be written down for the client to reinforce the information and help promote retail sales. Providing aftercare advice will also minimise or prevent possible **contra-actions** and inform clients of what to do in the event of a contra-action.

Communication techniques

Treatment objectives

During the consultation, your aim is to:

- identify what the client's needs and expectations are
- discuss the possible treatment options and prices
- discuss the treatment effects
- discuss the benefits of regular treatments
- identify any contra-indications — if they are not contagious, then the treatment can be **modified**
- state what the realistic treatment outcomes will be.

Top tip

Demonstrate good time management and never be late for an appointment, as it will look unprofessional, be a bad advertisement, will affect the treatment results and affect your relationship with the client.

Key terms

Modified – a treatment can be adapted or changed to take into account a contra-indication. For example, a bruise can be worked around, or if a client has bitten nails then adding a heat treatment with massage will help to stimulate growth.

Repetitive strain injury (RSI) – pain from bad posture.

The nail studio	
Manicure	£12
Luxury manicure	£18
Pedicure	£15
Luxury pedicure	£18
Nail art from:	£5
Fibreglass nail extensions	£25
Infills and maintenance	£18

Treatment list with prices

Using consultation techniques

You will need to use your communication techniques during a consultation to aid understanding between you and the client.

- Help the client to feel relaxed by positioning them in front of you.
- Use appropriate body language, verbal and written skills.
- Complete the record card and check for any contra-indications.
- Ask the client what they want from the treatment. For example, it could be to improve a condition such as split and dry nail plates or to make their nails look attractive for a special occasion. In this case, it could be either a manicure to repair nails and improve the condition or fibreglass nail extensions for an instant effect. This will depend on whether they want natural nails or artificial, and you will need to explain the advantages of each and the maintenance required for artificial nails.
- Establish whether the client's requirements are achievable:
  - If they are, discuss effects such as colour of enamel, use of heat treatment, length of extensions.
  - If not, explain why and offer alternatives.

Top tip

Don't sit on the couch while your client sits on a chair – you will be higher than them and this can be very intimidating. It may also put you at risk of **repetitive strain injury**.

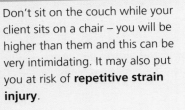
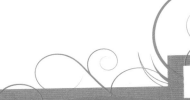

NAILS RECORD CARD

Name:	Date:	
Telephone no:	Medical history (treatment, comments):	
Address:		
	Appointments:	Weekly	
Date of birth:		Monthly	
Occupation:		Other	

Condition of nails

	Left hand:	Right hand:	Key:
Thumb			BR – broken
Index finger			BI - bitten
Middle finger			F – fungus
Ring finger			L - lifting
Little finger			N - normal

Record card used during a consultation

- Discuss the treatment plan and ask the client questions to check that you both understand what the plan will include.

The importance of using effective communication to identify client needs and expectations

Good communication will establish the client's needs and expectations, which need to be realistic. If you do not establish what effects are achievable, at the end of the treatment the client will either be very disappointed and will never return or they will complain to you and the manager. If the client is dissatisfied, this will cause a delay with your next client and they might overhear what has happened, which could impact on your next treatment. Use the communication skills discussed above to help you prevent this type of situation from occurring.

If you believe you cannot achieve what the client wants, it is important to tell them, as you might be able to recommend something else. For example, if a client with excessively bitten nails and a small nail plate wants fibreglass nail extensions, it is better to recommend a way to improve their nails so that may be able to have nail extensions as a treatment in the future. Below is a suggested alternative treatment plan.

Top tip

For clients who are nervous, hearing impaired or where English is spoken as a second language, you could use **visual aids** to ensure you understand fully what the client requires.

Key term

Visual aids – pictures or images to help understanding

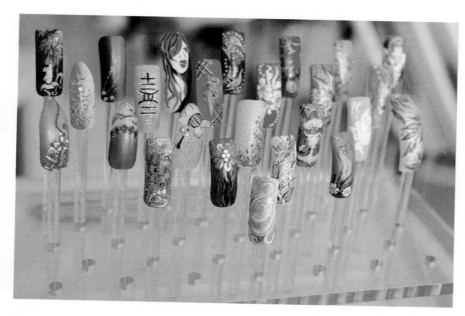

Visual aids such as examples of nail art can be used to help understand your client's needs

Client care and communication in beauty-related industries

Treatment plan and recommendations for a client with bitten nails and a very small nail plate

- Weekly manicure to speed up nail growth and improve the condition of the nails.

- Use a hand cream at home and massage skin, nails and cuticles.

- Wear gloves when using chemicals or gardening to protect the area.

- Use hand soaps that are pH balanced and moisturising.

- Buff the nails to stimulate growth.

- Use a cuticle cream.

- Gently file any rough edges to avoid the need to bite the nails.

- Do not bite the nails – use unpleasant-tasting clear enamels, wear gloves at home.

What is 'personal space'?

It is important to provide enough personal space for the client to feel comfortable when you are performing a treatment. Ensure your working space is not too small, allowing you enough room to work comfortably and safely. If you are uncomfortable when working, you may start to suffer from repetitive strain injury (RSI) — and having muscular aches and pains will affect your performance.

Some clients, especially those who are nervous or anxious, will not feel instantly relaxed when having a treatment and might find it difficult being touched — their stress levels might increase if you are too close. Be aware of your clients' feelings and do not invade their personal space — this will ensure a successful treatment and instil client confidence in your abilities.

The importance of providing the client with clear advice and recommendations

The consultation enables you to establish the client's individual requirements and then to consider their future treatment needs, appropriate aftercare advice, homecare advice and retail products to maintain the effects of the treatment and to improve any areas of concern. (For information on specific recommendations, see Skin analysis and the Practical skills units.)

When to provide advice and recommendations

You can provide advice and recommendations at certain points during your time with the client — during the consultation, if the client asks you a question during the treatment, and at the end of the treatment. It is better not to provide advice during the treatment, as the client will want to relax and enjoy it and they might feel you are trying to pressure them into rebooking or to purchase retail products. However, if you do not provide advice and recommendations to improve a

Top tip

If a client has a contra-indication, do not name what you think it is, as you might be wrong. Nail technicians are not medically qualified to assess a condition and you could cause unnecessary worry. The client might decide to treat it themselves, which could make the condition worse and cause discomfort. Instead, advise the client to see their GP, but remember to be tactful as the client could be very embarrassed. Perhaps offer them an incentive to return, such as a money-off voucher.

Check it out

Select a Practical skills unit and read about the different types of client needs, for example hard calluses. Think about the advice and recommendations you would give them, in preparation for your assessments.

condition, your client will be unaware that they have these options. Below is a suggested treatment plan for a client with excessively dry skin on their hands.

Treatment plan and recommendations for a client with excessively dry skin, nails and cuticles on the hands

- Regular weekly manicures with a paraffin wax treatment.
- Use a rich hand cream at home and massage the skin, nails and cuticles.
- Wear gloves when using chemicals or gardening.
- Use hand soaps that are pH balanced and moisturising.
- Buff the nails.
- Use a cuticle cream.
- Avoid enamels and remover.

Professional ethical conduct

It is important that nail technicians apply a professional, ethical approach towards their chosen profession, by adopting a positive and proactive attitude. This is essential in creating the right environment to develop good client, colleague and employer relations and generate loyalty and respect. The simplest of actions, like good time management, punctuality, pride in work and personal presentation, will help to reinforce your position within the business. Professional conduct also includes confidentiality — you must not gossip or share confidential information about the business, your colleagues or the clients.

Provide client care

Maintaining client confidentiality in line with the Data Protection Act 1998

All employees must comply with the Data Protection Act when handling clients' personal information that is stored on the premises, such as record cards, computer files and accident report forms. Clients' personal details include their name, address, contact number, medical history and GP's details.

The Information Commissioner's Office (ICO), the UK's independent authority set up to regulate businesses that handle the public's personal information, is responsible for enforcing the Data Protection Act. Businesses must register with the ICO and can participate in **audits** to ensure that they are complying with current legislation. The act sets out eight principles that businesses must follow when handling information. Data must be:

1 fairly and lawfully processed

2 processed for limited purposes

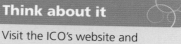

Think about it

Visit the ICO's website and research its purpose and role in the regulation of businesses.

Key term

Audits – checks performed to ensure procedures have been followed.

3 adequate, relevant and not excessive

4 accurate and up to date

5 not kept longer than necessary

6 processed in line with the individual's rights

7 secure

8 not transferred to other countries without adequate protection.

The importance of communication techniques to support retail opportunities

Retail sales are a way for businesses to boost their profits and employees should recommend retail products to all their clients. Not only does use of the correct products maintain the effects of the treatment and generally improve the appearance of the skin, nails and cuticle, it also identifies the business as one that offers the 'whole package', creating a more prestigious nail studio. Selling retail does not come naturally to everyone, so employers should provide staff training that covers:

- the use of role play to demonstrate selling techniques
- practise using the correct communication skills necessary
- appropriate timing of when to discuss retail
- reading the client's body language signals
- product training including **features** and **benefits** from the suppliers
- location when promoting a product — either at the workstation or at reception.

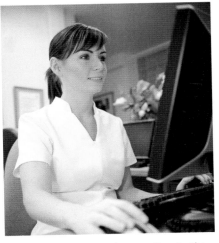

Store computer records according to the Data Protection Act

Top tips

Record cards and accident/illness report forms must be stored in a locked, secure cabinet, with access restricted to the client's personal nail technician(s) and manager. Any information stored on the computer must be stored securely and be password-protected. Only authorised individuals should be allowed access.

Key terms

Feature – what a product contains, for example cocoa butter.

Benefit – what the feature does, for example cocoa butter nourishes the skin.

Top tip

Appropriate timing is important to achieve retail sales and repeat bookings. Remember to use good communication skills and read your client's body language, especially if they do not appear to be interested.

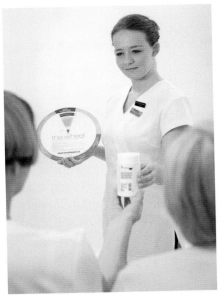

Staff training is important in areas such as communication skills and product knowledge

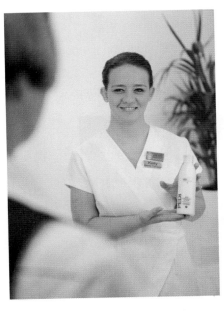

Provide accurate product information

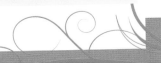

Client care and communication in beauty-related industries

Think about it

Look at the products you sell in your workplace or training establishment and select three examples. List their features and benefits. In pairs, practise your selling techniques, taking it in turns to be the technician and client.

Top tips

- When discussing a product with the client, allow them to handle it. This will encourage them to feel like it already belongs to them.

- Display retail products and information leaflets with special offers, as this will gain the interest of the clients and they can see exactly what you sell.

Top tip

Get some advertising leaflets printed so that during quieter times at work you can hand out leaflets in the salon, outside the premises, in local shopping centres or local businesses. This is a good way to promote the business and generate new clientele.

Below are some suggested ways to generate and increase retail sales.

- Display a range of products suitable for the type of clientele. This will depend upon the location of the business. For example, city centre salons may be able to offer more expensive products than those in towns or villages.

- Offer at least a couple of brands, with one cheaper than the other — if a client is unsure, they may want to try the cheaper alternative, which might persuade them to buy the more expensive product next time.

- Offer a range that has a good selection of products for all types, such as all ages, gender, ethnic backgrounds, vegans.

- Display stock in an eye-catching way using a range of visual props (see also Display stock and promote products and services to clients in a salon, page 55).

- Maintain stock levels — if a technician achieves a sale but the product is not in stock, this amounts to lost earnings for the salon and loss of commission for the technician.

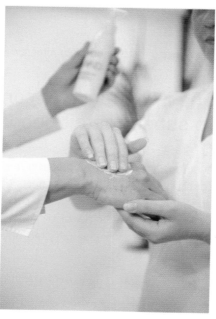

Testers are popular, especially hand creams, as clients can instantly feel the benefits

- Provide targets and offer bonus incentives for employees — incentives can create friendly competition between staff and inspire a stronger personal drive to sell.

- Special offers and promotions — these will entice clients to purchase and generate sales.

- Fully trained employees — employees need the knowledge to sell effectively.

- Good marketing strategy and advertising — hold regular team meetings to discuss these; use posters, website advertisements, mail shots, demonstration events, radio and newspaper advertising, leaflets/brochures, packaging and carrier bags with company logo and information to help promote the salon's services and products.

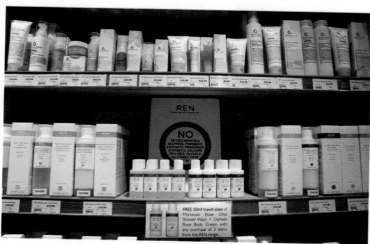

Display products in the reception area

The importance of client feedback and responding constructively

Clients might comment generally on how they enjoyed a treatment, but they do not usually give feedback on client care. However, understanding if you or other employees have provided excellent client care is important, as this will affect repeat booking and retail sales. Ways to gather this information can sometimes come from managers asking clients in person, but some clients might find this uncomfortable and will not give their true opinion. Surveys can be used to find out the information; for example, you could ask 'How good was the client care you received today?' and 'How could it be improved?' The survey's findings can be used in staff training sessions to improve communication skills of the nail technicians. The table below summarises the advantages and disadvantages of different survey methods.

Designing a survey

Here are some things that you will need to consider when designing a survey.

- Check that the survey is clear and to the point, and contains no jargon.
- Make sure the design is attractive — it needs to be eye-catching.
- Explain in a covering letter or email why it is important that the client completes the survey and include an incentive for completion.
- Put the most important questions at the beginning.
- Pitch questions at the correct level — do not use technical terminology.
- Only include a few questions — the client may get bored if you ask too many.
- Include a balance of multiple-choice questions (easier to complete) with a few questions where clients have to write a more detailed answer.
- Perform a trial run to see how effective the survey is.

Respond to feedback in a constructive way

Gaining feedback on your performance is the way you learn to become more professional and an outstanding nail technician. While training to become a nail technician, you will need to encourage constructive feedback, especially from clients, peers and trainers. Feedback on your techniques will help you to produce better effects, and feedback on your client care and communication will make you more attentive and understanding of your clients' needs. Do not be offended or become hostile or defensive when you are told the areas that require improvement — it will help you to improve overall techniques or performance.

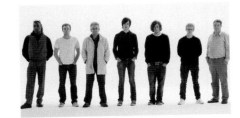

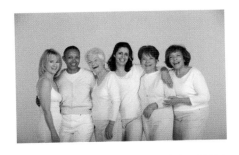

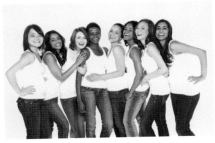

Target all types of people to increase your client base

Top tip

Learn about the features and benefits of products to help you sell them. For example, the feature of a hand cream may be that it contains a UV filter; its benefit is that it will protect the skin against UV damage and age spots.

Salon life

My story

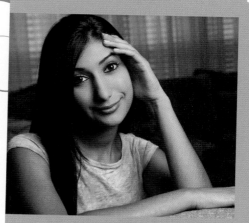

My name is Shailini. I am a newly qualified nail technician and recently started work in a large, prestigious city-centre studio. Everything was going well, except that I was failing to reach my retail targets. I just did not feel confident selling retail. Fortunately, I have an excellent manager, who asked to see me regarding my retail sales. I explained that I had no experience in selling and as I was new to the studio I was unaware of what retail products they stocked or what they were used for. From this, my manager organised a training session on retail products and selling techniques, which gave me more confidence. I now realise the importance of retail sales to the business and the client.

Ask the experts

Q How many products and treatments should I recommend at one time?

A You need to determine this from the type of client you have. Regular clients, for example, are likely to purchase more and book in more frequently than walk-in clients. Assess a client's initial needs. If they are having fibreglass nail extensions, they will need to rebook for their infill. If the client has a problem growing their nails, then recommend they come at minimum once a month or maximum once a week and allow them to decide. When recommending retail assess your client, then start by suggesting one or two products and offer another on their next visit. Some clients are more confident and will initiate most purchases.

Q What should I do if a client asks me a question about a product and I don't know the answer?

A Be honest, excuse yourself politely and go and find a more experienced nail technician for help. Listen and observe them and use this opportunity to learn from someone with more experience.

Benefits of providing excellent client care and good communication

- Gives the client confidence in the nail technician's abilities.

- Creates a good rapport between client and technician.

- Client feels important and relaxed.

- Enhances the enjoyment of the treatment.

- Client is more open to recommendations of future services and retail sales.

- Promotes a professional nail technician and studio.

Top Tip

When you are quiet at work or at home, read the product manual to increase your product knowledge. Try the testers or samples to see how the products feel and what their effects are. You need to be confident, which will grow the more you practise your selling skills.

Type of survey	Advantages	Disadvantages
In person (existing or new clients)	Can target new clientele who will be more honest about client care from other businesses.	Passers-by do not often want to stop. Existing clients might not feel comfortable saying anything critical.
By telephone	Clients might explain in more detail verbally than they would in writing. Can encourage clients to make an appointment if they have not been to the salon for a while. If a client was previously unhappy and has not returned, this might encourage them to discuss the issues and rebook.	Costly and time-consuming. Can only target existing clients.
Postal	Can target the whole client base. Can be completed when clients have the time.	Costly and most people ignore this type of mail. Old clients might have moved address.
Business website	Surveys can be completed at any time during the year and are less time-consuming to complete online. Can be a cheaper option.	Clients would need to have access to the Internet and know the business had a website. Clients would not necessarily want to complete a survey without being enticed with an incentive.
Emails	Can easily be sent out to client base. Cheap option.	Would need to have clients' email addresses. Clients might not regularly read emails. They might want an incentive to complete. Junk emails are often ignored.

Survey methods – their advantages and disadvantages

How to refer and assist in client complaints

When a client wants to make a complaint, take them somewhere quiet away from other clients so that it does not create an embarrassing and awkward situation for others. Often when a client complains they can become loud, distressed and hostile, which is not a good advertisement for a business. The salon manager should deal with a complaint and involve the nail technician if necessary. Be professional, demonstrate a calm, pleasant manner and be objective while discussing the complaint.

Reasons for complaints

When a client complains there can be a mix of emotions — they may feel angry, disappointed, in pain, confused, upset, impatient and anxious — depending on what has happened. There are various reasons why a client decides to complain, including:

- poor quality of treatment or results
- inexperienced nail technician
- products or tools used incorrectly
- no or little preparation of the nail and cuticle before applying nail extensions or nail art

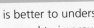
Top tips

- Offer an incentive to complete the survey, such as a discount or free treatment.

- By making the survey anonymous it will be more appealing to complete, as clients can be very honest in their answers.

Top tip

It is better to understand what you need to improve while you are training rather than when you enter the industry, as it will hold you back professionally and may affect your enjoyment and confidence later on. So encourage feedback, ask lots of questions and observe any demonstrations.

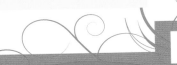

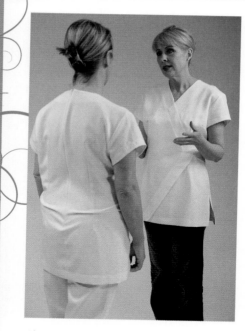

Always react positively to constructive feedback

- no pride in the nail technician's work — too tired or poor attitude
- poor communication regarding the desired effects
- treatment took too long or was not long enough
- parts of the treatment were not completed, for example no heat treatment in a luxury pedicure
- time restrictions or delays in starting the treatment
- salon too hot or too cold, which affects product's results
- injury or damage to client's belongings
- theft of client's valuables
- client had an allergic reaction — no skin test performed
- unidentified contra-indications that result in cross-infection — client in pain or the condition made worse
- client unhappy with a product they purchased or has had an allergic reaction
- unsafe environment or obstruction in the workplace leading to a client having an accident.

Resolving a complaint

If the nail technician or business is at fault, it is up to the manager to try to resolve the issue. If an accident or injury has occurred to the client and the business is at fault, it may be sued by the client. If a client is unhappy with their treatment results or effects, the manager may offer a refund or to correct the error. Occasionally, clients do not have a genuine complaint but do so because they do not want to pay for their treatment. If the manager cannot find fault in the nail technician or treatment results, they will often challenge the client and the client does not return.

Product returns

A client may be unhappy with a product they have purchased and request a refund. For example:

- they may have suffered an allergic reaction
- the product may already be out of date when they purchased it
- they may have chosen the wrong product
- the product has not had the desired effect
- the product smells unpleasant and is of the wrong consistency (possibly out of date or stored incorrectly)
- the product is damaged.

What you must do next:

- Evaluate the situation for the best course of action.
- You could offer the client an exchange or credit note.

Check it out

In pairs, create a script for a short play, in which a client makes a complaint. You choose what the complaint will be and how it should be correctly resolved.

Remember to include:

- where the complaint takes place
- procedures for dealing with complaints
- verbal communication and body language of the characters – manager, client and nail technician
- how it is resolved.

- Perform an allergy test before suggesting any further products.
- Contact the suppliers if the product is damaged or has caused a reaction.
- Seek advice from more experienced colleagues.
- Keep a record of refunded goods.

Complying with consumer legislation when selling and refunding products

There are several laws that protect consumers when buying and returning goods. You will need to understand these when selling and refunding products.

Sale and Supply of Goods Act 1994

Under this act, goods must be:

- of good quality with no defects
- fit for purpose
- described correctly.

If a product sold by your salon does not comply with this act, the consumer is entitled to a full refund.

The Sale and Supply of Goods to Consumers Regulations 2002

The regulations protect consumers who have purchased faulty goods within the European Union – they are entitled to a repair or replacement.

Trade Descriptions Act 1968

This act covers the false description of goods. It is illegal to mislead consumers by incorrectly describing a product or making false statements about it, so goods should have clear and accurate labelling.

Supply of Goods and Services Act 1982

This act protects consumers against bad workmanship or poor provision of services. It covers contracts for services and materials, but also applies where no contract is required, such as having your nails done at the nail bar. Services should be carried out with reasonable care and skill, within a timescale and at reasonable cost.

Consumer Credit Act 1974

This act helps to safeguard consumers who enter into a credit agreement (purchase on credit) which does not exceed £25,000. It is unlikely that a salon would provide this service. However, a salon owner might wish to purchase goods or equipment using a **hire purchase agreement**.

Businesses which allow consumers to purchase goods or services on credit agreements must be licensed by the Office of Fair Trading (OFT).

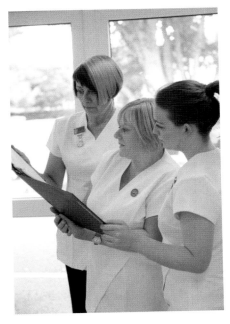

If in doubt, ask for guidance from a more experienced nail technician

Top tip

Local authorities' Trading Standards departments regulate and monitor local businesses to check if they are following consumer laws and will investigate any complaints.

Key term

Hire purchase agreement – the owner rents equipment to a purchaser and if all payments are made over a set period of time, the purchaser will then become the owner of the equipment.

Top tip

If your salon sells products via its website, you could be supplying to consumers globally, so ensure you are complying with all legislation.

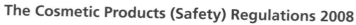

The Cosmetic Products (Safety) Regulations 2008

Products must be safe for their intended use and labels must be clear and accurate, including ingredients, weight, storage information, disposal methods, how to use.

The Consumer Protection (Distance Selling) Regulations 2000

The regulations refer to goods not purchased in person, for example on the Internet or via telephone, fax, TV or mail order catalogue. Goods and services must be clearly described. The supplier must also display their delivery procedures and costs, business details and the procedure to cancel orders (consumers have seven days to cancel an order).

Prices Act 1974

Prices must be clearly labelled or displayed to prevent the consumer from being misled.

Resale Prices Act 1976

This act made it unlawful for suppliers to set the retail price of goods. The recommended retail price (RRP) could be used only as a guideline.

Consumer Safety Act 1978

This act protects consumers from unsafe or defective goods/services, which do not reach safety standards. Employees must be trained fully to use such goods or services. Goods should be stored correctly, with accurate labelling and the prices must be clear and up to date.

Disability Discrimination Act 1995 and 2005

It is unlawful for businesses to discriminate against people on the grounds of disability — everyone should receive the same quality of service. Businesses must also provide easy access for disabled people.

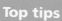

Top tips

- Hand-written price labels are easily damaged, so invest in a good pricing gun.

- Check the sell-by date and condition of the products before you sell them to the client.

Check your knowledge

1. What is an active listener?

2. When you ask a question and receive a detailed answer, what type of question has been asked?
   a) open
   b) closed

3. What do the terms 'feature' and 'benefit' mean when discussing retail products?

4. What are the three types of communication?

5. Read the description of how a client reacts while they are being recommended retail products and choose the answer that reflects how the client is feeling.
   The client is not asking any questions, gives little or no eye contact, is playing with their hair, looks nervous/confused and is frowning.
   a) The client does not want to buy the product.
   b) The client is in a rush and wants to buy the product.
   c) The client does not understand what you are saying.

6. Who deals with client complaints?

7. A client comes back to the salon after buying a nail enamel and has had an allergic reaction. What do you do?
   a) Give a full refund.
   b) Call the client a liar, as she must have used enamels in the past and probably doesn't like the colour she has bought.
   c) Ask her if she has any allergies and check other products' ingredients for differences or find a range for sensitive skins as an alternative, before offering a refund or exchange.

8. How should you react to feedback that identifies areas for improvement?
   a) It's their fault if you have done something wrong, as they haven't shown you properly.
   b) Embarrassed and annoyed
   c) Constructively, as this identifies areas that need to be practised

9. What law states how we are to handle a client's personal information?
   a) Consumer Safety Act
   b) Data Protection Act
   c) Consumer Protection (Distance Selling) Regulations

10. How should we store a client's personal information?

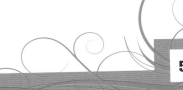

Getting ready for assessment

VRQ	
City & Guilds	**VTCT**
Service times: Not applicable to this unit Evidence: • You can take either the online test or complete knowledge tasks in the assignments • There is no particular time limit set for the completion of an assignment (tasks) • Knowledge tasks can be awarded a pass, a merit or a distinction grade • Practical tasks are graded pass, merit or distinction • You must carry out one consultation Knowledge and understanding will be assessed by: • a knowledge task or • an online GOLA test	Service times: There are no maximum service times that apply to this unit Evidence: • It is strongly recommended that the evidence for this unit be gathered in a realistic working environment • Simulation should be avoided where possible • You must practically demonstrate that you have met the required standard for this unit • All outcomes, assessment criteria and range statements must be achieved • Your performance will be observed on at least three occasions for each assessment criteria Knowledge and understanding will be assessed by: • oral questioning • portfolio of evidence

Display stock and promote products and services to clients

What you will learn

- Create displays to promote products and services
- Manage and dismantle promotional displays
- Promote products and services to the client

Display stock and promote products and services to clients

Key terms

Services – treatments that are available within the establishment for clients to experience.

Products – retail products and equipment that clients can use at home to maintain their nail service. These may differ from the professional products used within the salon as these are not always suitable for untrained people to use.

Commission – amount earned by nail technician through sales of products and services. Commonly a percentage, for example 10 per cent on total amount sold.

Introduction

The nail **services** industry has grown dramatically over the last few years. It offers a wide range of services to people from all areas of life and is easily accessible through an ever-increasing number of nail bars on the high street.

When a client first comes to your salon or nail bar, you will want them to become a regular, loyal customer. This will involve much more than the standard of the treatment they receive — you will need to inform them about the different services your salon offers and the retail **products** that they can buy.

With so much choice and information available, your clients will be very knowledgeable on the benefits of the products and services, and the price to pay for them too. Everyone likes to feel they have bought a bargain and promotions are an excellent way to expand on the services and products your client currently uses.

For any business, the ability to sell products is vital and, as a nail technician, you will be expected to perform and hit sales targets. This not only increases the salon's income but it will also increase yours by means of **commission**. In an industry known for its low pay, this is an excellent way to top up your monthly earnings. You will also increase your client base, as being a confident seller will show what a knowledgeable and experienced technician you are.

This unit looks at all areas of promotion and how to ensure they will work successfully within the business. When you begin your career in the nail industry you will need to show your employers that you can promote and sell confidently and successfully. Many people are put off selling as they do not like the 'hard sell', but it does not have to be forced in this way. By educating your clients, selling additional products and services will be a natural part of your working day.

Ensuring clients choose suitable products and services means they will be maximising the effects of the treatments at the salon and at home. The products used at home should enhance the results achieved by you and maintain them until the next appointment.

Create displays to promote products and services

Identifying the purpose of displays

When a client enters a salon, they are likely to see a display and/or promotional stand which aims to inform them of the types of service and products available. Displays are used to promote the business and to increase sales. They are an advertising tool designed to attract the eye and leave clients wanting to know more, and they can range from a small leaflet stand to a larger display cabinet, filled with information and visual props.

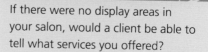

Think about it

If there were no display areas in your salon, would a client be able to tell what services you offered?

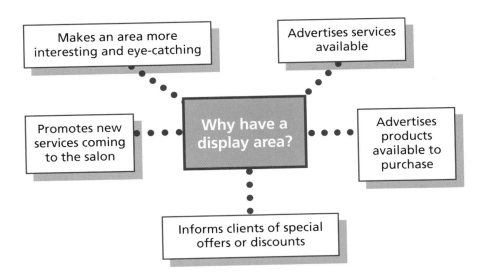

Makes an area more interesting and eye-catching

Advertises services available

Promotes new services coming to the salon

Why have a display area?

Advertises products available to purchase

Informs clients of special offers or discounts

A display area may simply provide information materials for clients to read. It does not always have to be about selling — reading about the latest trends in nails services can be enough to entice clients to try new services or at least start asking questions, which will give you the opportunity to introduce them to something new or different.

Before creating your display, make sure that you are clear about the message it is to put across. Too many different materials and visual aids can confuse a client and they will walk away. You may decide to work with a theme in mind, such as a seasonal display for summer. You will need to be sure that the theme is suitable for your salon and the time of year; for example, no one wants to see Christmas gift sets in the middle of the summer.

Selecting appropriate products and display materials

A wide range of materials can be used within a display, but they need to work together to make an eye-catching arrangement. Most of the products and equipment that you select will come from within the salon. However, it may also be appropriate to purchase materials to help enhance the display.

Products

As product companies invest time, money and effort in creating packaging that looks professional and attractive, products can work extremely well in a display. If displaying boxes, it is a good idea to remove the product and use only the empty box. You may decide to display the actual container. If so, you will need to take care where you place the product, as certain conditions can cause the product to **denature**; for example, the ultraviolet (UV) rays in strong sunlight can damage both the packaging and the product itself.

Top tip

Empty boxes in the display area will reduce the risk of theft. Actual products can be kept in a more secure area until the sale is made.

Key term

Denature – the chemical structures within the product may change and become more unstable, potentially leading to an ineffective product or a reaction on a client's skin.

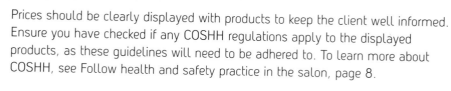
Prices should be clearly displayed with products to keep the client well informed. Ensure you have checked if any COSHH regulations apply to the displayed products, as these guidelines will need to be adhered to. To learn more about COSHH, see Follow health and safety practice in the salon, page 8.

Promotional materials

These consist of leaflets, posters, images and so on. They may be created by you; alternatively, many product companies will supply appropriate materials. The supplied materials will be of a high standard and very visual, so anything you create should try to match that standard. Posters and leaflets should be produced using computer software to ensure they look professional. The information given needs to be basic — the aim is to attract clients' interest so they then ask you questions about what is on offer.

Stationery

Stationery materials, such as tissue paper, card and glitter pens, can be used to make the display more visually appealing and attractive. Choose colours that complement the colour scheme of your products and promotional material.

Top tip

Any stationery created for a display must enhance and not overpower it.

Planning and preparing the display

Preparation is an essential aspect of planning a display so that it can be assembled safely and with all the necessary components. During your planning, write a comprehensive list of everything you will need and where they will be obtained from. Be sure to highlight any health and safety issues that need to be considered. An example is given below.

Check it out

To help you plan your display, answer the following questions:

- What is the purpose of the display?

- What features will be most suitable?

- What materials will you require?

- Who is the display aimed at?

- What will the display be placed on?

Items	From who	Health and safety
Nail varnishes	Technician	Do not display in sunlight as it will change the colour of the varnish
Promotional posters	Product company	Display securely on unit
Gift sets	Receptionist	Check COSHH regulations and manufacturers' instructions on storage

Planning your display

Your display will not be effective if the standard of your materials is not consistent. You may decide to create labels yourself to give information on specific areas of your display. When creating labels and promotional material you will need to ensure that you comply with the relevant legislation (see page 60).

Locating the display to maximise its impact

Most salons have an area where promotional materials are displayed, usually in the reception area where they will be clearly visible to clients. Nail bars are often in smaller premises so space may be limited, but this does not mean that you cannot create displays. The following spider diagram shows options for suitable display areas.

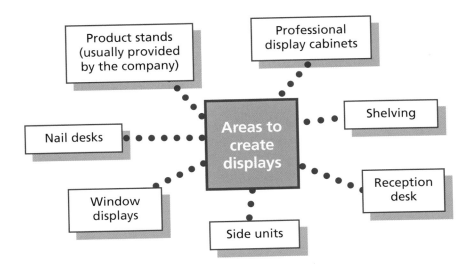

Each of these can be very effective. However, you will need to adapt your display to suit each one. For example, displays in areas of high traffic will need to be neat and sturdy to reduce the risk of items being knocked over.

Your display should have an immediate impact on clients. It should attract their attention and persuade them to enquire about the items on display. Where you choose to place the display will be affected by the purpose of it. For example, seasonal displays would be better placed in the reception area to tempt visitors, while specific treatment displays could be placed within the treatment areas. If the display is hidden away in a corner of the salon, it may go unnoticed and fail to have any impact. Placing it in a suitable area has the ability to increase sales and revenue for the business and boost commission for you as a technician. The following table identifies the consequence of suitable and unsuitable areas for displays in the salon.

Suitable display areas	Unsuitable display areas
• Attract clients' attention • Cause them to ask more questions • Could lead to sales of products • Could lead to clients trying new nail services • May attract new clients to business	• Fail to stand out from other salon furniture • May look old and tired as they are forgotten about • Products may go out of date while on display • New equipment for new services will go unused

The consequences of selecting suitable and unsuitable display areas

If the layout of the salon prevents the movement of furniture, you may be limited to a specific area(s) when creating displays. Since the display area is static, it is important to regularly change and update the display — clients will stop noticing the display if it stays the same.

Top tip

You are creating a visual display, so use your artistic skills.

Top tips

The following issues may be specific to individual salons and nail bars, but should always be considered.

- Are there any risks of cross-contamination?

- Ensure the display area is thoroughly cleaned prior to use.

- Be careful when handling equipment and stock – any breakages will cost the salon money.

- Check manufacturers' instructions when displaying products – there may be guidelines on storage and factors that may affect the shelf life of the product.

- If new display cabinets have been bought, follow instructions on assembly and work safely with any tools required.

Top tip

Remember, a promotional display reflects the image of your business. Old and untidy displays may mean that clients think all areas of the salon are like that.

Assembling the display carefully and safely

Once you have completed the planning, the display can be created. This section looks at how to assemble the display area safely and in accordance with the salon's rules.

Complying with legislation

When creating your display you will need to take account of the following legislation.

- The Control of Substances Hazardous to Health (COSHH) Regulations 2002. Due to the chemical ingredients in many nail products, you may be prohibited from using the actual containers in the display. You may, however, use the outer packaging such as the box to promote the product or service.

- The Personal Protective Equipment (PPE) at Work Regulations 1992. When creating the display be sure to protect yourself from injury. You may be moving boxes and furniture around, so appropriate footwear is essential.

- The Manual Handling Operations Regulations 1992. Most workplaces have posters on display to show how to lift and carry large items correctly, and you should also have been made aware of the regulations. Be sure to adhere to these guidelines to prevent any injury to yourself. It is advisable to carry out the activity with another colleague so you can support each other.

(To find out more about the above legislation, see the unit on Follow health and safety practice in the salon, page 1.)

Manage and dismantle promotional displays

Managing and maintaining the display area

Promotional displays need to be changed and updated regularly so that clients know what is available. For example, your salon may decide to run monthly special offers on products and discounts on treatments that are less popular. The display itself will need care and maintenance throughout its life to make sure that it looks as good as possible and does not start to look tired and forgotten. Below are ways to help you maintain your display in first-class condition.

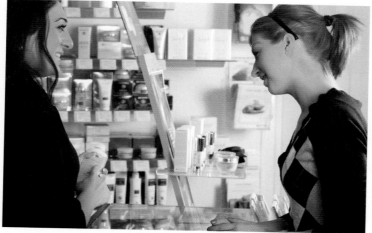

Keep your displays simple but eye-catching

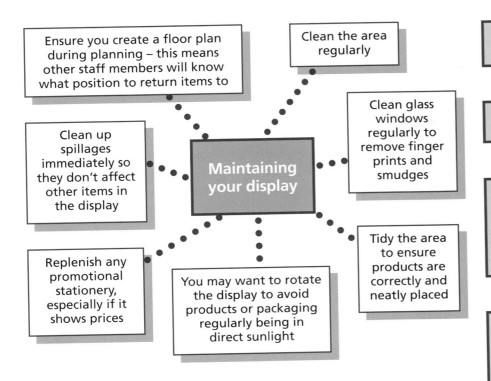

Ensure you create a floor plan during planning – this means other staff members will know what position to return items to

Clean the area regularly

Clean glass windows regularly to remove finger prints and smudges

Clean up spillages immediately so they don't affect other items in the display

Maintaining your display

Replenish any promotional stationery, especially if it shows prices

You may want to rotate the display to avoid products or packaging regularly being in direct sunlight

Tidy the area to ensure products are correctly and neatly placed

1. Remove stationery from area – this could be reused later

2. Remove and dispose of decorative items

3. Return leaflets and educational material to storage. They can be kept in the reception area (if applicable) or somewhere that is easily accessed

4. Remove products: dispose of empty boxes; inspect products for damage – dispose of damaged items appropriately, return intact products to the appropriate storage area (following COSHH)

5. Dismantle furniture, if used. Store all parts together and be sure to pick up discarded screws and nails to prevent them becoming a hazard. If furniture is being moved, ensure this is done safely. You should not try to move anything that is too heavy or tall (follow the Manual Handling Operations Regulations)

6. Clean empty display area and the surrounding floor and surfaces, ready for the new display

7. Dispose of waste using appropriate methods. Place cards and paper in the designated area for recycling waste.

Using appropriate techniques to dismantle displays

When the time for the display has ended, everything will need to be dismantled, packed away and the area cleaned and prepared for the next display. The changeover can sometimes be disruptive, and in a nail bar, where space is already limited, you will need to keep this to a minimum. It may help to change over the display during a quieter time in the salon when fewer clients are present or, better still, when the salon has closed – in particular, this will reduce the risk of clients and staff tripping over furniture and boxes temporarily left on the floor.

Follow the seven-step process for dismantling a display as shown opposite.

As discussed earlier, all relevant legislation should be followed and adhered to during the dismantling process. There will be a high risk of injury if carelessness occurs.

Top tip

When dismantling your display, try to recycle as much as possible. Follow your salon's guidelines on recycling.

Check it out

Which products or services do not sell well in your salon? Plan a display aimed at increasing the sales of these items.

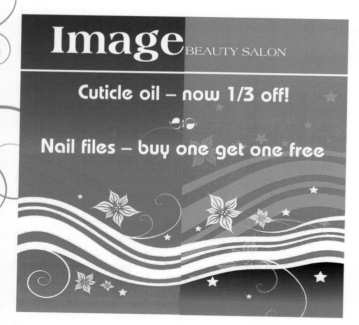

An example of a promotion

Key legal requirements relating to the display of stock

Prices of products and services should be clearly highlighted to clients. During a promotion, clients may be confused by the new prices. Any discounts should be clearly marked, showing the original price and the current selling price. Products need to be labelled with the price before they are put within a display. The labels can be either handwritten or computer-generated, as long as they are legible. Try to avoid using only fractions or percentages without showing the final price — leaving clients to calculate prices could cause errors and confusion and may cost the salon money.

This is the main legislation that you will need to consider when displaying stock:

- Trade Descriptions Act 1968. Information about products and services provided by the retailer (the salon) must be accurate and not misleading. Do not exaggerate the effects of a product or service to try to increase sales.

- Consumer Protection Act 1987. The products available for clients to buy need to be safe and suitable for use. Careless storage could cause the product to deteriorate, making it unsafe to use. This is particularly important if trying to sell products near to the end of their shelf life.

- Data Protection Act 1998. Any sale made must be kept between the client and the retailer. Information on what services and products the client purchases must be kept confidential by the retailer.

- Prices Act 1974 — you will need to ensure that all products and services have a price clearly attached to them so there is no confusion on the clients' behalf, particularly if running discounts.

- Sale and Supply of Goods Act 1994. The retailer forms a contract with the buyer which gives them the right to return a product if it is defective and to supply the buyer with a refund. The issue can then be taken up with the supplier.

- Consumer Safety Act 1978. The retailer must only sell reputable products to ensure they are safe for the clients to use.

Promote products and services to the client

Benefits to the salon of promoting services and products

When working within the industry, your salon may set the nail technicians targets for the promotion and sale of products and services. Setting achievement targets is a commonly used method of motivation and aims to ensure you attempt to increase your sales turnover. Your targets will be set according to the services you can offer and how many hours you are contracted to work. A member of staff who works 16 hours a week does not have as many opportunities to sell as a full-time member of staff, for example.

Targets are set not only to help technicians increase their earnings but also to boost the income within the salon. By encouraging clients to use professional products at home, you will see a sharp increase in the monthly takings. Clients will also get the best results out of their treatments if they use professional products between visits.

Clients can fall into the habit of having the same treatment at each visit and never trying anything new. Promotions help to prompt clients to experience new services which they then book in for regularly. The salon will look current and up to date, keeping clients interested.

Ensure you are aware of what your target is and identify the amount of commission you will receive. This is normally highlighted in your contract. Many establishments also offer rewards for achieving targets, such as free products or complimentary treatments. If you feel your target is unachievable, you should discuss this with your salon manager, as an unachievable target is unlikely to motivate you into selling.

Your salon may have its own policies and guidelines on selling and promoting, so ensure you are familiar with them. Being an enthusiastic member of the team will be rewarding for both you and the salon. If you are complacent about selling, it may leave your manager with a negative opinion of you.

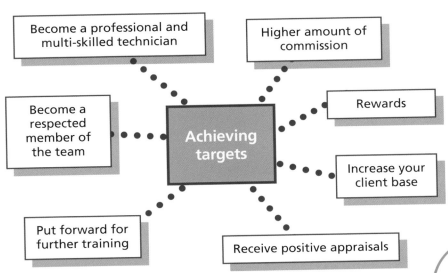

Become a professional and multi-skilled technician

Higher amount of commission

Become a respected member of the team

Rewards

Achieving targets

Increase your client base

Put forward for further training

Receive positive appraisals

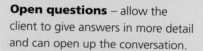

Think about it

It is important that target setting encourages a healthy amount of competition within the salon, but remember that you are part of a team.

Although it is important to try to achieve your targets, you need to be realistic about what you offer to clients. Always keep in mind how suitable the products and services are for individual clients. Sometimes technicians become so focused on hitting targets that they start recommending the most expensive items in the salon, whether they are suitable or not. This will only lead to an unhappy client who may complain or not return to the salon – not the outcome you were hoping for.

You need also to avoid stealing sales from other members of your team, as this will lead to tension and unhappiness in the workplace. Remember to treat everyone else in the same way you would expect to be treated. It is very common in the salon for a technician to spend time with a client, informing them about products, without the client purchasing anything. There could be several reasons for this. If the client were to return to the salon and purchase something that was recommended to her, the sale (commission) should go to the technician who advised the client in the first instance, as they did the work.

Listening and questioning techniques used for promotion and selling

Many newly qualified nail technicians find the idea of selling products very daunting. They are concerned that they will feel under pressure from their manager to demonstrate that they can promote products to clients. However, advising clients on appropriate products that complement nail services should occur naturally throughout the service they are receiving. There is no need to pressure the client into buying. Remember, a client will purchase a product or service if they feel that they will benefit from it and it is appropriate for their needs – educating clients about suitable products and services does not involve putting pressure on them.

Key terms

Open questions – allow the client to give answers in more detail and can open up the conversation.

Closed questions – usually only allow the client to answer 'yes' or 'no', which will prevent the conversation flowing.

Nail services allow plenty of time to communicate with the client, so it is advisable to use this to ask them questions to help draw out their needs. Use a variety of both **open** and **closed questions** to obtain the information that you will require to make your advice specific to them. (To learn more about communication techniques, see Client care and communication in beauty-related industries, page 38.)

Check it out

For your assessment, you will need to demonstrate that you can sell products and services to clients. Once a sale has been made, highlight it on the consultation card and use the receipt as evidence. Your assessor can then confirm the sale has taken place.

Having confidence will enable you to raise the subject of products and services, and clients will have faith in your knowledge. You will need to discuss the benefits to the client of purchasing the item – that is, the results they can expect to see from using it. If you lack confidence, the client will not take your advice seriously.

Clients need to understand the advice you give them, so it is important to use terminology they will recognise. Using technical terms (jargon) might prevent them from understanding why the product or service is suitable for them. Keep your explanation simple and always link the benefits of a product or service to the client's needs.

Consultation techniques used to promote products and services

During your initial consultation with the client, it is important to listen and record the information they give you accurately. This is when your client will begin to talk about their concerns and problem areas. Focusing on their needs when recommending products and services means your client will be more likely to show an interest in what you are suggesting. They will be able to see how the products and services will meet their needs.

There will be times throughout the client's service when you will be able to advise them on specific products. Choosing the right moment will ensure your client has the opportunity to listen to your advice. During a hand and arm massage, for example, the client will want to relax not discuss cuticle oil. Below are some suggestions on when might be an appropriate time to advise the client:

- while nails are soaking
- while feet are soaking in a foot spa
- when hands/feet are in mitt and booties
- when gel is curing under UV light
- as you complete the client's treatment log on their consultation card.

Remember, the client may bring up the topic themselves – do not ignore the opportunity just because you feel it is an inappropriate time.

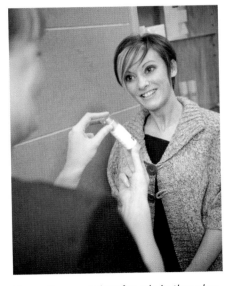

Promoting a product for sale in the salon

Top tip

Listen to the client – they will often discuss their concerns about their skin and nail condition throughout the treatment.

Spotting sales opportunities

One of the most common mistakes newly qualified technicians make is to miss opportunities and signs that a client is interested in something the salon has to offer. If you spot the right opportunity, it will make the sale much easier, as the client has already expressed an interest. Below are some opportunities to look out for.

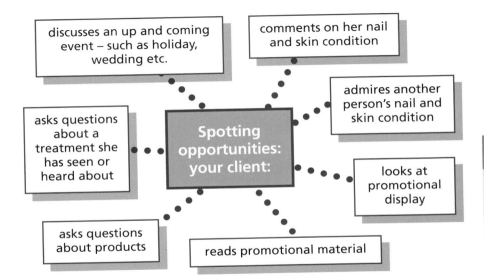

Think about it

In pairs, discuss what signs a client would show if they were interested in a product or service. Share them with the rest of the class.

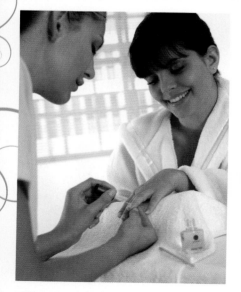

Talk to clients about new products during the treatment

Sometimes the client does not make it that easy for you, so it will be up to you to create the opportunities as the service takes place. This is when you will need to be confident in your approach. Generally, you can inform your clients of any new products and services and the promotions that are running in the salon at any point during the treatment – this means they will be more informed and might be tempted too. The table below suggests some links between the treatment the client is currently having and new products or services they could try.

Treatment	Links to new products and services
Acrylic nail removal	Deluxe manicures to help repair/promote healthy, natural nail growth, cuticle oil and strengthener for home use
Basic nail art	Matching nail art on toes/fingers (whichever is applicable), Minx or more elaborate nail art (airbrushing, 3D, etc.), top coat to protect varnish
Pedicure	Deluxe pedicure treatments, waxing treatments, foot exfoliants, heel repair creams, etc.

Links between client's current treatment and new products or services

Your client may not have the time after a treatment to talk about possible homecare products, but your salon should have a supply of literature and samples that you could give the client to try. At the next treatment, you can then discuss how she got on with them.

Features and benefits of services and products

The terms **features** and **benefits** should be used when informing clients about professional products and services. These are key points that should help the client to see why products and services are suitable for them. When attending product training, each product will be explained in detail, but a knowledgeable technician should be able to identify the key features and benefits easily. To help with selling, first identify the main features, which should entice the client to find out more. The benefits should then be explained so they can see exactly how the product or service will benefit them and solve the problem areas.

The principles of effective face-to-face communication

When dealing with clients face to face, you will need to use both verbal and non-verbal communication skills. Your facial expressions will help support your selling skills; a lack of confidence will be obvious to the client, and they will doubt the information you are giving them. Positive expressions such as smiling and nodding your head will ensure the client feels you are making the right decisions for them. (To learn more about verbal and non-verbal communication, see Client care and communication in beauty-related industries, page 38.)

Check it out

Look at the services your salon offers and identify which ones could be linked together for promotion.

Key terms

Feature – what will attract the client to the product; for example, cuticle cream helps keep cuticles soft and flexible.

Benefit – the advantage of using the product on the hands or feet; for example, rough skin remover helps dissolve dead skin.

Salon life

My story

My name is Ravneet and I have worked within the nail industry for 10 years. At the beginning of my career I found selling very challenging and would often avoid it if at all possible. My only sales came if a client specifically asked for something.

I moved jobs and found myself working for a reputable professional nail range. They provided me with excellent training and I began to fall in love with the products and became very impressed by the effects I saw when using them on myself. After the training I began to talk to my clients about my training and what I had learned. My clients became interested in the products and wanted to try them for themselves. My sales shot through the roof! I couldn't believe it as I wasn't trying to sell anything, I was just talking to them. I realised that my confidence in the product's ability and knowledge of the effects was capturing their attention. They trusted my opinion as a professional nail technician and followed my recommendation. I became the best seller at the salon and even went on to win an award from the nail company itself. I was completely transformed from when I first came into the industry. If you are passionate about your products, your client will be too!

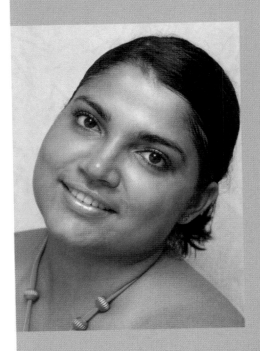

Ask the expert

Q Does it matter how many products go into a display?

A No, but if you put too many different types of product on display your customers may be confused about what is on offer. Remember to keep it simple but effective.

Top Tip

People like to touch displays – check glass doors regularly for fingerprints.

The importance of effective personal presentation

When assisting clients with products and services you will need to ensure your presentation reflects the standard of the salon. A client will have more faith and trust your advice if you present yourself in a professional manner. (To learn more about personal presentation requirements, see Follow health and safety practice in the salon, page 18.)

The importance of good product and service knowledge

At the beginning of your career in the nail industry, you will be required to attend a wide range of training courses. Attending training on the services and products supplied within your salon will make you a more confident seller. The following table outlines the advantages of attending product and treatment training.

Product training	Treatment training
In-depth knowledge about effects and benefits of product Knowledge about use of product Confidence in matching product to client's needs Knowledge of product's key ingredients and their functions	Confidence in carrying out treatment Matching treatment to needs of client In-depth knowledge of results achieved from treatment Ability to adapt treatment to meet specific needs of client

Advantages of attending product and treatment training

By attending training, clients will notice your knowledge in the advice you give them – this will give them confidence that you have recommended correctly. You will need to use your knowledge and expertise to discuss products and services with clients. Clients tend to ask lots of questions before they will commit to a sale. As discussed earlier in the unit, displays can be used to raise clients' awareness of what the salon has to offer.

As a professional technician, it is your duty to be well informed about the products and services on offer to your client. This should be a continual theme, as the industry changes so frequently that you will continually need to update your skills throughout your career. There are many ways to increase your knowledge:

- Attend regular training courses.
- Use the products yourself.
- Receive the treatments on offer.
- Keep up to date with new products and services on the market.
- Share information at team meetings.
- Read literature on products and services.
- Shadow a more experienced member of staff.

Product companies not only run sessions on using their range but they also often run sessions on how to increase sales. This is a valuable skill that everyone in the salon will benefit from.

Stages of the sale process

Ideally, all clients should use a wide range of homecare products to help maintain the service they have received, and then visit the salon regularly to

Top tip

Clients will spot if you are not telling the truth – this could discourage them from purchasing the item and returning to the salon in the future.

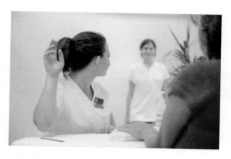

Ask a more experienced member of staff if you don't know the answer

receive treatments. But this can be unrealistic, so you will need to ensure you select items that can achieve the most for your client. Factors that will affect your recommendations include:

- the client's financial situation
- the client's commitment
- their nail and skin type
- how much time the client has to spend using products or visiting the salon
- how high-maintenance the service is that they receive
- the client's awareness of products and services that are available.

You might like the client to purchase five homecare products, but some clients may not wish to purchase as many as this and the quantity might put them off. Start with two key products that you know will make a visible difference and build up as necessary. Recommending products that achieve great results will win your client round and they will respect the advice you give them in the future.

The flow chart on page 70 shows the process of making a sale from the early signs of interest to closing the sale and the client making the purchase.

How to interpret buying signals

You will need to be able to interpret the difference between positive and negative buying signals and react to them accordingly. When a client shows positive buying signals you will need to start to close the sale. Examples of positive buying signals include:

- client nodding during conversation
- client asking more questions about the product and service
- client having a positive facial expression, such as smiling
- client identifying why they feel the product will work for them
- client describing themselves using the product or receiving the service
- client picking up products or trying out the samples.

Overcoming obstacles

Nobody likes to be pushed into making a decision, so if a client is clearly saying they are not interested, it is best to end that part of the conversation. There will be other opportunities for selling with other clients and sometimes the client just needs time to think about it before making a decision. Make sure they are aware that they can call back any time for more advice if it is needed.

Check it out

In small groups, list reasons clients may give for not making a purchase. Discuss ways of overcoming them.

Display stock and promote products and services to clients

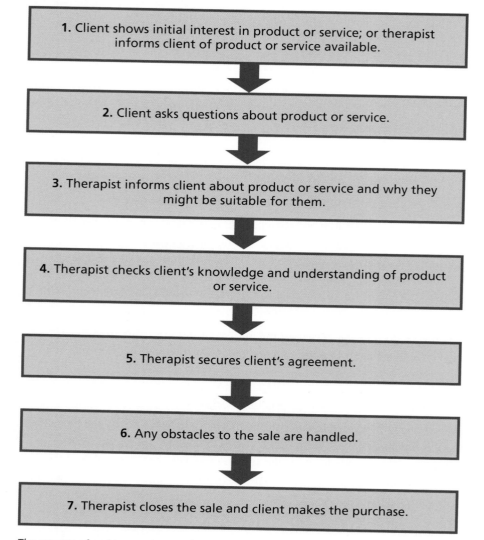

1. Client shows initial interest in product or service; or therapist informs client of product or service available.

2. Client asks questions about product or service.

3. Therapist informs client about product or service and why they might be suitable for them.

4. Therapist checks client's knowledge and understanding of product or service.

5. Therapist secures client's agreement.

6. Any obstacles to the sale are handled.

7. Therapist closes the sale and client makes the purchase.

The process of making a sale to a client

There may be times when the client is not saying no, but you are faced with objections such as 'I cannot afford to spend that much' or 'I don't have that much time to spend using products'. Here are some tips on how to turn an objection into a sale.

- Finances – if a client is wavering due to the cost of the treatment, explain how long the product will last and break the cost down into how much it will cost per week. Many of the high-street brands will cost less but not last half as long. Professional products have a higher concentrate of active ingredients, so a little goes a long way. There may also be a range of sizes, so perhaps you could suggest the client takes home the smaller size hand cream this time, for example.

- Lack of time – with this type of client it is important to select a product that is easy to use but has amazing results. Give suggestions to your client on efficient ways to use it, such as 'Keep your cuticle oil on your bedside cabinet, then apply once in bed'. This way the client will actually visualise doing it, and see that it will not take much time to do.

- Already has products at home – if the client is happy with the products they have at home, they are likely to be happy with their nail and skin condition. Look back at the client's key concerns on their record card and highlight them to the client again. Perhaps you could recommend a more suitable product that will give the results that the client requires.

- Out-of-stock item – this is an obstacle that may be beyond your control. As it can be very disappointing for the client, take the time to become familiar with the salon's stock. You may need to refer this to a senior member of staff for them to place the order, but you will still need to inform the client about when they can expect the item. Take responsibility to track the order, so that when it comes in you can contact the client and they can to come to the salon to collect it or you can forward it via the post immediately. To keep the client happy, provide them with some samples that they could use until the product arrives.

- Fully booked technician – again, this can be disappointing for the client. Once the client has shown an initial interest in a service, it is advisable to check the diary for availability. Make the client aware that there may be time constraints. Specialised services such as 3D nail art or Minx may only be offered by a small number of technicians – explain this to the client so that you can arrange a booking which is suitable for both client and technician.

- Referring clients – unfortunately, you may come across situations where you will need to refer your client either to another stockist or to another salon for a particular service. This does not always have to be a negative experience. Clients will appreciate your honesty and trust the advice you give them. A nail bar, for example, may not be able to offer generic beauty therapy treatments, so you might need to a recommend a salon that does. Likewise, your salon will not be able to stock every product available, so research where the client could purchase it from. It does not mean that you will lose the client to another business; if you were to turn them away without any advice you might, but by helping them you will show that you are truly professional.

How to secure agreement and close the sale

Securing agreement

Once the client has shown an interest in the product they would like to purchase, it is essential that they have a detailed knowledge of how to use it, including the amount, frequency and method of application. It is advisable to demonstrate the product, then ask the client to try it out too – this will also help in closing the sale, as the client can then visualise themselves using it at home.

When explaining the use of the product, keep making eye contact with your client. You need to be sure that they are still showing an interest in the product and are not getting confused with the instructions you are giving. The client needs to feel confident in using the product, as your aim is to get them to purchase it regularly. If they do not feel confident, the product will sit unused

Check it out

In pairs, each select one product from your nail range. Your aim is to educate each other as if you had never seen it before. How did you get on? Were there any aspects that you found challenging?

Top tip

Keep checking for signs that the client has become confused. Their facial expression may change; for example, they may start to frown.

Think about it

The information you give your client should contain enough details to answer the following questions: how, when, what, why and who?

Display stock and promote products and services to clients

Key term

Guarantee – a promise that the product will perform as is stated in the manufacturer's guidelines and is fit for purpose.

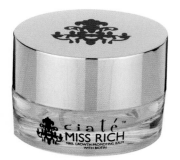

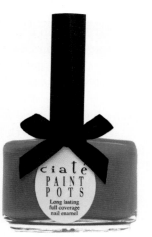

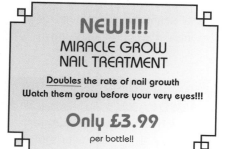

NEW!!!!
MIRACLE GROW NAIL TREATMENT

Doubles the rate of nail growth
Watch them grow before your very eyes!!!

Only £3.99
per bottle!!

Advertisements for new products must only show the facts and not exaggerate

at the back of their bathroom cupboard and they will be unlikely to purchase anything again.

Most product companies offer purchasers a **guarantee** that if they are not completely satisfied with their product they may return it without any cost to the salon. It may be advisable to check your supplier's policies on this matter. You should also reassure your client that they can return to the salon if they have any queries about their purchase.

Closing the sale

The next stage is to close the sale as, at this point, there is still a risk the client may change their mind. Keep things positive and ask the client which products they would like to take home today. Give them time to make the decision. Many technicians do not feel confident enough to ask the client to make a final decision, but as you have given the client all the appropriate information they may now need a final prompt from you to make the purchase. Below are some phrases you could use to close the sale.

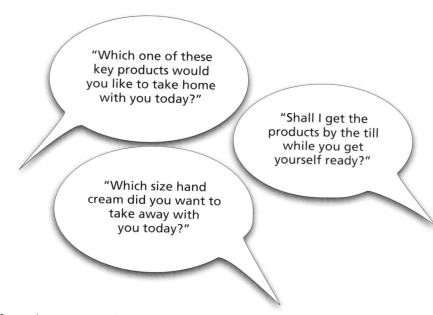

Some phrases you could use to close a sale

Evaluating selling techniques and their effectiveness

The way to know that you have successful selling skills is to see a rise in the amount you sell. During regular team meetings, targets for sales and treatments should be discussed to identify if there are any issues. It is also an appropriate time to identify the need for further training if you are still not confident. Your salon should support you and help you to develop strategies to increase your sales and meet your targets. If you are continually not hitting your targets, they may need to be negotiated, otherwise you may start to lose motivation.

Listen to your client's feedback — as a professional, you should follow up the sales you make to your clients. Check whether they are seeing results with the products they are using at home or that they enjoyed a new treatment they received. Positive feedback will confirm you are matching the products and services to the client's needs; negative feedback may highlight the need to refresh your skills.

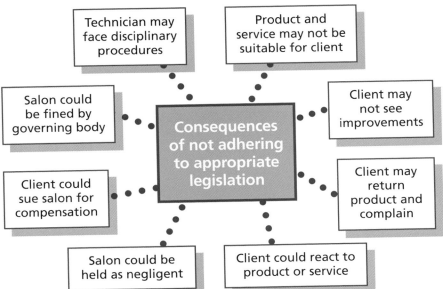

Legislation affecting the selling of services and products

Within this unit we have discussed how legislation affects the display of goods and services — it also affects the sales of products and services. (To learn more about relevant legislation, see Client care and communication in beauty-related industries, page 51.)

When promoting products and services to the client you must adhere to the legislation linked to the sale of goods and services. Whatever information you give to the client must be accurate and never exaggerated. Most clients will want to know what the product or service is going to do for them. The product's key features and benefits should be outlined to them. Show how it will meet their needs, but avoid getting carried away with what the product can or cannot do. Recently, some very well-known brands have been fined, as their adverts were thought to be misleading in what they claimed could be achieved with the product.

Although it is important to sell products to clients, the consequences of not complying with legislation may be serious.

Methods of payment for services and products

Taking payment for products and services will be the final stage in the sales process and shows your client's commitment. To learn more about payment methods, see Salon reception duties, page 93.

Check your knowledge

1. What is the purpose of a display?

2. List five items that could be used within a promotional display.

3. What is the main consequence of not placing a display in an appropriate area?

4. Why is it not always appropriate to display actual products?

5. What legislation is involved with promotional displays?

6. List five ways a client may show interest in a service or product.

7. Why is it vital to be well informed about the products and services available in your salon?

8. What are some of the obstacles clients may give?

9. What legislation covers the sale of products and services?

10. Why is it important clients are educated on how to use a product?

Getting reading for assessment

VRQs
VTCT

Service times: Not applicable to this unit

Evidence:
- Practical assessments will be internally assessed
- You will need to show competence in your practical assessments on three occasions
- Where at all possible, simulation should be avoided
- All outcomes, range statements and assessment criteria will need to be completed

Knowledge and understanding will be assessed by:
- written tasks to cover the criteria
- an internally-assessed portfolio of evidence

Salon reception duties

What you will learn

- Maintain the reception area
- Carry out reception duties
- Book appointments
- Deal with payments

Introduction

This unit looks at the various skills needed to run a successful salon reception area. This is the first port of call for all clients and visitors to the business, and first impressions count. Nail bars are often open plan, so the reception area may be part of the working area, which means that it is vital to ensure reception runs smoothly. When a client arrives it is important they have a positive experience so they leave happy and satisfied with their service.

Nail bar receptions are not always the same as beauty therapy salons. The two industries generally run the reception area in very different ways. Nail bars deal with existing clients who have pre-booked, but they also have walk-in clients who will expect a quick service. The reception area can be busy with waiting clients, so it can be a challenge to keep it neat and tidy throughout the day. It is important to have suitable **hospitality** to keep clients happy while they wait.

Each client needs to be dealt with politely and accommodated as much as possible. Receptionists need to work with nail technicians to plan their time effectively. It is a very competitive industry – clients have plenty of other salons to choose from if they are unhappy with your service.

Individual salons and nail bars will have their own guidelines for running the reception area. It is your responsibility to learn and abide by these guidelines and to attend training and support programmes throughout your time there.

As receptionist, you will be the first staff member clients come across, but you may not be able to deal with every enquiry. Knowing when to refer to another member of staff is essential, as failure to do so may lead to the client being dealt with ineffectively and having a negative experience.

Key term

Hospitality – the friendly welcome given to clients and visitors to the salon and items to make their wait more pleasurable, for example magazines, tea, coffee, etc.

Maintain the reception area

The reception area is often part of the working area, which can make it more difficult to maintain due to the lack of space. The area needs to be well planned to optimise space – neat, compact furniture will stop it from looking cluttered. When there is lack of space it is best to keep things minimalistic (simple and basic), so look for clever storage ideas to store the reception stock.

Not all salons can afford to employ full-time receptionists, which from time to time may mean that another member of staff is responsible for looking after the area. Having clear systems and procedures for dealing with clients will reduce the risk of mistakes being made when staff change over.

Keeping the reception area clean and tidy

The reception area should be inviting, comfortable and make a statement to clients about the type of business you are. An untidy and dirty reception area will give clients the message that your business is unhygienic and unprofessional.

Reception desks do not need to be filled with stationery and paper – use cupboards and drawers to keep spare pens and pencils. There should be space on the working desk for the receptionist to work on, alongside the phone, payment system, computer system if applicable, appointment pages and stationery.

The surrounding area where clients are waiting needs to be monitored throughout the day and any litter left by clients removed. Small coffee tables are ideal to display magazines and newspapers and for clients to put their drinks on, but they need to be kept as tidy as possible. It is acceptable to sweep or pick up debris from the floor, but try to avoid vacuuming during clients' treatments. This should be kept for the very end or the start of the day. Many salons provide a coat and umbrella stand for their clients – the best place for this is in the reception area if there is enough room. Otherwise, it could be placed at the back of the salon to avoid the reception area looking cluttered.

It is a good idea to have a checklist of the daily tasks that need to be carried out on reception, so if there is a changeover of staff on reception, everyone will know what their responsibilities are. Having a box in which staff sign their name once the tasks are complete means the salon manager can have confidence in what staff are doing. An example of a daily checklist is given below.

Daily tasks	Time and signature	Time and signature	Time and signature
Sorting post			
Getting out record cards			
Checking supplies for refreshments			
Vacuuming/sweeping floors			
Polishing/tidying displays			
Tidying magazines/ newspapers			
Checking answerphone/ voicemail messages			
Prepare float money for till			
Cashing up			
Switching on lighting, equipment, etc.			
Switching off lighting, equipment, etc			

Reception maintenance tasks: daily checklist

Maintaining levels of reception stationery

In a successful salon the receptionist can be extremely busy, as they have such a variety of jobs to undertake. They need to stay at the reception area to deal with enquiries, whether from walk-in clients or phone calls. In order for the reception area to be well run, everything the receptionist requires should be easily accessible. For example, the appointment book should not be moved away from the area, as the receptionist may not be able to access it when needed.

It is important to keep the reception area stocked with the appropriate stationery, with spare stationery kept in the stockroom so it can be topped up as necessary. Below is a checklist of what should be present:

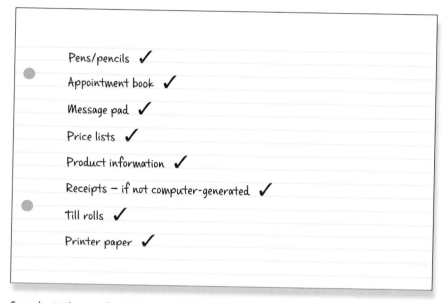

Pens/pencils ✔
Appointment book ✔
Message pad ✔
Price lists ✔
Product information ✔
Receipts – if not computer-generated ✔
Till rolls ✔
Printer paper ✔

Sample stationery checklist

Think about it

A client kept waiting while the receptionist looks for a pen could easily find another local salon to provide them with a nail service.

Ensuring display areas have the correct level of stock

Reception areas will often have display areas to promote the salon's products and services. Displays should be eye-catching and entice clients to look closer. Retail is very important in the nail services industry, as it can help to boost the salon or nail bar's income – and your earnings by way of **commission** – but it will also ensure your client is using the correct products to look after their nails in between treatments. Below are the items that should be on display in the reception area.

It is the receptionist's responsibility to ensure the area is not only kept clean but is also well stocked and secure. Keep the display areas neat, uncluttered and eye-catching. It is better to have a few key products than so many that the client cannot easily look through them.

You will need to find time during the day to monitor stock levels in the reception area and replenish stock. Clients may become frustrated if they are unable to

Key term

Commission – amount earned by nail technicians through sales of products and services. Commonly a percentage, for example 10 per cent on total amount sold.

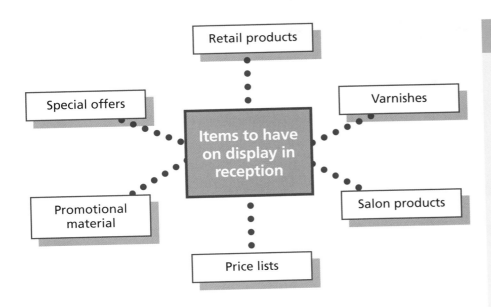

Retail products

Special offers

Varnishes

Items to have on display in reception

Promotional material

Salon products

Price lists

Salon reception duties

Top tips

The more products you have on display, the more dusting and cleaning you will have to do – so keep it simple.

- It is a good idea to have a plan of your stock display area in reception so that if there are any gaps, you can easily find out which item needs replenishing.

- Varnished nail tips make excellent display material as they can be very colourful. You could also display different enhancement finishes to encourage your client to try new things.

purchase their desired product. Varnishes, although they may seem low in cost and unimportant, can help a client maintain their nails at home and can also introduce them to the salon product range. Stock checks should take place at regular intervals and a record kept for the salon manager. It will help you to monitor what products sell well and what may need some extra promotions.

(To learn more about how to display stock and promotional material in the reception area, see Display stock and promote products and services to clients, page 56.)

Offering clients hospitality

All clients like to feel special and looked after during their nail service. The type of hospitality offered by salons can vary greatly, as it depends on how much money the salon owner wishes to invest in it. When the client arrives, the receptionist should greet them warmly and make them feel comfortable. The types of hospitality that should be offered as standard are:

- magazines and newspapers to read while waiting

- tea/coffee

- water.

Some salons also offer hot chocolate, fruit juices and biscuits/chocolates to make the client's visit more memorable.

It is part of your role to take care of clients when they arrive and ensure that there are refreshments available for them. Before opening in the morning, you will need to check that there are enough refreshments to last the day and that the magazines/newspapers are updated regularly. Who wants to read last year's news and gossip? It may also be a good idea to have information on the services that the nail technicians offer. A small brochure or leaflet alongside the magazines often encourages clients to try different services, which will boost the salon's takings.

Top tip

Although the initial cost may be higher, it is worth investing in your clients. They are more likely to return if they feel that they are getting good value for their money.

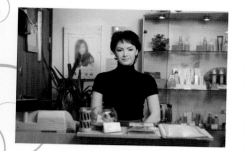

Carry out reception duties

In this section, you will look at the roles and responsibilities of the receptionist when dealing with clients in the reception area. The receptionist is an ambassador for the business, and clients will get to know them well. It is vital that the receptionist can handle the many different enquiries/clients that contact the salon.

Dealing with clients effectively and appropriately

The nail industry has never been so competitive – it is not uncommon to see three or four different nail salons on one high street – so every person who contacts the salon should be given the highest standard of service possible at all times.

Clients wanting nail services often change salons frequently. Unlike beauty therapists, nail technicians tend not to have regular clients, but once a client finds a nail technician who offers them the best service they will become very loyal. Any client who comes into your salon or makes another type of enquiry should be treated equally and with respect. It is not uncommon for salons to offer clients who spend more money a better service – this is very unfair and should not happen. New and existing clients should be treated the same. Some guidelines to help you deal with clients are given below.

Think about it

In groups, discuss one good and one bad experience that you have had in the retail industry, for example when you bought an item or received a service. What made these experiences memorable? The bad experiences are the ones you tend to remember most and the ones you will tell all your friends about.

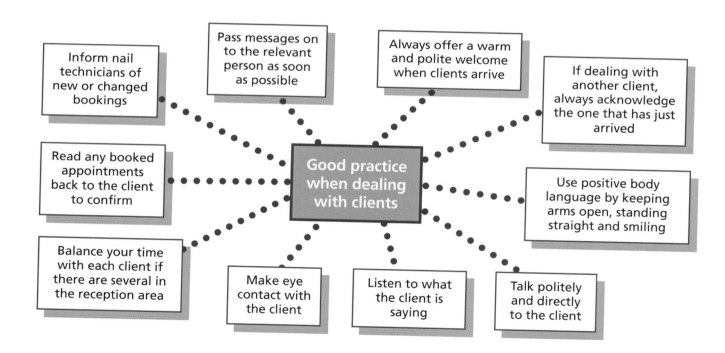

- Inform nail technicians of new or changed bookings
- Pass messages on to the relevant person as soon as possible
- Always offer a warm and polite welcome when clients arrive
- If dealing with another client, always acknowledge the one that has just arrived
- Read any booked appointments back to the client to confirm
- Use positive body language by keeping arms open, standing straight and smiling
- Balance your time with each client if there are several in the reception area
- Make eye contact with the client
- Listen to what the client is saying
- Talk politely and directly to the client

Good practice when dealing with clients

Handling a variety of enquiries

Every enquiry that comes into the salon will be different and needs to be handled in a variety of ways. Being flexible will ensure your clients feel satisfied with the outcome. This section looks at the different types of enquiries you may be faced with and gives guidance on how to deal with each one.

When working on the reception area, enquiries may come via the telephone, email or from a person walking into the salon.

A good receptionist will be knowledgeable about the services available in the salon, but they should also know when to pass on an enquiry to another suitable member of staff.

Telephone enquiries

Some people feel nervous and anxious when answering the phone in a busy salon. As a receptionist, you will need to be confident and have good communication skills. Here are the best ways to handle a telephone enquiry:

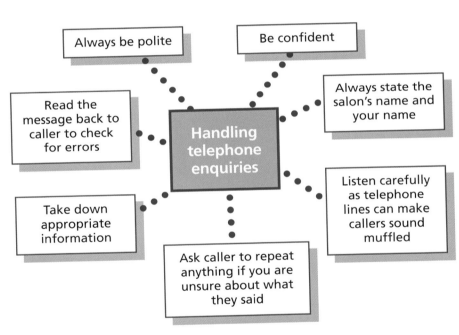

- Always be polite
- Be confident
- Always state the salon's name and your name
- Listen carefully as telephone lines can make callers sound muffled
- Ask caller to repeat anything if you are unsure about what they said
- Take down appropriate information
- Read the message back to caller to check for errors

Handling telephone enquiries

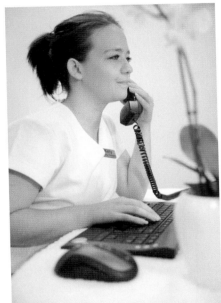

Email enquiries

Many salons and clients are increasingly using email to communicate with each other. It is also an excellent and fairly inexpensive way to promote the salon and its services. You will need to check emails regularly throughout the day. Email replies should be polite and professional and the salon's information – name, address and telephone number – included, for example as a footer. If you cannot deal with the enquiry yourself, print out the email and give it to the appropriate member of staff.

> **Top tip**
>
> Remember the key word PLEASE whenever you deal with an enquiry:
>
> **P**osture
> **L**isten
> **E**xpression
> **A**ppearance/attitude
> **S**peech
> **E**agerness to help others.

Think about it

In pairs, discuss what you would do in the following situation:

You are a receptionist in a busy nail bar. Mr Smith has come in as he wishes to treat his fiancée to a nail treatment before their wedding. He knows that she has been to the salon before. He has asked for a voucher for acrylic nail enhancements but has commented that his fiancée has long, natural nails. What would be your response?

Top tip

Do not show any anger when faced with a negative enquiry as this could lead to a confrontation. You do not want this to happen in the business, as there may be many witnesses to your unprofessionalism.

New clients

Not all enquiries will come from existing clients. These enquiries can be more challenging, as the visitor will be unfamiliar with the nail services offered and may be unclear about what they want. This type of visitor will need lots of guidance — you will need to display your excellent knowledge and communication skills to make a good impression.

Walk-in enquiries

All the factors for handling telephone enquiries should be considered, but the visitor will also have a visual experience of the salon and receptionist.

Handling a negative situation

Unfortunately, not every enquiry that you deal with will be a positive one. Sometimes you will have to handle negative situations and even confusing ones. It is vital that you maintain your professionalism throughout and stay positive.

Remember, you can never please everyone. Working in a customer service industry means that you will have to deal with both positive and negative feedback. From time to time, a client may feel the need to complain about the service they have received. Give the client time to express their feelings and explain what they are unhappy about. Be understanding and sympathetic. Many salons will have a policy on how to deal with complaints, which should be adhered to. Hopefully, there will be a way to resolve the situation, but it may be that the complaint needs to be handled by a more senior member of the team. Usually, decisions regarding refunds are taken by the manager.

If a client appears angry, keep calm and do not raise your voice. Make sure the information you give is clear and accurate. It is often better to deal with the client away from the reception area to avoid attracting other clients' attention. Often the client will find it difficult to stay angry if you are very accommodating. However, you may need to refer the client to a more senior member of staff — there should be someone available to support you.

Dealing with clients with disabilities

Clients with disabilities may need assistance around the salon and nail bar areas. Always offer to help, but do not patronise the client, as they may well be able to manage on their own.

Dealing with a confused client

There may be several reasons for a client's confusion. For example, they may speak English as a second language, or they may be unsure of the nail services on offer, or there could be confusion about appointment times (this is very common). Always try to ascertain the facts first and clarify information with the client. It's important to remain calm and never become frustrated during this type of enquiry.

Salon life

My story

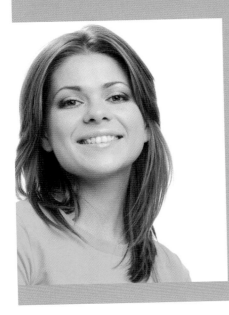

My name is Christine and I have worked in a busy nail bar as a receptionist for six years. I took a part-time course in manicure and pedicure but worked mainly in retail before starting here. I love the buzz of being on reception. I am constantly meeting different people and work on a number of tasks at the same time. There are challenging moments, particularly when clients make difficult enquiries, but due to my experience I find these moments to be positive, as I am constantly learning. When dealing with awkward clients I have found the best way to handle them is to stay calm and listen carefully to what they are asking. Where at all possible you should try to accommodate the client. They will find it hard to stay annoyed when you are positive and helpful. It really helps to diffuse the situation.

The team I work with is very supportive and I have been placed on training courses to ensure my knowledge of the nail bar is up to date. I take pride in being the ambassador for my nail bar and I am often complimented on my customer relationship skills.

Procedures for taking messages for a variety of enquiries

Sometimes, when dealing with an enquiry, you may be required to take a message. When writing down a message it is important to ensure that the information you give is accurate.

Every salon will have its own guidelines on how to take messages and which members of staff deal with different enquiries. Failure to follow these may result in the enquiry being dealt with ineffectively and incorrect information being given to the enquirer. The salon manager will be disappointed to discover that guidelines were not being adhered to. In the nail industry, clients are spoilt for choice and an unsatisfactory service could result in that client moving salons and potentially taking other clients with them.

It is not always appropriate to interrupt a nail technician when they are providing a client with a service. The client may find this rude and feel that it takes up time they are paying for. If you know the nail technician will not be available for another hour, for example, mention this to the person making the enquiry so they know not to expect an answer straight away. This would also apply to enquiries that need to be passed to the salon manager. The message should be detailed and accurate and the client given a time frame for when the enquiry will be dealt with. It is also best if the message can be handed to the appropriate member of staff by the person who took the message, so that they can clearly explain the message.

Wheelchair access

Deaf person

Customers with special needs may require extra assistance

Message for: **Louise**	Person who took message: **Carol**
Date: **Tuesday 12th Sept 2010**	Time: **9:54am**
Message: **Mrs Whitlow telephoned regarding advice needed about possible repair on thumb nail. Is going on holiday and if repair is needed, must be before the 16th Sept.**	
Follow up: **Ring back ASAP**	
Action completed (date and time): **12.9.10 , 10:33am**	Staff member: **Louise**

Sample message on a pad

Top tip

Written messages must be neat. Illegible messages may be misinterpreted.

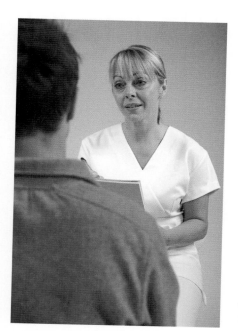

If a client is unhappy, always give them your full attention and make a note of relevant information

How to communicate and behave within a salon environment

When working in a salon environment your behaviour will be observed by everyone who enters the establishment. You are constantly representing the salon, so you will need to put across a professional image. Whether you are treating clients, on reception or taking a break, you need to use appropriate language within the salon. Raising your voice or using slang terms is never appropriate. Similarly, your behaviour should be consistently professional and respectful to everyone within the workplace. Clients are very observant and will quickly notice unprofessional behaviour, which could lead to a complaint. (To learn more about effective communication, see Client care and communication in beauty-related industries, page 42.)

Salon services – duration and cost

As mentioned above, the receptionist needs to be knowledgeable about the nail services available within the salon, not only to deal with enquiries from clients but also to discuss business matters with representatives from product or equipment manufacturers, particularly if the salon owner or manager is unavailable.

The range of services available within the nail industry is growing all the time and a good salon will update its treatment list constantly. As a receptionist, you should know the types of treatments available, their cost and the duration needed for an appointment and be able to promote treatments if required. Services include:

- manicure/pedicures
- deluxe manicure/pedicures
- nail art
- nail enhancement maintenance
- repairs
- removals
- nail enhancement full sets (method used — acrylic, gel and fibreglass)
- free-hand nail art
- air-brushed nail art
- Minx
- cured varnish finishes
- nail piercings
- tooth gems.

The importance of dealing with enquiries promptly and politely

When on reception you will deal with a variety of enquires from many different people. To ensure the salon has a professional and respected reputation, each enquiry must be dealt with as quickly as possible and politely. Enquiries coming from product manufacturers will need to be referred to the salon owner or manager and may be very important. If you are perceived as being impolite to another business it could give a very negative impression of the salon. It could mean they are unwilling to work with you again. Even though you cannot deal with the enquiry, it still needs your full attention.

Check it out

In pairs, obtain a list of the nail services offered in your establishment. Try to memorise as many as possible. Test each other the next day to see how well you did.

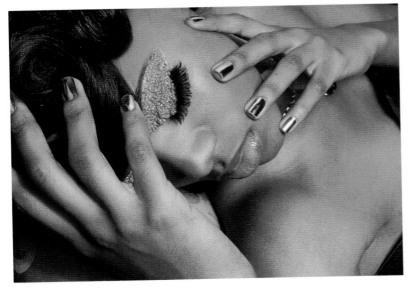

You can promote popular services at reception

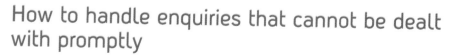

How to handle enquiries that cannot be dealt with promptly

There may be times when an enquiry cannot be dealt with as promptly as you would like. In such cases, you will need to inform the enquirer when their enquiry will be dealt with and when they might expect a response. There is always a risk that an enquiry could be forgotten about when it is not dealt with immediately. It is a good idea to have a system set up for a reminder, either by email or written in the appointment book.

Book appointments

In this section, you will look at how to make and record appointments, using paper-based or electronic booking systems, and the consequences of not doing this accurately. As a receptionist, you will be expected to pass on messages and appointments details to colleagues and to abide by the legislation designed to protect clients' personal details. You will also need to know the consequences of breaching this confidentiality.

How to make and record appointments

An effective appointments system will ensure that the day-to-day operation of the salon runs smoothly. The receptionist may be solely in charge of the system. However, the team also needs to be able to follow the salon's guidelines when booking appointments. Failure to have an effective system will lead to mistakes and the whole working day may be thrown into chaos.

As a receptionist, you should be able to independently book appointments for new and existing clients. You will be given training so that you know what services are available and, in time, you will also learn treatment prices and timings. Occasionally, you may need to refer to the nail technician if the client has a specific query.

You will need to be sure of the service the client requires before making the booking. Some clients may be unsure — checking regular clients' record cards should confirm their usual service. For new clients, the services may need to be explained to them first before they make a decision. A knowledgeable receptionist will be able to run through the different options with them.

Setting up an appointments system

Traditional methods of booking appointments into a book are still very popular in many salons, but increasingly salons are using computer-based appointments systems. There is no right or wrong way — it is whatever suits the individual salon best.

The appointment systems should be set up a couple of months in advance as many clients will want to book treatments further into the future. This helps the salon to plan ahead and can aid nail technicians when it comes to booking time off. The salon should have clear guidelines on how appointments should be scheduled. Paper systems leave more room for error such as double-booking and allowing insufficient time for treatments. Computer systems are designed to flag such errors and do many other tasks to keep the salon running smoothly — however, you will need to be able to use the computer software confidently to make the most of its features.

Scheduling appointments and making the booking

Whichever method your salon uses to book appointments, the information that needs to be recorded will be the same. Here is an example of an appointment page for a busy nail bar.

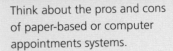

Think about it

Think about the pros and cons of paper-based or computer appointments systems.

Date: **Tuesday 13th October 2010**

	Lindsey	Priya	Lina	Mark	
AM **9.00**	Mrs Anderson		Miss Turner NC		**9.00** AM
9.15	Pedicure		Minx toe nails		9.15
9.30	0123445678 NC		01329 815242		9.30
9.45					9.45
10.00			Mr Karlsson		**10.00**
10.15	Miss Smith		Basic manicure		10.15
10.30	repair 1 nail 357928		335215	Miss James	10.30
10.45			Mrs Rashid	Removal	10.45
11.00	Mrs Jones	Mrs Osborne	File and paint	221335	**11.00**
11.15	Basic manicure	Full set gels	447812		11.15
11.30	with nail art	223335 NC	BREAK	Mrs McCarthy	11.30
11.45	02392815815			File and paint,	11.45
12.00	LUNCH	NC	Miss Coulson	hands and feet	**12.00**
12.15			French manicure	02271881578	12.15
12.30			and luxury	Miss Palmer	12.30
12.45			pedicure	Rebalance	12.45
PM **1.00**	Miss Barnett	Mrs Stewart	213122	07807577211	**1.00** PM
1.15	Full set acrylic	Luxury			1.15
1.30	413927	pedicure			1.30
1.45		01235 771540			1.45
2.00					**2.00**
2.15					2.15
2.30	NS				2.30
2.45					2.45
3.00		BREAK			**3.00**
3.15					3.15
3.30					3.30
3.45	Ms Smith				3.45
4.00	Repair, 2 nails				**4.00**
4.15	08729815111				4.15
4.30		Miss Hill			4.30
4.45		Acrylic infills			4.45
5.00		445877 C			**5.00**
5.15					5.15
5.30		Mrs Pearce			5.30
5.45		Full set			5.45
6.00		gels			**6.00**
6.15		315579			6.15
6.30					6.30
6.45					6.45
7.00					**7.00**
7.15					7.15
7.30					7.30

An appointment page – can you work out the different codes that have been used?

These are the codes used in the appointment page above:

C — cancellation
N — new client
E — exisiting client
L — client was late
NS — no show, client failed to arrive.

To make a booking you will need to have the following information:

- client's name

- service required

- contact telephone number

- if they are a new/existing client

- nail technician who will carry out service

- date and time of appointment.

If using a paper-based appointments system, it is best to write in a pencil so that changes can be made easily. Any information written down should be neat and legible so all members of the team can read it. Be careful not to overload the nail technician — it can be difficult when a client is standing over the appointment book and sees space — but every member of the team needs their breaks. It may help to fill in the set break times so that no one can book a treatment at these times.

When using a computer-based booking system, ensure that you have all the necessary information. Since all the available services are programmed into the software at the start with the time required for each, the computer should recognise the service required and automatically allocate the appropriate amount of time to the desired nail technician. The computer will also manage stock levels by alerting you when there have been lots of the same treatment, meaning some products may be running low. The downside of the computer system is inflexibility. It can be difficult to fit in short treatments such as an emergency repair, as the computer will not recognise enough time for the service. If break times for the technicians are programmed into the system, it may not allow these to be changed during the working day.

Once the appointment is made, read back the information to the client to double check all the details. It is advisable to provide clients with appointment cards which they can keep as a reminder.

Date	Time	Treatment booked	Therapist
14.9.10	3.30pm	Nail enhancement maintenance with nail art	Melissa

An appointment record card

Consequences of failing to record appointments accurately

If you fail to get all the information for an appointment or enter it inaccurately into the booking system, many issues may arise. For example, should the appointment time need to change, the salon will be unable to alert the client if no contact telephone number is available, or if the nail technician is unsure of the service required, they will be unable to prepare for their client. Below are some consequences of failing to record appointments accurately.

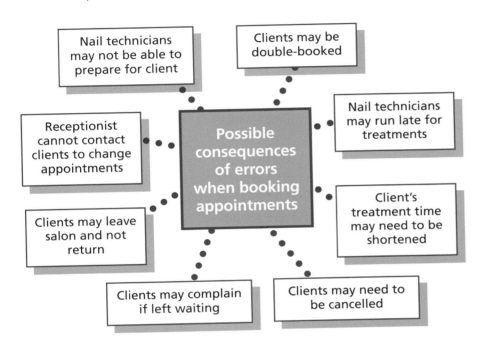

Nail technicians may not be able to prepare for client

Clients may be double-booked

Receptionist cannot contact clients to change appointments

Possible consequences of errors when booking appointments

Nail technicians may run late for treatments

Clients may leave salon and not return

Client's treatment time may need to be shortened

Clients may complain if left waiting

Clients may need to be cancelled

Missed or cancelled appointments

Missed and cancelled appointments can be very frustrating and may lose the salon money. Many salons will have guidelines and policies on what to do when these situations occur. A receptionist needs to be able to manage the appointment system so that the nail technicians are working productively throughout the day.

Missed appointments can sometimes be the result of a simple misunderstanding or the client may be ill. Nowadays, many salons charge clients a small fee if they miss an appointment; others charge the service amount if the treatment is cancelled without notice. If a client cancels their appointment well in advance, it gives the receptionist time to allocate the time to another client. There may even be a waiting list if it is a particularly busy time such as Saturdays and evenings. This means the salon does not lose out on any income. Ideally, reminder phone calls can be made to clients the day before, but this is not always realistic in a busy salon.

Top tip

If the salon has a cancellation policy, ensure that it is well advertised and explained to clients. A client may complain if the policy is suddenly pointed out to them.

Late arrivals

This can be very frustrating for a nail technician, especially if they have a busy day with clients back to back. It can cause them to run over and be late for their next client, which is poor customer service. If a client arrives late, remain calm and explain that the technician may not be able to provide them with the full treatment they were booked in for. It is reasonable to adapt the treatment to fit into the time that remains so that other clients are treated on time.

Walk-in clients

Clients who walk in without an appointment can boost the salon's takings and may become regular clients. However, not all nail technicians view walk-in clients in a positive way. If the nail technician has a quiet time, they may begrudge a client being suddenly booked in. This is a very negative attitude to have. Where possible, walk-in clients should be accommodated and will be impressed with the service they receive if they can have treatment they require. With nail enhancements, damage and breakages can occur at any time and the client will not want to wait long for a repair. The client could easily go elsewhere for an appointment.

Passing on messages and appointments details to colleagues

Keeping your colleagues up to date with appointments will help the salon run smoothly. Any changes that are made need to be passed on to the technicians, as it may affect their set-up. It is quite common for clients to be running late or to change their treatment at the last minute. Passing on any messages will ensure technicians are always prepared for clients and will avoid them getting frustrated by being ill-informed. Salons are very busy environments, so the receptionist needs to work very closely with their colleagues.

Legislation designed to protect the privacy of client details

When booking appointments you are dealing with clients' confidential information, which is protected by the Data Protection Act. The appointment pages should only be viewed by people working within the salon and should not be on display to other clients. If using a computer system to book appointments, the computer should be password-protected so that only authorised people can access it. (To learn more about the Data Protection Act 1998, see Follow health and safety practice in the salon, page 11.)

Here are some guidelines to help you adhere to the legislation's requirements:

- Keep record cards in a lockable cabinet and keys secure.

- Do not leave record cards lying around the reception area.

- Password-protect computer systems so only authorised people have access to client information.

Think about it

Client record cards may contain sensitive information regarding the client's medical history. Would you want this personal information to be accessed by anyone?

- Do not read out clients' details in front of others at the reception area.

- Remove clients' details from paper-based and computer systems if they have not been to the salon after three years.

- Appointment pages should be kept in the reception area and only basic client information should be written down.

Consequences of a breach of confidentiality

The consequence of not adhering to data protection legislation may mean that sensitive information about your clients is leaked to the public. If the salon were found to be negligent with clients' data, it could be liable to prosecution and have to pay compensation to the client involved. This could have a potentially devastating effect on the business, one it may not recover from. Clients are very aware of the consequences of someone getting hold of their personal information, which could ultimately lead to identity theft. Ensure you do everything possible to keep clients' information safe and protected.

Deal with payments

Having good customer service skills will always ensure a smooth exchange of money at the end of the client's service. It is important to check that the client is happy with the service and that no errors occur with the payment, as this is the client's final experience of the business before they leave. A good business will have a clear and appropriate payment system to suit the size and operation of the salon.

Totalling the cost of services

Do not assume that every salon will have a till to calculate the overall costs of treatments. It will often depend on the size of the salon — some smaller salons may prefer to use a manual method. As mentioned earlier, computer software can work as a till too, calculating sums and working out discounts, but be prepared to calculate these manually too.

When working out payments for clients it is vital that you are accurate. Overcharging a client will not encourage them to return to the salon, while undercharging them will lose the salon money and potentially reduce your commission. In either case you will not appear very professional to the client, who may lose faith in the business. Once you have identified the correct cost for the services, clearly state the amount to the client. When taking the payment from the client you will need to be polite and courteous and never demand payment. Ensure you use the terms 'please' and 'thank you'. This is the final stage of the client's experience within the salon, so it should remain positive and make them feel that they are a valued customer.

Special offers

To encourage clients to try different nail services within the salon, your manager may decide to run special promotions from time to time. Special offers are

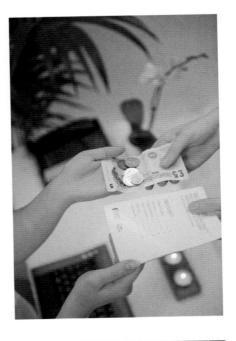

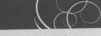

Check it out

Look at your establishment's price lists and produce a grid of all the nail services that are available. In pairs, manually calculate different combinations of treatments.

Top tip

It is up to the salon manager to decide whether to run promotions – do not suddenly start offering discounts to any client that walks in, as this is not an appropriate way to run a business.

Think about it

When you see an item of clothing with a 25 per cent discount, does it tempt you to buy it?

a great tool for promoting products that are not selling or advertising new treatments. (To learn more about promotions, see Display stock and promote products and services to clients, page 63.)

Promotions will cause the cost of the service to vary. Below are some examples of how to calculate discounts using fractions, decimals and percentages.

Fraction	Decimal	Percentage:
$\frac{1}{4}$	0.25	25%

Diagram	Fraction	Decimal	Percentage
1/4	$\frac{1}{4}$	0.25	25%
1/2	$\frac{1}{2}$	0.50	50%
3/4	$\frac{3}{4}$	0.75	75%

Fraction	Divide using the calculator	Decimal	· by 100	Percentage
e.g. $\frac{1}{5}$	(1, 5)	= 0.2	(0.2 · 100)	20%

Fraction		Decimal		Percentage
e.g. $\frac{1}{8}$	(1, 8)	= 0.125	(0.125 · 100)	= 12.5%

Converting fractions to decimals and then percentages

Cost of treatments and price increases

When dealing with payments in the reception area, it is helpful to understand why treatments cost the amount they do, in case a client queries it. This information comes from the product manufacturers – they will have calculated how much product is used in each treatment and therefore the cost of the treatment. Also be aware that many salons will put up their prices once a year to keep up with inflation. Price increases need to be managed carefully and clients should be advised in advance – do not just surprise them. Signs or notices in the reception area and around the salon will help keep clients informed.

Inspecting purchases before payment

When a client purchases a product you will need to check that it is in good condition and suitable for sale as you package it. Check that any outer packaging is undamaged and that any seals have not been broken. When products are on display within the reception area other clients may have opened the product to try without anyone noticing. Check for splits or cracks within the packaging as this could lead to the product leaking when the client takes it home. The client would then have to return to the salon to exchange it and this is not good business.

Methods of payment and how to process them

The types of payment a salon will accept vary. Some methods such as card payments may actually cost the salon money to offer. In this section, you will look at all the methods available and how to deal with each of them.

Methods of payment include:

- credit card
- debit card
- cash
- cheque
- salon/nail bar gift voucher.

Card issuer — **Current Account** — **NEW BANK** — Card number — XXXX XXXX XXXX XXXX — Name of cardholder — Mrs S Bloggs — Valid from date — 06/07 — Expiry date — 06/10 — Signature of card holder — S Bloggs — Cumulus — Magister — £100 — Network — Cheque guarantee limit

A credit card

Credit cards

Increasingly, clients prefer to use this method of payment for their nail services, as it is convenient. The salon will decide which credit cards it will accept as it will need to take out a contract with the credit card company, which will charge them for using the service. Most salons will accept the main types of credit cards, but this will vary due to the cost factor. The introduction of chip and PIN, whereby the salon is able to get authorisation directly from the card provider that the card holder has enough credit to pay for the service, has made this method of payment more secure.

As the receptionist, you will need to enter the details of the amount due into the chip and PIN machine and then ask the client to enter their PIN (personal identification number). This should be done discreetly, especially in a busy reception area. It is advisable to check that the name on the card matches the client who is paying. Once the payment has been taken, give the customer their receipt and keep a copy for the till.

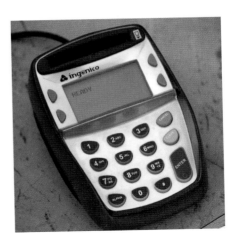

A chip and pin machine

Debit cards

The payment is made electronically from the client's bank account directly into the business's bank account. The process is similar to credit cards using a chip and PIN machine, but in this case the authorisation comes from the client's bank. It is a very popular choice with clients, as it is the equivalent of carrying cash around.

Cash

Paying with cash means the business will benefit immediately. The receptionist is responsible for managing the cash levels in the till throughout the day and ensuring there is enough change. Salons will have a **float** to help them to do this.

When giving the customer their change you will need to be vigilant to ensure no errors have been made. Physically counting the change back to the client will help to reduce the risk of the customer being short-changed or given too

Key term

Float – an amount of cash that is put in the till first thing in the morning and left last thing at night ready for business the next day.

Salon reception duties

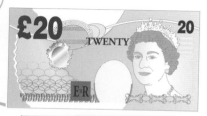
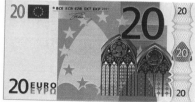

£20 and 20 euro notes

much money. A receipt should also be issued to the client so they can check the accuracy.

Counterfeit money can be an issue if you are given large denominations of cash such as £20 and £50 notes. There is equipment that the salon can buy to check the notes' authenticity, which should be done every time. Equipment ranges from pens that you mark on the notes to machines that will scan the note to check for inaccuracies. If the salon does not have any of this equipment, there are some manual checks you can do as well.

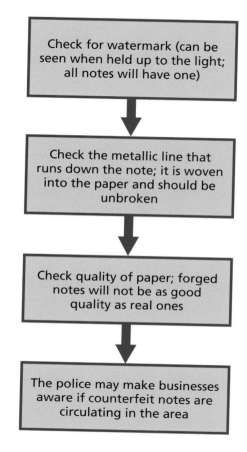

Check for watermark (can be seen when held up to the light; all notes will have one)

Check the metallic line that runs down the note; it is woven into the paper and should be unbroken

Check quality of paper; forged notes will not be as good quality as real ones

The police may make businesses aware if counterfeit notes are circulating in the area

It is important to carry out all of the checks, but they should be done discreetly, as it can make the client feel like they are being scrutinised. Below you will look at how to deal with any discrepancies with cash payments.

Over the course of the day, the till may become full with cash. You will need to monitor this and, if necessary, remove some to the safe until the end of the day. A poorly managed till could result in cash going missing and the takings not balancing. It will also be harder to calculate the total takings for the day.

Cheques

Some salons no longer accept cheques, as it is one of the more unreliable methods of payment — cash or credit/debit cards mean that the business is guaranteed to receive its money.

Currently, when a client pays with a cheque they must present a cheque guarantee card. This will ensure the bank honours the amount the cheque is written for. When accepting a cheque the following should be checked:

- The cheque and the guarantee card have the same name.
- The amount written on the cheque does not exceed the amount stated on the guarantee card.
- Check all the points highlighted in the picture of the cheque below.

However, the cheque guarantee card scheme is due to end on 30 June 2011 and after this date, it will no longer be possible to use a cheque guarantee card.

If a cheque is filled out incorrectly, the bank may not pay the salon the money. This would mean the cheque is returned to the business and the client would have to be contacted to supply another form of payment. This can be embarrassing for the client and a nuisance for the salon, especially if it is not a regular client.

Where a salon decides no longer to accept cheques, it is important to announce this to clients well in advance, so they are fully aware of the change in policy. This can be done by putting up notices around the salon and in the reception area.

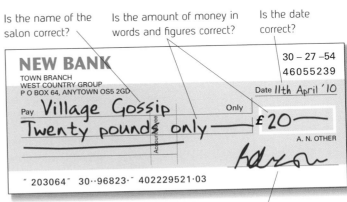

Is the name of the salon correct?

Is the amount of money in words and figures correct?

Is the date correct?

Does the signature on the cheque match the signature on the guarantee card?

A cheque

How to deal with problems that may occur with payments

There may be occasions when there are problems with the payment you are taking from a client. Remember that this can potentially be very embarrassing for them, so be as discreet as possible. The most common problem when dealing with non-cash payments is when a card payment is declined. You will need to inform the client that their card has not been accepted, which may be because:

- there are not enough funds in the account
- the card is out of date
- the bank or credit card company has put a block on the card
- additional authorisation is required (see below).

In this case, politely ask your client for another form of payment, either another card or cash. In the worst-case scenario, if they have no alternative methods of payment, you may need to obtain advice from a senior member of staff. Sometimes, for regular clients your manager may be happy for another form of payment to be dropped into the salon later. You should never make the decision alone; always gain authorisation first. The client needs to be made to feel as comfortable as possible in a very awkward situation.

When taking a card payment, there may be times when you need to gain further authorisation for the card payment to go through. You will be prompted by your card payment system. This most commonly involves ringing through to the service centre; the customer will then need to speak to the centre and go through a series of security type questions. If at all possible this should take place in a more private area, so other customers do not overhear. Where possible the card payment will be authorised and the payment accepted.

Here are some examples of problems with payments you may come across when working in the reception area and how to deal with them:

- Invalid **currency** — politely ask the client for the difference that is needed.

- Invalid card — it may be out of date. Apologise and ask the client for another form of payment. In some cases, you may have to contact the provider so the client can authorise the payment.

- Incorrect completion of cheque — be polite and ask the client to write another cheque. If errors are not corrected, the bank will not accept the cheque.

- Suspected **fraudulent** use of payment card — this should be passed to the salon manager to deal with as it is a criminal offence. Stay calm and polite while dealing with the client.

- Payment disputes — stay calm as your client may well be frustrated. This is why it is vital that the correct price is clearly advertised to the client. If they are still unhappy, it may be advisable to pass the problem to a more senior member of the team.

Gift vouchers

Salon gift vouchers are very popular as family and friends can purchase them for clients instead of giving them the cash alternative. Every salon should provide a gift voucher service and it should be advertised around the salon.

Vouchers are sold throughout the year, with an increase in sales at Christmas time, which will boost the salon's takings during November and December. The downside to this is that people usually use the vouchers within the first three months of the year, and when the client uses a voucher the salon does not receive any payment for the nail service, as this was banked when the voucher was bought. January can be a tough month for salons — not only are people cutting back on nail services but there will be an increase in the redemption of vouchers. As a business, it may be advisable not to use the takings from voucher sales until the quieter months.

Most vouchers will have a redeem-by date, which will encourage the client to use it sooner rather than later. It is also sensible to give the customer a choice of either having the voucher for a specific nail service or for a sum of money. When a client uses a voucher the following steps should be taken:

- Check the voucher has not expired.

- Check the amount covers the service, or matches the service the client had.

Key terms

Currency – payment clients use in exchange for their service, for example cash.

Fraudulent – client being dishonest with their payment.

Bliss Salon
This voucher is for the value of **£20**
Redeemable against any treatment
Valid until September 2011

A salon gift voucher

- Treat it as a cash payment.

- If the client has not used the full amount, mark on the voucher how much is left to spend (it is a good idea to sign or initial this too).

- If the full amount is used, draw a line through the voucher and place your initials or signature on it.

How to keep payments safe and secure

Keeping the daily takings secure

In many salons the reception area will be where the exchange of money and payments takes place. It is vital that all staff are trained in the salon's security procedures and understand the importance of following them. This is a big responsibility and the consequence of not following them can be devastating for the business.

Whatever the size of the salon, there must be a secure way of accepting payments and then storing them. Throughout the day the till will fill up with receipts from card payments, vouchers and cash. The receptionist should remove large sums of money from the till and place them in a safe within the salon until it can be taken to the bank. It is advisable to have a safe on the premises for this purpose. Any money removed from the till needs to be recorded to ensure the till balances up at the end of the day.

Tills need to be locked and only one or two members of staff should have a key. Too many keys greatly increase the chances of one going missing. If that happened, the lock system would have to be replaced and this can be expensive.

Ideally, the takings should be banked at the end of the day. However, this is not always possible. It is important for salon staff to be discreet about the takings and not to discuss them with customers. Being open with information about the takings may lead to it being exploited by people who could see the salon as an easy target. This could also happen if the takings were deposited at the same time every day – the person making the drop-off could easily be targeted by thieves. Some salons prefer to use security firms to collect the takings and take them to the bank. Their employees are specially trained in security procedures and this removes the responsibility from the salon's staff.

Totalling the day's takings and preparing the float

When working on reception you may be responsible for totalling up the day's takings and preparing the float. This is done at the end of the working day so that you can calculate how much the salon has earned. The takings should be divided into cash payments, card payments, cheques and vouchers. Once you have calculated the cash takings, you will need to prepare the float for the next working day. This should contain a variety of notes and change – the salon owner will decide how much the float should be. If you left no float in the till, you would not have any change to give to your clients.

Similarly, you will need to monitor the change levels within the till throughout the day. If you let levels fall too low, you may be unable to give clients their

Check it out

Gather evidence when you have taken different methods of payments, such as photocopying the receipts. This will show that the ranges were covered in a realistic environment and were naturally occurring.

Check it out

In pairs, discuss the pros and cons of members of staff or a security company delivering the takings to the bank.

change. Once you notice a shortage, you will need to inform the salon manager so they can replenish the till. In most cases, the salon should have a supply of change within a safe, but if levels drop too low they may need to visit the bank to pick up some more. This may take time if there is not a bank close to the premises, so be vigilant.

Petty cash

There may be times when you will need to replenish small items from the reception area, such as milk for drinks and stationery items, or to replace magazines with more current issues. Some salons like to use **petty cash** for this purpose. The amount required is taken out of petty cash and replaced with a receipt as evidence of the purchase. Other salons prefer to use the main till to pay for these items. It is vital that receipts are obtained and that these are clearly identified, otherwise when cashing-up takes place at the end of the day the takings will appear to be less than they should be.

Consequences of not following salon security procedures

If you do not follow security procedures when handling payments, there could be serious consequences for the salon. For example:

- there may a higher risk of theft
- cash may go missing
- cheques, card payment receipts and vouchers may go missing
- the till may not balance at the end of the day
- the total takings may be inaccurate.

Key term

Petty cash – a small sum of money that can be used by members of staff to purchase items for the salon, for example refreshments, stationery.

Top tip

It is advisable to avoid lending staff members money from the till for them to pay back later. This can be confusing and runs the risk that the takings will not balance.

Check your knowledge

1. List five skills a good receptionist should have.
2. Why is it important to keep the reception area clean and tidy?
3. Identify five key items that should be on the reception desk.
4. What does PLEASE stand for and why is it important?
5. Why is good hospitality important in a salon?
6. Identify two ways of using the reception area to promote the nail services and products
7. What are the consequences of not recording a message accurately?
8. What six pieces of information should be recorded when booking an appointment?
9. What is the consequence of not adhering to the Data Protection Act?
10. Give two reasons why a card payment may not be accepted.

Getting reading for assessment

VRQs	NVQ
City & Guilds	
Service times: Not applicable to this unit Evidence: You will be required to carry out a range of practical tasks to show you can: • carry out reception duties • book appointments • deal with payments Knowledge and understanding will be assessed by an: • assignment or online test	Service times: There are no maximum service times that apply to this unit Evidence: • The evidence for this unit must be gathered in the workplace or a realistic working environment • Simulation is not allowed for any performance evidence within this unit • You must practically demonstrate in your everyday work that you have met the required standard for this unit • All outcomes, assessment criteria and range statements must be achieved • No mandatory written questions are required with this unit • You must be observed demonstrating competence performance on all practical outcomes on at least three occasions

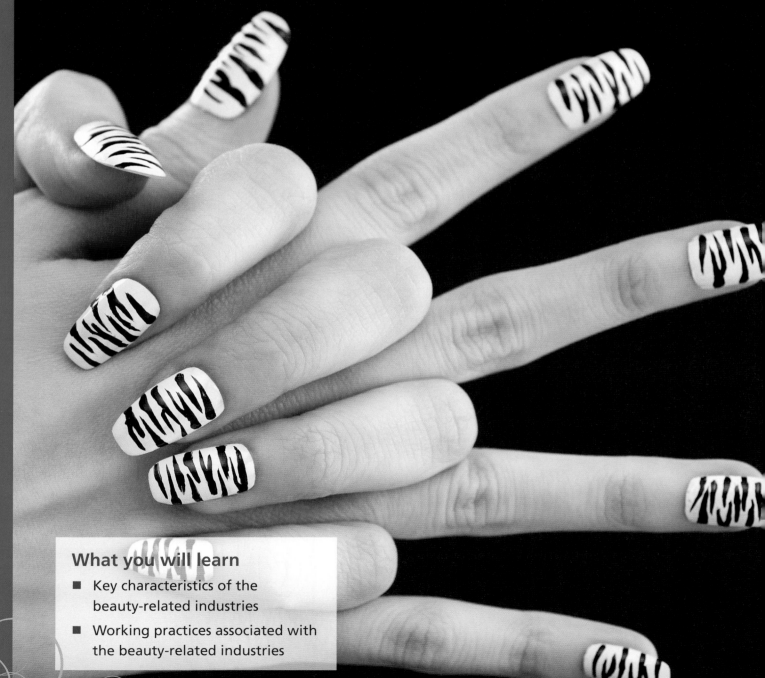

Working in beauty-related industries

What you will learn

- Key characteristics of the beauty-related industries
- Working practices associated with the beauty-related industries

Introduction

This unit is designed to help you prepare for work within the nail industry by outlining the skills and knowledge you will need to progress. With such a diverse industry no two people's career paths will be the same and that is what makes the industry so exciting. The unit will look at the many pathways and also the skills you will need to work alongside your colleagues. Your time at college is just the start of a thrilling and challenging journey through your career.

Gone are the days when a therapist would be limited to the town's local salon, treating the same clients day in day out. There is so much choice available to you now, that every day of your career will bring you different experiences. When you become fully qualified, a whole world of further training will be open to you, taking you from being a novice to working as an expert in the nail industry.

Whether you decide to work in a large salon or perhaps become self-employed and work by yourself, you will constantly be communicating with other people from the profession. It is important to build these relationships – they will help you to establish yourself and the business within your local nail community. Having the skills to work with a variety of people is essential. It is not just about your relationships with clients – your colleagues and peers are equally important.

Legislation and employee rights play a vital part in creating a healthy and productive working environment. Every salon owner is responsible for ensuring that their employees are treated fairly and that correct precautions are taken to keep them safe at work. As an employee you will be responsible for adhering to the guidelines that have been set out. Even as a self-employed nail technician there are many laws and regulations that you will need to become familiar with to ensure your business operates legally.

Now that you have chosen a career in the nail industry you will be surprised at the number of options that are available. This industry links with many different sectors, from sports to healthcare. Making a leap between the sectors is not as difficult as you might at first think; there is a lot of flexibility surrounding you. Your career within the industry can be as exciting and varied as you want it to be. Your determination and imagination are all that are needed. There are no rights and wrongs when it comes to your progression – so, welcome to your new career!

The key characteristics of the beauty-related industries

In this section, you will learn about the types of organisation and the main services offered in the nail and beauty industries. You will also look at the variety of occupations, education and training opportunities available, as well as what it is like to be employed in the beauty-related industries. Finally, you will learn about the legislation that you will have to comply with when at work, the basic principles of finance and selling and the main forms of marketing and publicity.

Types of organisations within the beauty-related industries

There are many areas that make up the nail industry, which will give you a variety of choice when looking for employment. Throughout your training you will have discovered your likes and dislikes, enabling you to focus your career in an area that particularly appeals to you.

The organisational structure of the nail industry is rather like a family tree, with many branches you can explore. However, you will need a starting point, and the best place to gain experience of the industry will be in a busy, successful salon. To develop your professional skills and become more employable, it is best to work with as many types of nail enhancement systems as possible.

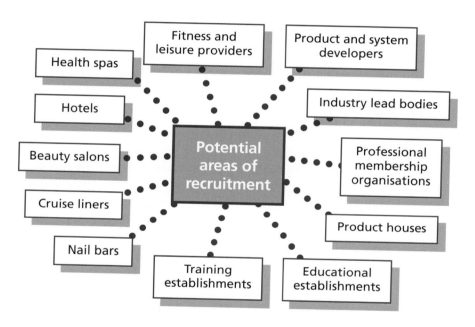

The spider diagram demonstrates the many potential areas of recruitment available to you. Nail bars, beauty salons, hotels, cruise liners, fitness and leisure providers and health spas will all give you the opportunity to apply the practical knowledge you have gained throughout your training. Working with a variety of clients who have different nail and skin types can be challenging but also rewarding. Many nail technicians are content working within these environments, as it allows them to be creative and use the skills they have learned. Working in these types of organisations also enables you to develop your skills as a team member, as you are likely to be working with a variety of therapists and staff who may not all specialise in your area.

Training and educational establishments

These provide learners with the opportunity to complete nationally recognised qualifications within the nail industry. The types of course on offer may differ slightly, but these establishments should be your first port of call when considering a career in nails. Likewise, once you have gained experience within

Check it out

In pairs, make a list of all the establishments that offer nail services in your area. Are any two the same?

the industry you may decide to become a trainer/lecturer, which will give you the chance to help train new technicians coming into the industry and can be particularly rewarding. To progress in this area of the industry, you would be required to undertake a professional teaching qualification.

Product houses

Product houses provide training for the products that they supply. Reputable salons should ensure that you are given product training within the first few months of joining a salon. This will equip you with the knowledge that you need to use specific products effectively and safely.

Professional products are developed and marketed to meet the demands of the industry and companies will support any salon that uses their range by offering training, marketing and promotional materials, and financial rewards. This may include money off when first taking on a product range, and so on.

Awarding bodies

The awarding bodies design the qualifications offered by training and educational establishments. They ensure the courses on offer meet the requirements of the industry and also set the assessment criteria — that is, what you will need to do to pass the course. This usually involves a variety of practical and written work. Some examples of awarding bodies are VTCT, City & Guilds and Edexcel.

Product and system developers

The developers are the brains behind the products you use on clients. It can take years to develop a product to an acceptable standard before it can go on sale. The developers continually assess and adapt products to ensure that you, as a nail technician, get the best results for your clients. Providing nail services involves using complex chemicals that, if not used safely, could cause harm. Developers need to ensure that the products adhere to the relevant health and safety legislation as failing to do so could have severe consequences for the salon.

Over the years, many chemical formulae have had to be changed as the law has changed. For example, methyl methacrylate (MMA) used with acrylic systems has been banned in the USA and by many local authorities within the UK. So this ingredient has been removed from all the products and replaced with ethyl methacrylate (EMA).

Professional membership organisations

Professional bodies were established to help regulate and standardise the industry by giving guidance to therapists and technicians on appropriate conduct and behaviour. There are many different bodies and some are specific to the treatments you offer. You are not legally obliged to become a member of a professional body, but when you first start out in your career they are a good source of support in what can be a challenging industry.

Membership organisations often charge a subscription fee, so you may wish to shop around first to ensure you get the best deal and a professional body that suits the services you offer. Examples include **BABTAC**, **FHT** and Habia.

> **Key term**
>
> **Product houses** – companies or manufacturers that are responsible for the production of the professional products, packaging them ready for distribution.

> **Key terms**
>
> **BABTAC** – British Association of Beauty Therapy and Cosmetology.
>
> **FHT** – Federation of Holistic Therapists.

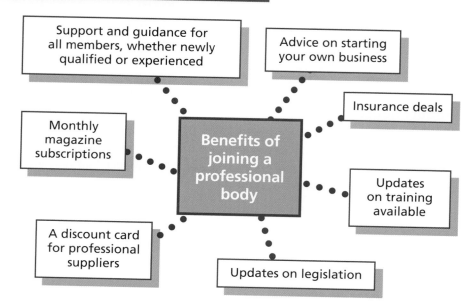

As a nail technician, you will need to keep up to date with what goes on within the industry. Similarly, a salon will not attract new clients if it continues to offer the same types of treatment that it provided ten years ago. There are many ways to access the latest information on the organisations described earlier.

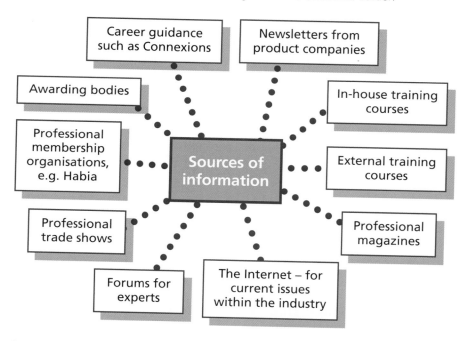

Journals

Professional journals or magazines such as *Scratch* and *Professional Nails* are available on subscription. They are an excellent way to keep in touch with issues within the industry and also provide information on new and upcoming treatments and products that you may wish to offer in your salon. Their articles can help you to overcome common problems and provide other sources of advice. Most journals have a job recruitment section, highlighting vacancies all over the UK and even Europe.

Training providers and further education colleges

Any type of training course will give you information on the industry. In-house courses such as those offered by further education colleges and training providers may help develop existing skills, but from time to time you may be required to update your qualifications. For example, technicians who trained 20 years ago may not have worked with the latest high-tech equipment and to ensure they can use it safely and effectively, they may be required to retrain. Retraining should never be seen as a negative thing — even the most qualified and experienced technician can always learn more.

Newsletters from product companies

These are similar to magazines but may come directly from a product company. They will help to keep you informed about:

- new products available for professional or retail use
- training courses available to your salon
- hot topics and current issues from the industry
- advice and guidance that the company can offer.

Newsletters tend to be advertising tools, so will not include information on any other product range, but they can still be beneficial.

Having a good relationship with your supplier will also enhance the services you offer. Many suppliers have representatives who regularly visit salons to keep the communication and relationship positive. These visits can be very beneficial to the business, as they can motivate and inspire you.

The Internet

The Internet is a source of a vast amount of information and will often be a person's first port of call when seeking information about the nail industry. Professional bodies, awarding bodies, training and educational establishments and so on will have websites you can access. The Internet is also an excellent way to communicate with other professionals and experts in the field through **forums**.

Trade shows

Throughout the year, exhibition halls hold professional trade shows for the beauty and nail industries. New and established technicians can benefit from these exciting events, as they are an excellent way to gather information on all aspects of the industry from the different types of organisations represented there. Product and equipment suppliers and professional and awarding bodies will have stands at trade shows, which also run conference and training sessions giving you the chance to see the latest treatments before anyone else.

Key term

Forum – discussion of questions on a professional topic, commonly taking place through the Internet.

Top tip

What better way to solve a problem than to hold discussions with other professionals from your industry? Ensure you demonstrate your own professionalism when communicating with them, as they may not want to be associated with someone who is letting the industry down.

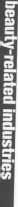

Services available in the industry

There are so many different services available within the nail services industry that it may not be possible to offer all of them in one salon. It is also unrealistic from a business perspective for the following reasons:

● The wider the range of products and services offered, the greater the initial cost to the salon to provide them.

● Staff members may need more training, which can be an additional expense for the salon.

● Less popular treatments may lose the business money.

The range of services offered will often be decided by the salon manager, although most managers will be open to suggestions as technicians deal with clients on a day-to-day basis and might have a greater understanding of what clients want. The location of the salon may also affect the services available due to the area's **demographics**.

The role of service and training organisations

Whatever the service your salon offers or the products it uses, you will need to communicate and build relationships with service and training organisations. They play an essential role in creating well-trained, professional nail technicians. Service organisations deal with a specific professional product range, while training organisations such as further education colleges are more general.

Key term

Demographics – the age range, ethnic background, financial circumstances and so on of a range of people living within an area.

Services available:

Manicures – £18; 45 mins

Deluxe manicures – £ 22; 60 mins

Pedicures – £20; 60 mins

Deluxe pedicures – £24; 1 hr 15 mins

Nail art – prices vary; up to 30 mins

Nail enhancements – £25–£45; 1 hr 30 mins to 2 hrs

Infills/maintenance – £20; 1 hr

Rebalance – £25–£30; 1 hr 30 mins

Repairs – approx. £5 per nail; 15 mins

Removals – £20; 1 hr

Sample price list of nail services

Think about it

What nail services would a city-centre salon offer compared to a salon in a village?

Service organisations	Training organisations
● Provide product and treatment training ● Offer refresher courses ● Provide updates on changes within companies ● Ensure products are of the highest standard and are fit for purpose ● Support salons and establishments that have invested in the products ● Keep up to date with changes within the industry ● Develop new products and treatments to reflect these changes	● Provide learners with professional qualifications for nail services ● Provide learners with skills required for working within the industry ● Ensure delivery of courses matches requirements laid down by the awarding body ● Ensure teaching staff are current and up to date with their own skills ● Pass on knowledge and skills so learners achieve ● Keep up to date with changes within the industry and qualification framework

Occupational roles within the nail services industry

Once you have achieved your nail service qualifications, you may wish to research the employment options available to you. Some people have a very clear idea of where they would like to work, while others may need to try a few different roles before settling into one they are truly happy with. Remember that working within the industry is demanding and also very competitive. If you want to progress far with your career, it will take a lot of determination and dedication, but equally this will bring you immense job satisfaction.

When most technicians leave college they start work within a salon, to gain experience. They will be considered a junior member of staff. Junior does not mean that they are any less valued than other members of the team. It simply refers to a technician's experience within the salon. You can quickly progress up the salon **hierarchy** by showing your professionalism and commitment and by attending training courses. As a nail technician you will provide a wide range of services, including nail enhancements and manicures and pedicures. Due to the fast-growing nature of the nail services industry it is possible to find employment using such a specialised skill.

Experience will be needed before you can progress, so you will need to work hard to increase your **client base** and work on a wide range of people. Once the salon manager has seen your skills and you have completed further training, you will become a more senior member of the team. This may mean your responsibilities increase, something that should not be taken lightly. The business and the manager trust you to fulfil these responsibilities. At this time, you may also be asked to look after and mentor newer members of staff. This can be very rewarding, as you will remember how daunting those first few weeks can be.

Working in a salon, whether as a therapist or a nail technician, is a good stepping stone into the industry, but there are many other roles that you may wish to explore. Spas, cruise liners, health farms and so on will all help develop your practical skills and increase your experience. Working for these types of establishment may be beneficial if you are keen to travel and seek employment outside the UK.

Experienced therapists and technicians who are thought of highly within the industry may have the opportunity to help develop products and courses by working alongside awarding bodies and professional membership organisations. These types of organisation rely on input from therapists and technicians who are working within the industry to see what changes and updates are needed.

Becoming a salon manager or salon owner

Some nail technicians are keen to develop their managerial skills and become a salon manager and perhaps even the salon owner. This may involve training that is not directly linked to the industry and practical skills and will include learning management techniques, relevant legislation and the principles of finance. The salon owner and manager are two completely different roles. A manager looks after the day-to-day running of the salon and supports members of the team,

Key terms

Hierarchy – a system of people ranked one above another.

Client base – clients who come and see the salon/therapists specifically, on a regular basis.

Top tip

Shadowing a more senior member of staff will show initiative and help you learn about other roles. You will see what their responsibilities are.

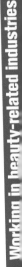

Working in beauty-related industries

Working in beauty-related industries

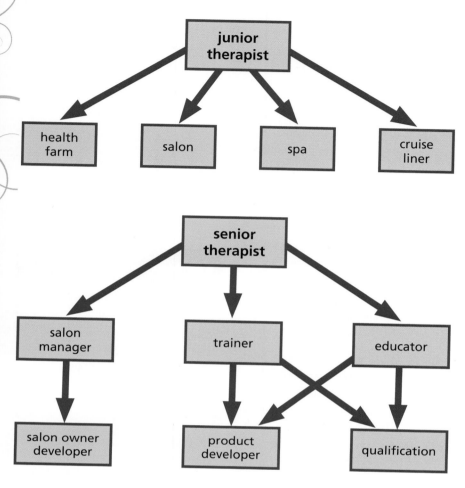

Career progression paths

while the salon owner looks after the business finances and is responsible for the upkeep of the premises, equipment, staff wages and so on.

Becoming a tutor or trainer

This can be extremely rewarding and is another potential career path. Information on the qualification requirements can be found on the Internet but may vary slightly, depending on the establishment. Tutors more commonly work in a further or higher education establishment, while trainers may work in a private academy or for a specific product house, training nail technicians who are already qualified. A sales representative would support salons with product ranges and will often have to do lots of travelling. The job involves working with a wide range of businesses as you promote a professional product range.

The diagram opposite demonstrates the many career paths available to you. You may decide to stick to one or experiment and gain experience in many different areas.

Employment characteristics of working in the beauty-related industries

With all the different types of role available to you, there is also a choice of how you are employed:

- full-time

- part-time

- freelance

- on contract.

Full-time and part-time employment often depends on an individual's personal choice and circumstances. For example, mothers with young children may decide to work part-time so that they can spend time at home with the family. Some people need to work full-time for financial reasons. There is no right or wrong, and you will find the pros and cons are different for everybody. What should be clear in your contract is the number of hours you are required to work each week. The amount of holiday and sickness pay entitlement are then calculated on a **pro-rata basis**.

An employer must provide all employees with a contract, which you will need to read and check carefully before signing. Any inconsistencies should be discussed with your manager and then changed where appropriate.

A freelance therapist is usually self-employed and provides their services for a fee. For example, make-up artists are rarely directly employed by any one company. When their services are required, a company will pay the make-up artist for their time. Being a freelance nail technician will give you some flexibility over your working hours and your choice of work. However, the amount of work and when you work might not be consistent.

How suitable employment characteristics can open up opportunities

In order to progress in your career there are certain attributes — qualities — that you will need to have. In this section, you will look at the ones that may help you with either promotion within your existing salon or perhaps applying for a more senior role elsewhere.

Promotion does not come automatically, nor is it necessarily linked to the number of years you have worked for the company. In fact, it is common to find therapists and technicians who have never progressed within a salon, even though they have worked there for several years. Promotion must be earned and you will need to demonstrate that you are capable of taking on new challenges. For example, in the table below, technician A increases their job opportunities while technician B decreases them. There is a big difference between technicians A and B — they are, of course, two extreme cases. However, your employer will be constantly watching and assessing your performance.

> **Key term**
>
> **Pro-rata basis** – for employees who do not work full-time, their holiday and sick pay entitlements are calculated as a percentage of a full-time member of staff; for example if you work 70 per cent of a full-time post, your holiday entitlement will be 70 per cent of full-time.

Technican A – increasing job opportunities	Technican B – decreasing job opportunities
<ul><li>work with a positive 'can do' attitude</li><li>attend staff training</li><li>attend and participate during staff meetings</li><li>perform treatments to the highest of standards</li><li>show enthusiasm with all tasks</li><li>shadow senior members of the team</li><li>research and gain knowledge on the requirements of the job</li><li>be knowledgeable on the industry</li><li>increase client base</li></ul>	<ul><li>failing to update skills with new qualifications</li><li>attend staff meetings but not participate or communicate with other members of the team</li><li>lack motivation and enthusiasm when given tasks</li><li>carry out poor treatments of a low standard</li><li>receive customer complaints</li><li>show no interest in other job roles or increasing responsibility</li></ul>

Increasing and decreasing job opportunities

Education and training opportunities within the beauty-related industries

Developing your professional skills is a vital part of your career. To learn more, see the Continual professional development section, page 116.

Opportunities to transfer to other sectors or industries

The nail industry is classified as a commercial and service industry. As the industry has developed over the years, links have been made with many other industries. This is valuable, as you can learn a lot from the way that other people work.

The beauty and nail industry can link with:

- healthcare
- sport and leisure
- complementary and holistic therapies
- management and finance.

Therapists often work alongside healthcare professionals, and it is becoming increasingly common for recommendations to come from either side. These two industries can then work alongside complementary and holistic therapies to improve the health of a client. For example:

- nail services and **chiropodists/podiatrists**
- therapists and patients suffering from life-threatening illnesses
- therapists trained in massage have the basic knowledge and understanding to train in sports massage. Sports massage is a vital part of keeping an athlete healthy and injury free. Many of the top football teams incorporate sports massage into their post-match wind-downs.

If you wish to own a business or become a manager, you will need specialised training. It takes a lot of hard work and business knowledge to make a success of it. There are many management and finance companies that can support you when running a business. You are likely to need the expertise of legal teams, financial advisers, accountants and so on at various times throughout your management career.

Main legislation affecting the beauty-related industries

Information about legislation affecting the beauty-related industries can be found in other units, as shown in the table below.

Think about it

In pairs, discuss when you might need to refer a client to another industry. Feed back your findings to the rest of the class.

Key term

Chiropodist/podiatrist – a member of a healthcare organisation who is trained to deal with and treat medical conditions of the feet.

Top tip

Being a nail technician does not qualify you to become a manager. You will need to attend further training to educate yourself and develop managerial skills.

Legislation	Unit name	Page number
Disability Discrimination Act	Client care and communication	52
Health and Safety at Work Act	Follow health and safety practice in the salon	5
Data Protection Act	Follow health and safety practice in the salon	11
Trade Descriptions Act	Client care and communication	51
Consumer Protection Act	Display stock and promote products and services to clients	62
The Performing Rights Regulations	This act protects artists and their songs. If a company wishes to play music in their premises, they will need to inform the Performing Rights Society. They will then need to pay a fee to cover the radio and/or CDs they play. This ensures that artists get financial reward for their work – royalties.	

Basic principles of finance and selling within the beauty-related industries

In order to create a successful business, the salon owner will need to have a thorough knowledge of suitable financial and marketing techniques. For information on finance and selling, see the unit Display stock and promote products and services to clients, page 55.

Main forms of marketing and publicity used by beauty-related industries

Advertising is very powerful and it is unusual to find a salon or nail bar that does not use some form of marketing to promote itself. Even relying on word of mouth is a form of marketing – you just don't need to pay for it.

There is no right or wrong marketing tool to use, but some are more suitable for different types of salons then others.

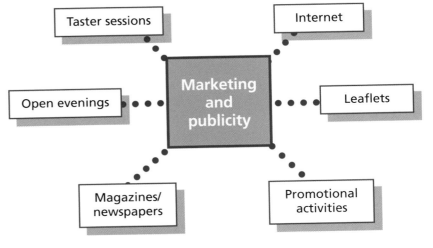

The Internet

More and more people now have access to the Internet, and it has become an everyday tool for organising people's lives. Having a salon website allows clients to access information about its services 24 hours a day, 7 days a week. They no longer have to wait for opening hours to find their answers. Information on a salon website should include:

- contact details
- opening hours
- services and prices
- products used and retailed
- images of the salon
- treatment information
- special offers
- customer feedback.

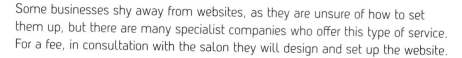
Some businesses shy away from websites, as they are unsure of how to set them up, but there are many specialist companies who offer this type of service. For a fee, in consultation with the salon they will design and set up the website.

Leaflets

Leaflets that provide treatment and production information and price lists should be available in your salon for clients to look at and take home. But how would people access leaflets if they never visit the salon? Leaflet drops can be used in the surrounding areas to promote the salon. Again, there are companies that can do the leaflet drop for you or you may wish to involve members of staff during quiet periods. Building professional relationships with other businesses in the area could help encourage them to display your leaflets, for example GPs' surgeries, community centres and so on.

Promotional articles in magazines and newspapers

Local magazines and newspapers can be used to promote the salon to the surrounding community, through advertisements or promotional articles. This may include new promotions or services available within the salon. Advertising rates are usually quite reasonable. Professional magazines can be more expensive, so it would depend on the salon's marketing budget. However, professional magazines can help to promote the salon to other professional companies. This helps build professional relationships between companies – networking events are often advertised within magazines.

Promotional activities, taster sessions and open evenings

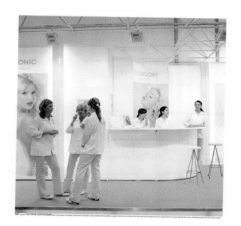

Promotional activities may involve setting up information stands in busy commercial areas, such as trade events or in shopping centres. They may help to increase the salon's client base by attracting potential new clients. The cost of a promotional activity will vary depending on the location, but they have proven to be very effective.

Taster sessions and open evenings are aimed at both new and existing clients, giving them a chance to perhaps try new treatments and gain advice from professional therapists and nail technicians. They are also very effective if the salon is launching a new product, treatment or promotion.

Working practices associated with the beauty-related industries

To be a successful nail technician, you will need to have good working practices and excellent personal presentation. This section looks at opportunities for developing and promoting your own professional image and discusses the importance of **continual professional development (CPD)**. You will also learn about employment rights and employer responsibilities.

Key term

Continual professional development (CPD) – updating skills in your professional area throughout your career.

What are good working practices?

Everybody would like harmonious working conditions but this requires effort from the whole team. Your personal actions will contribute to the effectiveness of the salon and the effectiveness of the team. Working safely also contributes to an effective working environment — to learn more about PPE, COSHH and methods of sterilisation, see Follow health and safety practice in the salon, page 1.

As a nail technician, you will mainly work independently with clients, which may cause you to become detached from the rest of the team. Directly carrying out treatments on clients does not involve a lot of teamwork. However, your behaviour and actions throughout the day may affect other staff members. For example:

- Running late with a client may prevent another technician using the products and equipment or the working area.

- Poor service will reflect badly on the whole salon, not just you, causing a decrease in the client base, which will affect everyone.

- Failing to tidy up after your treatment, leaving it for someone else to do, is not good teamwork. It could cause your colleague to run late or mean the equipment is not prepared for their client.

During a busy salon day, when you have clients back to back, it is easy to be busily occupied with your own tasks. However, take the time during gaps to check on your team members. Look to see if they need help setting up, seeing a client out, taking payments and so on. There is nothing worse for team morale than one technician sitting down doing nothing while everyone else rushes around getting tasks done.

Each workplace will have its own set of guidelines for professional expectations. As a new member of staff, be sure to familiarise yourself with the policies and ensure you adhere to them at all times.

To learn more about professional ethical conduct, see Client care and communication, page 35.

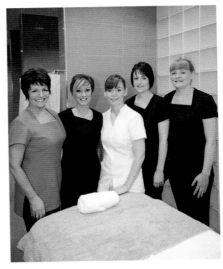

Working in a nail studio needs a lot of teamwork

The importance of personal presentation in reflecting a professional image

To promote yourself as a professional nail technician, you will need to show you can present yourself appropriately. This will help to build working relationships with other companies. Other professionals will form a negative opinion of you and your establishment if you are dressed inappropriately. To learn more about personal presentation requirements, see Follow health and safety practice in the salon, page 17.

Opportunities for developing and promoting your professional image

To progress in the nail industry, you will be required to build as many professional relationships as possible. This will involve promoting yourself to companies, organisations and other professional people in order to build an image that reflects your dedication and determination to succeed.

When progressing from job to job you will need an up-to-date **curriculum vitae (CV)** which can be used during the application process. Your CV gives you the opportunity to promote the skills you have acquired during your career. In such a competitive industry, any additional skills and qualifications that show your dedication can help you win a job opportunity.

Ways to create professional links include:

- working with professional healthcare advisers for the treatment of clients
- working with the local community
- attending regular continual professional development (CPD) events (see below)
- building a large and successful client base
- taking part in professional competitions, for example nail technician awards
- building relationships with other professionals from a wide range of organisations, for example professional membership organisations and product companies.

> **Key term**
>
> **Curriculum vitae (CV)** – a document showing the history of education, employment and professional skills; often required when applying for jobs.

Basic employment rights and employer responsibilities

As an employee or an employer, you will need to know about the following legislation and regulations, which are designed to protect both employees and employers so that everyone is treated equally and can work in a safe environment.

The Working Time Regulations 1998

These regulations set standards for working hours and holiday entitlement. This is to ensure everyone is treated fairly and enables staff to work safely. The regulations cover:

- hours of work per week (no more than 48 hours averaged over a 17-week period)
- rest entitlement (a break of 11 hours between working days)
- short break entitlement (working over six hours entitles you to a 20-minute break)
- days off (a minimum of one day off a week)
- holiday (four weeks' paid holiday a year).

The law is slightly different for employees under the age of 17, and more information can be found on the Directgov website.

The National Minimum Wage

The National Minimum Wage is the minimum amount per hour that most workers in the UK are entitled to be paid. Employers are responsible for keeping staff informed of any updates and changes to this. Many therapists who first start out in the industry will start at the minimum wage. Following are the minimum wage rates (as of 1 October 2010):

£5.93 – the main rate for workers aged 21 and over

£4.92 – the 18–20 rate

£3.64 – the 16–17 rate (for workers above school leaving age but under 18)

£2.50 – the apprentice rate (for apprentices under 19 or 19 or over and in the first year of their apprenticeship).

Employment rights

The following table summarises the responsibilities of employers and employees.

Employer responsibilities	Employee responsibilities
<ul><li>provide a **contract of employment**</li><li>give clear **job specifications** and responsibilities</li><li>provide appropriate amount of wage</li><li>provide a safe working environment</li><li>provide safe and appropriate equipment</li><li>adhere to employment legislation</li></ul>	<ul><li>adhere to salon's policies and guidelines</li><li>work in a safe and responsible manner</li><li>adhere to job specifications and contract</li><li>inform employer of any inadequate policies</li><li>adhere to employment legislation</li></ul>

Key terms

Contract of employment – a legally binding contract that sets out the specification of your job, it will outline working hours, holiday and break entitlement, sick pay etc.

Job specification – this will outline your roles and responsibilities within your job role so you will know exactly what is expected of you.

Employment Act 1997

This act was intended to bring equality to employment and ensure people are treated fairly. It covers:

- pay
- working time and leave
- termination of employment
- variation on basic conditions.

More information can be found on the Directgov website.

Check it out

In pairs, write a job description for a nail technician. Remember to include their roles and responsibilities.

Working in beauty-related industries

Consequences of failing to act professionally

Everyone in the workplace is accountable for their own actions and there may be times when consistently poor behaviour has to be dealt with by the salon manager or owner. As a nail technician, you represent a multi-billion pound industry, which has an excellent reputation. Failing to act professionally can damage a salon's business and may affect the public's positive attitudes to the industry. The consequences of unprofessional behaviour are shown in the diagram following.

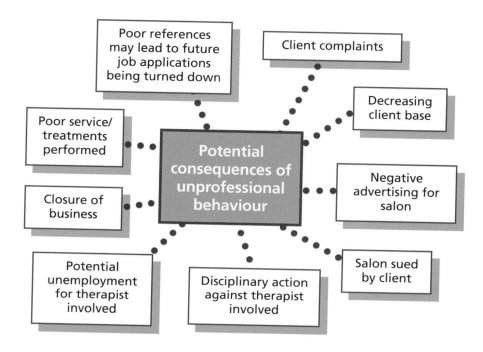

The importance of continual professional development

Your training within the industry should never end — it should be a continual part of your career. You work in an ever-changing industry where new products and services are being developed all the time, so there will always be something new for you to learn. Continual professional development (CPD) should be a part of your contract of employment. It is an integral part of your career and should always be thought of as a positive opportunity. Unfortunately, some technicians believe CPD to be a waste of time or unnecessary — that kind of attitude will not allow you to progress in your career.

Attending regular CPD training will show you are up to date and knowledgeable about everything happening in the nail industry, from new treatments to changes within codes of practice. The knowledge you gain will be passed on to your clients, who will be impressed by your dedication, and this can lead to an increase in your client base. It may also inspire other members of your team, as you demonstrate your knowledge and skills in the salon environment. Your enthusiasm to learn will also be reflected in the **appraisal** system.

Key term

Appraisal – assessment of someone's performance within the workplace.

Techniques that were developed in the early years of the nail industry were effective and professional, and updating your skills does not mean that what you had been doing previously was wrong. However, as research is carried out and technology advances, there are even more effective techniques available to achieve incredible results on clients. Treatments are also developed to make them safer for the client and technician and to help ensure that you comply with the latest health and safety legislation.

Organisations that can provide training

The diagram below shows the many types of organisation that can provide you with CPD training.

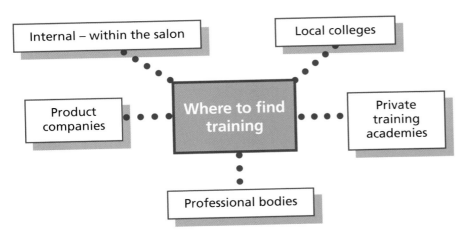

Internal training

Internal training may be provided by your employer. When you join a salon, you should be trained in its guidelines and policies. In some cases, you may also be offered treatment training by another member of staff. However, this does not always mean you are fully qualified to carry out the treatment. Where a salon uses a particular range of products, the product house may insist that every member of staff attends its training courses, without which you may invalidate your salon's insurance cover.

Product companies

Training provided by product companies varies from product knowledge (suitable for receptionists) to full-service and treatment training. Some also offer refresher training to update skills of technicians who have used their products in the past. Product companies should keep your salon notified of the training courses they are running.

The cost of training will depend on the product company. Some offer free training for all staff; others will train two members for free and the rest of the team at a cost.

Professional membership organisations

Professional bodies may not always provide practical training, but they are a good source of information for current issues within the industry. They may offer

Think about it

Would you visit a salon that offered treatments that were developed 20 years ago, or would you go to a more current one?

Top tip

Share your new skills with your peers by performing demonstrations. It could inspire them to undertake more training too.

Think about it

What training were you offered in your first place of employment? Compare it with the rest of the class.

Working in beauty-related industries

courses on changes within qualifications, legislation and so on. Attending them will ensure you have an insight into all areas of the industry.

Training establishments

These offer nationally recognised qualifications. If you have been enrolled by your employer, then they will normally cover the cost of the course. If it is something you personally are interested in, then you may be expected to pay the cost. An advantage of having a nationally recognised qualification is that all organisations within beauty therapy will recognise it, so you will be given credit for the qualification wherever you go.

Why update my skills?

You should never assume that once you become a qualified technician your training ends. For example, if you were to compare the techniques used for manicuring 20 years ago with techniques used today, you would find they are very different.

The diagram opposite looks at the potential consequences of not updating your skills throughout your career.

Building your client base is essential to a successful career. Clients nowadays are very informed about the industry — they read magazine articles, research the

Check it out

Using the Internet, research manicuring tools that were used in the past, and compare them to yours. How different are they?

Salon life

My story

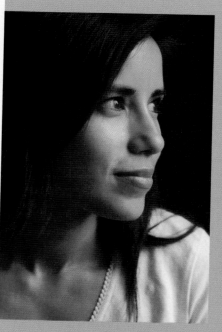

My name is Melissa and I currently teach beauty and nail services with a FE college. I fell in love with nails at college, so as soon as I was qualified I found employment within my local salon. I expected to start on clients straight away and be considered as fully qualified, due to my college certificate. This wasn't the case. I was put in as a 'rookie' and they monitored my performance very closely. After months of hard work I was told I could attend the training to become a nail technician. I had to attend the salon's own training academy, where I had to sit an exam and then perform a practical assessment. They would then decide if I was of a technician standard. Thankfully I passed, but this was not the end of my training. I then had to do the assessments to become a senior technician and then an advanced technician. At each stage I received a certificate and a pay rise. Overall it took me three years to get to that level! It was hard work but it was very rewarding when I was told I had passed. We also had product and treatment training on top of that, whenever new systems came into the salon. When I left the salon I had a portfolio filled with evidence of my training, which helped me get the role I have today. It gave me a excellent experience and taught me that you can never have too many qualifications. There is always something new to learn!

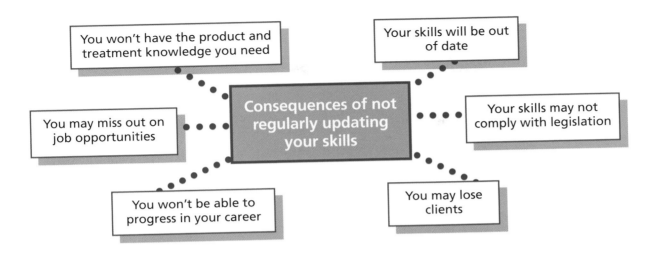

You won't have the product and treatment knowledge you need

Your skills will be out of date

You may miss out on job opportunities

Consequences of not regularly updating your skills

Your skills may not comply with legislation

You won't be able to progress in your career

You may lose clients

Internet and so on, which means they are very aware of market trends and the new treatments becoming available. If your salon fails to take an interest in new treatments, clients will eventually go elsewhere. As new products and services are being developed all the time, it would be too expensive for your salon to invest in them all, but it is important to do research and find out what is creating the most interest. Listen to your clients as well and ask their opinion on what services they would like to see in the salon.

When applying for a job, you will need to be able to sell yourself and show the new company all the skills you can offer. If your skills are too dated, it may not be interested in employing you. Potential employers will look at the cost of taking on new staff — paying for all the new training courses to update you may be too expensive for them. There will also be plenty of other candidates applying with the latest, more relevant qualifications.

Recording and evidencing continual professional development

Documenting your training is an essential part of your CPD, as this is your evidence to say you have undertaken courses to develop your skills. Depending on the type of business, there may be specific criteria for recording your CPD. It should be seen as a portfolio of evidence that could be shown to new employers, clients and so on, to promote your skills.

Within a salon environment, certificates should be on display either in the reception area or in treatment rooms. They should always be visible to the clients. This not only promotes how skilled you are as a technician but it also rewards you for the hard work you have done by completing courses. Displaying certificates is a way of sharing the achievement with clients and other members of the team.

Within training and education establishments, there are strict policies on how much CPD a member of staff should undertake. This is usually a combination of in-house and external training courses, but should always link to the member of staff's skill area. The professional membership organisation for educators in further education, Institute for Learning (IfL), promotes professional good practice and CPD. Lecturers are required to record annually how much CPD they

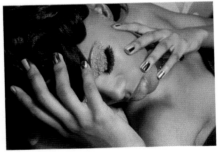

Be aware of the new products that are causing the most interest

Top tip

Clients like to know how qualified their technician is, as it gives them a sense of security that they will do a good job.

have undertaken and give details. Awarding bodies have also followed suit, for example VTCT. This ensures that people responsible for training and educating new nail technicians are training them in skills that are current and relevant.

Check your knowledge

1. Where would you access information on organisations within the industry?

2. What are the advantages of being a member of a professional membership organisation?

3. State the hierarchy of staff within a salon.

4. Describe the Working Time Regulations 1998.

5. Identify ways of promoting yourself as a professional nail technician.

6. List five ways to market and promote a new treatment available in your establishment.

7. Why should nail technicians keep their skills current and up to date?

8. What does CPD stand for?

9. List four responsibilities of an employer.

10. List four consequences of not updating your skills.

Getting reading for assessment

VRQs
City & Guilds
Service times: Not applicable to this unit

Evidence:
You will need to show that you can access sources of information on organisations, services, occupational roles, education and training opportunities within the beauty-related industries.

Knowledge and understanding
will be assessed by an:
* assignment or online test

Anatomy and physiology

Think about it

If you understand that a client with very dry skin on their hands has a lack of **sebum**, then as a technician you can investigate why. Is the cause an internal factor such as poor diet (lack of nutrients in the blood) or does the client suffer from eczema (underactive sebaceous gland)? Or is it the result of an external factor such as dermatitis caused by chemical irritants such as household cleaners? Before performing a treatment on a client, practise your questioning techniques during the consultation. You could find out the answer to this question.

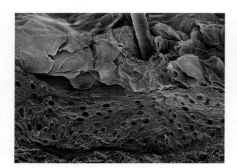

The skin surface magnified x600

Key terms

Desquamation – dead skin cells on skin surface lifting away naturally.

Mitosis – the process by which new cells are made.

Introduction

As a nail technician, you will treat the hands, arms, legs and feet, so it is essential that you have an understanding of **anatomy** — that is, the **structures** of the body and how they relate to each other — and **physiology** — the body's **functions**. This knowledge will help you to become a successful nail technician, as it is important to know how a treatment may affect the client's body. For instance, a hand and arm massage will stimulate the blood supply, bringing **nutrients** to the skin tissue and improving the condition and colour of the skin. Understanding anatomy and physiology will give you the knowledge to identify contra-indications or a flaw, such as bitten nails or **eczema**, and enable you to make all-important decisions when creating the client's treatment plan.

Key terms

Anatomy – the study of the structures of body parts and their relationships to one another.

Structure – how something is made up.

Physiology – the study of the functions of the body.

Function – what something does.

Nutrients – substance that provides energy.

Eczema – underactive sebaceous glands, which leaves the skin dry.

Sebum – oil produced by the sebaceous gland.

The skin

Skin is the largest organ of the body — it covers an area between 3.5 and 7 square metres — and with its many functions (which are explained later in this unit), it is an incredibly versatile organ that is essential for our survival. Healthy skin appears smooth and soft to the touch, but a closer look reveals a different picture — skin is covered in dead, scaly cells with deep ridges and grooves. Skin accounts for 12 per cent of an adult's body weight and is approximately 1.5 millimetres thick. New cells constantly replace old cells that are lost as they are naturally shed from the skin's surface — a process known as **desquamation**.

Cells

Skin tissue is made up of many cells that have the same function (see page 126). All are able to reproduce themselves and old skin cells are continually being replaced by a process called **mitosis**.

Cells are the building blocks of life — when many cells join together, they form tissue. An organ such as the skin or the heart is made up of several types of tissue, which work together to perform a specific function. There are different types of cells located in the human body, including skin, blood, nerve, muscle, bone, gland and reproductive cells, all of which have specific functions.

The cell consists of many structures. Each structure has a specific task to perform. The following table will explain the functions of each of the main structures.

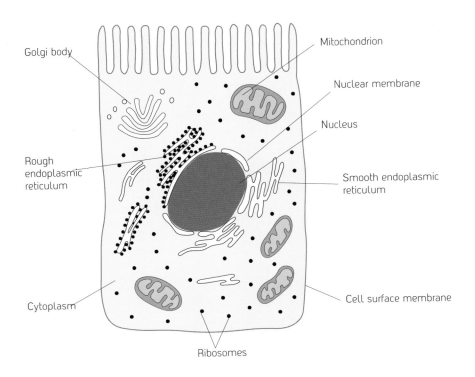

Golgi body

Mitochondrion

Nuclear membrane

Nucleus

Rough endoplasmic reticulum

Smooth endoplasmic reticulum

Cytoplasm

Cell surface membrane

Ribosomes

A basic cell structure

Cell surface membrane	The outer cell wall surrounds the cytoplasm and allows nutrients to enter and waste products to exit the cell.
Cytoplasm (protoplasm)	The protoplasm surrounding the cell nucleus is known as cytoplasm. It is a clear gel-like substance that all cells contain, which helps move materials around the cell and also dissolves any cellular waste produced.
Nucleus	This controls all cell functions. The **DNA** found in the nucleus contains specific instructions that the cell needs in order to form proteins and genetic information to be passed on during mitosis. The nucleus ensures that all functions are correctly carried out.
Mitochondrion	The 'power house of a cell'. Mitochondria generate energy for the cell's activities and are involved in mitosis.
Chromosomes	Chromosomes are located in the nucleus. They are the packaging for our **DNA coding** that gives instructions to our body on how to grow, develop and function.

The structure of a cell

Key terms

DNA – deoxyribonucleic acid is an important molecule that contains our genetic blueprint. This is our personal information which defines how we look, function and grow. The information is passed on to our children.

DNA coding – DNA information.

Cell mitosis

Mitosis is cell division, where new cells are created. It takes place in the lowest layer of the epidermis, known as the *Stratum germinativum*. A mother cell remains in this layer and creates an identical daughter cell, by splitting and dividing. The new cells move up through the layers of the epidermis, where they are eventually shed from the surface of the skin. This process continually occurs to renew the epidermis and keep the surface of the skin healthy.

The structure of the skin

The skin consists of three layers:

- epidermis (outer layer)
- dermis (middle layer)
- subcutaneous layer (bottom layer, also known as the hypodermis).

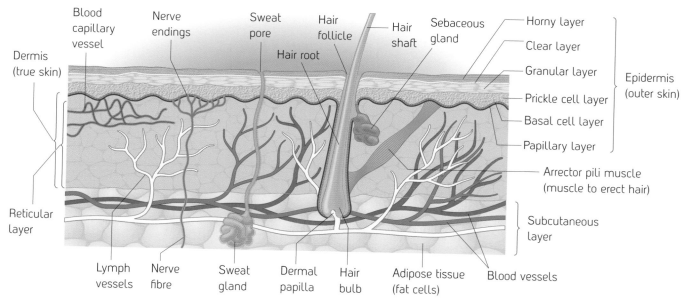

The structure of the skin

The epidermis

The epidermis is the top layer of skin and is 0.01–2 millimetres thick, with the thickest areas located on the palms of the hands and soles of the feet. It is made up of five layers – their Latin names are shown in brackets:

1 Horny layer (*Stratum corneum*)

2 Clear layer (*Stratum lucidum*)

3 Granular layer (*Stratum granulosum*)

4 Prickle cell layer (*Stratum spinosum*)

5 Basal cell or germinating layer (*Stratum germinativum*).

Layers 1, 3, 4 and 5 are located all over the body, except on the palms and soles where there is an extra layer, the *Stratum lucidum*.

The epidermis creates a waterproof layer that protects the underlying tissue from infection, dirt and injury. It also prevents the entry of foreign bodies by producing **keratin**, a hard protein that makes the skin tough, reducing the passage of substances in or out of the body. This layer does not have its own blood supply. Instead it receives nourishment from **interstitial fluid**, a liquid that is formed in blood plasma, which acts as a link between blood and cells. From mitosis occurring to desquamation takes approximately four to six weeks.

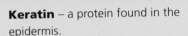

Key terms

Keratin – a protein found in the epidermis.

Interstitial fluid – also known as tissue fluid.

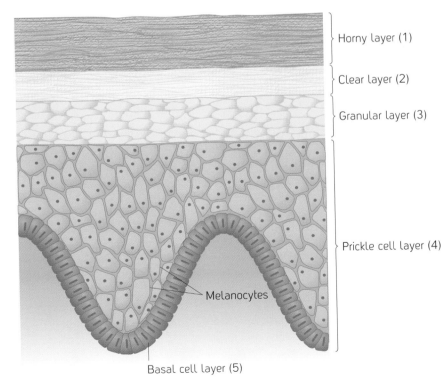

Horny layer (1)

Clear layer (2)

Granular layer (3)

Prickle cell layer (4)

Melanocytes

Basal cell layer (5)

Layers of the epidermis

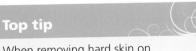

Top tip

When removing hard skin on the feet during a pedicure, never remove too much. This would cause discomfort to the client, as feet require extra cushioning and protection that skin provides.

Key terms

Basement membrane – a thin supportive layer that anchors the epidermis to the loose connective tissue, the dermis, below.

Melanocytes – cells that create the pigment of the skin.

Melanin – the pigment of the skin, this determines the colour of our skin and how it changes colour when we tan.

Key terms

Lipids – fats , oils.

Langerhans cells – special defence cells that detect, absorb and remove foreign bodies. Also known as macrophages.

Lymphatic system – the system that removes waste from the body.

Layer	Function
Basal cell or germinating layer (*Stratum germinativum*)	• A single layer of column-shaped cells, joined to **basement membrane**. • Mitosis occurs in this layer. New cells are pushed upwards to the next layer. • The cells contain a nucleus and are filled with fluid. • **Melanocytes** are distributed throughout the layer and produce **melanin**. Melanocytes are stimulated by ultraviolet (UV) light to produce a skin tan. Melanin acts as an umbrella, protecting underlying tissues from UV damage. • With Caucasian skins, the melanocytes are usually destroyed when they get to the granular layer; however with UV stimulation, melanocytes can be present in the upper epidermis.
Prickle cell layer (*Stratum spinosum*)	• 2–6 layers of elongated cells. • Cells have soft spiky spines which connect to other prickle cells – the spines protect the cells by preventing bacteria from entering and will also prevent moisture loss. • Cells contain a nucleus and are filled with fluid. • Cells produce and retain **lipids** to retain moisture in the skin. • Contains keratinocytes, cells which produce keratin, a strong fibrous protein that also prevents moisture loss. • Contains **Langerhans cells**. They move from the epidermis to the dermis carrying foreign bodies to the lymph nodes to be removed by the **lymphatic system**. • Melanocytes can extend into this layer.
Granular layer (*Stratum granulosum*)	• 1, 2 or 3 layer(s) of cells that have started to flatten as the cells begin to die. • The nucleus begins to break down, creating the appearance of granules in the cytoplasm, and later form keratin.
Clear layer (*Stratum lucidum*)	• Made up of flattened dead cells that are translucent (clear). • No nucleus (because the cell is dead at this point), cell filled with clear substance (eledin) produced at late keratin stage. • Only present in non-hairy areas, e.g. soles and palms. • Melanin granules are destroyed as they are not present in this layer.
Horny layer (*Stratum corneum*)	• Outer layer of skin consisting of scale-like, overlapping, flat dead cells of keratin which are shed from the surface of the skin (desquamation).

Functions of the epidermis

The dermis

The dermis is found below the epidermis and is also known as the true skin. It consists of two layers:

1 papillary

2 reticular.

The two layers are positioned very close to each other, so it is hard to see clearly where one starts and the other ends. The dermis layer varies in thickness from 0.3 millimetres (eyelids) to 3 millimetres (back).

The dermis contains three types of tissue:

● collagen fibres — providing strength

● reticular fibres — providing support

● elastin fibres — giving flexibility to the skin.

These fibres are found throughout the two layers, although the papillary layer has more collagen fibres. Mast cells are present in the dermis and produce a chemical called histamine when the skin is either damaged or is having an allergic reaction. The production of histamine causes skin irritation (so you are aware of the reaction), swelling (from excess tissue fluid in the area, to cool the rise in body temperature) and erythema (increased blood circulation to bring nutrients, white blood cells and oxygen to repair the area).

Papillary layer

● Upper layer of the dermis.

● Has loose **connective tissue** which supports and binds to other tissues. It is loosely arranged so that it can move more easily.

● Contains a vast supply of tiny capillary blood vessels delivering blood to the basal layer of the epidermis. This blood supply provides food and oxygen essential for cell growth.

● Contains a thin arrangement of collagen fibres to provide strength.

Reticular layer

● Composed of thick collagen (white fibres) and elastin (yellow fibres) which give the skin its strength and elasticity.

● Criss-crossing collagen fibres create a strong support to the skin.

● Fibroblast cells produce collagen in this layer.

● Collagen fibres are embedded in a jelly-like **matrix**, which holds a lot of water and helps to make the skin firm.

● Contains **dense connective tissue**, which is composed of collagen and elastin fibres and makes up the **tendons** and ligaments that are arranged in bundles.

● Contains sensory nerve receptors, sweat glands, **lymphatic vessels** and hair **follicles**.

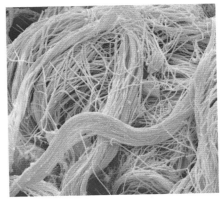

Collagen (thick fibres) and elastin (thin fibres)

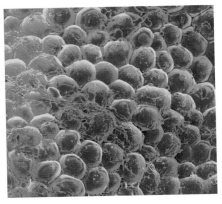

Adipose tissue in the subcutaneous layer

Key term

Connective tissue – has many types of cells and fibres; supports and binds other tissues together.

Key terms

Matrix – a thick, fluid-based substance.

Dense connective tissue – composed mainly of collagen fibres.

Tendons – attach muscle to bone.

Lymphatic vessels – remove waste products from body.

Follicles – holes in the skin which the hair sits in.

Anatomy and physiology

Key term

AHAs – (alpha hydroxy acids), molecules found in fruit and milk, usually products containing fruit acids, which are used as either an anti-ageing product or as an exfoliator.

Check it out

The next time you go shopping, take a look at the different types of hand and body creams available. Look at the ingredients, as many anti-ageing creams have collagen, **AHAs** and UV protection added. As a nail technician, you need to understand that as we age, collagen fibres start to break down and are replaced slowly, causing wrinkles to form. Creams with collagen will plump the skin up, AHAs will make wrinkles more superficial (not as deep) and UV protection will protect the skin from damage, giving a more youthful look. Take notes while you are researching and use them as a revision tool.

Subcutaneous layer

This layer contains mainly fat cells (adipocytes) — known as adipose — and is made up of loose connective tissue. It is the deepest layer situated below the dermis and has many functions.

- It acts as a layer of insulation to keep the body warm and maintain the correct body temperature.
- It protects underlying structures such as organs and bones by acting as a shock absorber.
- It is a major energy reserve, as the body stores water and fat.
- The loss of this layer can cause the skin to sag and deep wrinkles to form.
- It gives the body its shape and curves.
- Too much adipose can lead to the body becoming overweight.

Structures within the skin

Sebaceous glands

The sebaceous gland opens up into the hair follicle and secretes sebum, which lubricates the hair and skin's surface, making skin and hair soft, supple and adding lustre. It creates water-resistant protection and prevents infection.

Key terms

Acid mantle – an even balance of dead skin cells, sebum and perspiration which acts as a barrier against infection.

pH – indicates whether a substance is acid, neutral or alkaline. A pH of 7 is neutral; with a pH of 5.5, the skin is naturally acidic.

The **acid mantle** is made up of an even balance of dead skin cells, sebum and perspiration to maintain a natural **pH** of 5.5, preventing bacterial infection and maintaining a normal skin type.

- Too many skin cells and too much sebum cause oily skin.
- Too little perspiration causes dehydrated skin.
- Too few dead skin cells and too little sebum cause dry skin.

Sudoriferous glands

There are two types of sudoriferous glands — eccrine and apocrine — that produce **perspiration**. Their functions are to:

- cool the body, as part of heat regulation

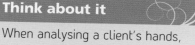

Think about it

When analysing a client's hands, try to assess what might have caused a particular problem such as very dry skin, cuticles and nails. Think about internal and external causes, for example using household chemicals without wearing protective gloves. What else could be the cause?

- excrete waste products, e.g. urea
- hydrate the skin, preventing dehydration.

Eccrine glands are found all over the body and open on to the skin surface via a duct. They begin in the dermis as a coil-shaped tube that straightens as it goes up through the epidermis. These glands are found in abundance in certain areas of the body such as the soles and palms.

Apocrine glands are larger than eccrine glands. They are coil-shaped tubes that are located in the dermis and then, as they reach the epidermis, they form a straight section before opening up into the hair follicle. The glands are located in certain areas: the axillae (armpits), the areola (around the nipples) and the genitals. The glands become active at puberty and are stimulated by many factors, including a nervous response, stress or anxiety, excitement and sexual attraction, which trigger a hormone response producing adrenaline that is carried in the blood to produce apocrine sweat.

Hair

Hairs cover the whole body except the palms of the hands, soles of the feet, lips and parts of the sex organs. Hairs have many functions:

- Protection — from dust particles entering via the eyes, ears and nose. Eyebrows reduce the amount of UV light entering the eyes.
- Warmth — hairs become erect when the body is cold to maintain a warm body temperature and create insulation.
- Friction — hairs reduce friction and irritation of the skin.
- Touch receptors — hair helps with nerve responses to things such as touch.
- Smell — hairs retain an individual's personal smell, which occurs when the body releases pheromones.

Types of hair

Hairs are made up of tightly packed, dead skin cells containing keratin. There are three types of hair.

- Lanugo hairs are soft, fine hairs with no medulla (see diagram of cross-section of a hair, below) and are usually unpigmented. They are found on unborn babies (or premature babies) and are replaced by vellus and terminal hairs in the later stages of pregnancy, around 7–8 months.
- Vellus hairs are soft, downy hairs found all over the body and face. They are either unpigmented or slightly pigmented hairs that can be stimulated externally (by shaving) or internally (hormonal response) to become terminal hairs. A medulla is not present and the bulb is not well formed.
- Terminal hairs are strong, coarse, pigmented hairs found on the head, pubic regions, axillae, eyelashes, eyebrows and in male pattern growth areas: face, chest and back. They are located deep in the dermis and have deep-seated follicles with a rich blood supply.

Key terms

Perspiration – (sweat) fluid secreted by the eccrine glands containing water and sodium chloride with small amounts of urea, uric acid, ammonia and lactic acid, and traces of amino acids, sugar and absorbic acid (vitamin C); or fluid secreted by the apocrine glands which is a more milky fluid containing organic substances like fats, sugars, proteins and **pheromones**.

Pheromones – chemicals produced by the body that act as signals to the opposite sex.

Top tip

Shower daily to prevent body odour, as bacteria feed on sweat and excrete a strong odour. Sweat itself does not have a distinct smell but if left will become unpleasant. Feet alone have more than 250,000 sweat glands and produce more than a pint of sweat per day. Generally, the body has 2–5 million sweat glands.

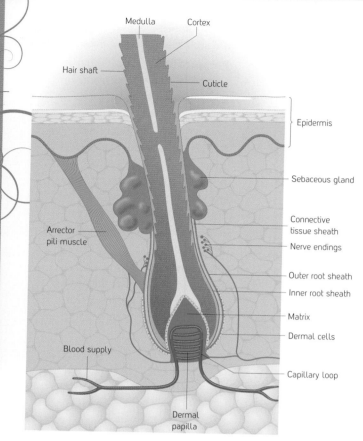

Medulla Cortex

Hair shaft

Cuticle

Epidermis

Sebaceous gland

Connective tissue sheath

Nerve endings

Arrector pili muscle

Outer root sheath

Inner root sheath

Matrix

Dermal cells

Blood supply

Capillary loop

Dermal papilla

Cross-section of the skin and hair

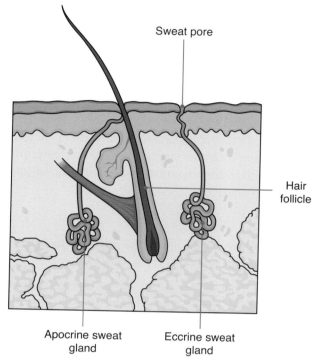

Sweat pore

Hair follicle

Apocrine sweat gland

Eccrine sweat gland

Eccrine glands are found all over the body. Apocrine glands develop during puberty and are found in the armpits, areolar, genital and anal areas

The hair's structure

The visible part of the hair is known as the hair shaft.

- The cuticle is the outer layer and is made up of overlapping, transparent, interlocking scales that protect the cortex and give hair its elasticity.

- The cortex consists of several layers of thick, closely packed, **keratinised** cells, making it the largest layer, and gives the hair its strength. Melanin is present and gives hair its colour.

- The medulla is found in the middle of the hair. It contains air pockets that allow light to reflect through, providing colour and sheen to the hair. It is only found in coarse or thick hair.

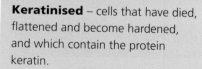

Key term

Keratinised – cells that have died, flattened and become hardened, and which contain the protein keratin.

Anatomy and physiology

Structure	Description and function
Hair follicle	A depression in the skin, where the hair grows from.
Hair bulb	The largest part of the hair at the base. Mitosis occurs here to produce new cells.
Hair root	The part of the hair that is not visible and lies beneath the skin, within the follicle. The root is made up of the hair bulb and dermal papilla.
Inner root sheath (IRS)	The root is surrounded by the inner and outer root **sheath**. The inner root sheath is moulded to the root and dissolved when it reaches the sebaceous gland, so it is not visible on the shaft. The IRS and cuticle of the hair are interlocked, to secure the hair in the follicle and guide the hair out of the follicle.
Outer root sheath (ORS)	The function of the ORS is unknown; however, the ORS cells can leave the follicle and enter the epidermis to aid cell renewal, if superficial damage occurs to the epidermis. It is multilayered and thicker next to the arrector pili muscle. The ORS surrounds the IRS and is next to the epidermis/dermis.
Dermal papilla (matrix)	The lowest part of the bulb where mitosis occurs. This is also where the blood supply brings nutrients and oxygen to nourish the hair.
Arrector pili muscle	Attached to the hair follicle, it contracts when stimulated by strong emotions like fear or as a reaction to low body temperature. To retain body heat when cold, we shiver and the arrector pili muscle contracts. This closes the follicle opening and traps warm air next to the skin. We can see this happening – when goose pimples appear on the skin's surface and the hairs stand erect.

Structure and function of hair

Nerves

The body is made up of trillions of nerve cells known as neurons, which are cells of the nervous system. There are two types of nerves — sensory and motor — which are made up of whitish bundles of fibres surrounded by a sheath. The cells carry messages from sensory nerve **receptors**, found in the skin, eyes, tongue, ears and nose, to the central nervous system (spinal cord and brain). There are different types of nerve sensors in the skin and they are found in abundance in certain areas such as the hands, face and genitals. These receptors detect pressure, touch, pain, heat and cold, acting as warning devices to protect the skin from harm. Motor neurons send messages from the central nervous system to a muscle or a gland.

Key terms

Sheath – a protective covering.

Receptors – detect pressure, touch, pain, heat and cold. They act as warning devices to protect the skin from harm.

Check it out

In pairs, test your skin's sensitivity. Collect a cotton wool ball, an orange stick and two test tubes – one filled with warm water and the other with cold water. The first person closes their eyes and their partner runs each item over the skin – the first person states whether they feel a soft, sharp, hot or cold response.

Functions of the skin

Each letter of the word SHAPES is the first letter of a skin function.

Function (SHAPES)	Description
Secretion	• Sweat is secreted to help regulate body temperature and hydrate the skin to prevent it becoming dehydrated. • Sebum is secreted by the sebaceous glands to create a water-resistant barrier to protect the skin and to keep the skin soft and supple.
Heat regulation	• Vaso-dilation – this occurs when blood vessels expand and blood flow is increased to allow heat to escape from the skin's surface. This cools the blood and, in turn, the body. • Vaso-constriction – blood vessels narrow and blood flow is reduced to retain heat. • If the body is cold, we shiver and the arrector pili muscle contracts. This closes the follicle opening and traps warm air next to the skin to help keep the body warm. This causes goose pimples on the skin's surface. • Perspiration occurs when the body is too hot, as sweat covers the skin's surface and evaporates to cool the body.
Absorption	• The skin absorbs UV light to produce vitamin D that absorbs and uses calcium within the body, e.g. for bone growth and repair. • Medications, drugs and chemicals can be absorbed through the skin. • Skin can absorb water, e.g. after swimming the skin can look like a prune (wrinkled) because the skin has absorbed excess water through the pores. • The skin can absorb products with very small molecules much deeper into the skin. This includes things like AHAs (alpha hydroxy acids) which are found in anti-ageing products and exfoliators. AHAs speed up skin renewal, which helps to reduce wrinkle depth. • Vitamin E or vitamin E cream can be absorbed through the skin.
Protection	• Langerhans cells are special defensive cells that detect, absorb and remove foreign bodies. • Skin has a water-resistant barrier (sebum) that prevents absorption of harmful substances. • A healthy acid mantle protects the skin from bacterial infection. An equal balance of dead skin cells, perspiration and sebum helps to maintain the skin's natural pH 5.5, which helps to prevent harmful bacteria multiplying on the skin's surface. • Skin contains melanin that is stimulated by UV light to create a tan and create an umbrella effect protecting underlying tissues.
Excretion	• The sweat gland excretes sweat, which contains waste products such as urea, water and salt that the body does not require.
Sensation	• Nerve endings sense (detect) heat and cold, touch, pressure, vibration and tissue damage.

Nails

The nail is an **appendage** of the skin and is located at the ends of the fingers and toes. The nails have more than one function:

● They create a protective covering for the ends of fingers and toes.

● They help when grasping tiny objects.

● They can be used as tools, although this could cause damage to the nail and surrounding tissue.

Key term

Appendage – something that is attached to something else.

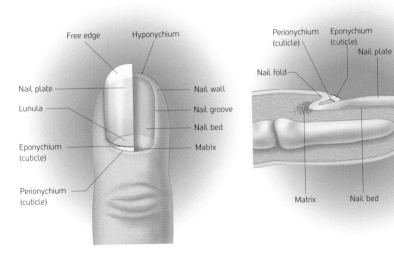

Free edge   Hyponychium

Nail plate

Lunula

Eponychium
(cuticle)

Perionychium
(cuticle)

Nail wall

Nail groove

Nail bed

Matrix

Perionychium   Eponychium
(cuticle)   (cuticle)

Nail fold   Nail plate

Free edge

Matrix   Nail bed   Hyponychium

Structure of the nail

Think about it

- Toenails are thicker than fingernails.

- It takes about 4–6 months for fingernails to grow from the matrix to the tip.

- Toenails take 12–18 months to grow from the matrix to the tip.

When working on a client who has lost a nail or one who has recently stopped biting their nails, make a note of this and observe how long it takes for their nails to regrow.

Structure and function of the nail

Structure	Location/description	Function	Relevance to nail technician
Nail plate	Main part of the nail, which grows from the matrix and moves down to form the free edge.	To protect the nail bed, fingers and toes.	Broken or bitten nails, especially exposing the flesh line or hyponychium, could cause infection.
Cuticle	Part of the *Stratum corneum* that overlaps the nail plate.	Protects the matrix from infection.	Prone to infection if excessive removal occurs or is accidentally cut with the nippers. Dry and overgrown cuticles are prone to tears.
Lunula (half moon)	Curved shaped area visible on the nail plate. The front end of the matrix (the visible part of the matrix). Not present on all nails. Whitish lunula are keratin cells which have not completely flattened.	The shape of the lunula determines the shape of the free edge	Injury or pressure to the lunula could damage the matrix located beneath.
Nail bed	Lies beneath the nail plate. Made up of the epidermis and dermis layers with nerves and blood vessels.	Has interlocking grooves that keep the nail securely in place. Contains sensory nerve endings to help protect the area and blood vessels to provide nourishment.	If nail plate is not in contact with the bed, it is prone to infection.

Anatomy and physiology

Anatomy and physiology

Structure	Location/description	Function	Relevance to nail technician
Perionychium	Cuticle that surrounds the nail border.	Protects the matrix from infection.	Prone to infection if damaged.
Free edge	The nail plate that has grown beyond the nail bed.	To protect the fingers and toes. Helps with grasping tiny objects.	Damage or infection could occur if not present.
Matrix	Found under nail plate, beneath the lunula. Contains blood vessels, nerve endings and is where mitosis occurs.	Cell division occurs here to create new nail cells.	Excessive pressure to the matrix can cause damage; for example, temporary or permanent ridges on the nail plate.
Hyponychium	Underneath the nail plate, just before the free edge begins. A raised wall of skin that is in contact with the nail.	Protects the nail bed from infection.	If the nail is damaged, exposing the hyponychium, it is prone to infection.
Eponychium	A thin layer of skin attached to the nail plate. An extension of the cuticle.	Protects the matrix from infection.	The area is prone to infection if excessively removed, dryness or damage occurs.
Lateral nail folds (nail mantle)	A fold of skin that is located at the base of the nail, just before the cuticle appears.	Protects the matrix from external damage.	Too much pressure can damage the matrix and could affect how the nail grows.
Nail grooves	Grooves located down the edge of the nail plate	Direct the nail so it grows in the correct direction toward the free edge.	Damage could cause the nail to grow in the wrong direction.
Nail wall	Folds of skin that run over the sides of the nail plate.	Protects the area from external damage.	Cuts or bitten skin can cause infection.

Think about it

The longest fingernail recorded was on an Indian man who grew a nail 120 centimetres long.

Key terms

Voluntary muscles – muscles we can control, for example skeletal muscles that allow us to run or jump.

Involuntary muscles – muscles controlled by the brain over which we have no control, for example the heart.

Nail growth

Cell division is called mitosis. It is the process where new cells are made and occurs in the matrix. As the cells move away from the matrix they begin to harden and flatten, by the process of keratinisation, to start forming the nail plate. The nail begins to grow over the nail bed, along the nail grooves toward the end, to eventually create the free edge.

Muscles

There are more than 600 muscles in the human body and their functions vary from pumping blood around the body to helping us lift heavy objects. There are **voluntary muscles** that we control, for example leg muscles, and **involuntary muscles** that we do not control, such as the muscles of the heart. They are made up of bundles of elastic fibres, surrounded by a sheath. When muscles contract they shorten and when they relax they lengthen. Muscles always work in pairs, so when one relaxes, the other contracts. In fact, muscles never completely relax, as a few fibres will contract to create muscle tone.

Types of muscle

There are three types of muscle:

- Smooth muscles – these are involuntary muscles. As they are controlled by the brain, you have no control over them. Smooth muscles are found in the stomach or digestive system, bladder, uterus and behind the eyes. They contain layers (like sheets) of muscle.

- Thick cardiac muscle – the muscle that forms the heart and pumps blood around the body. This is also an involuntary muscle.

- Skeletal muscles – these are voluntary muscles. They are attached to a bone by a tendon, giving the body power and strength.

Structure and functions of the muscles in the hand and lower arm

The muscles of the hand and lower arm create movement in the arm and the fingers. The 12 muscles of the hand and lower arm are referred to as flexors and extensors. They perform the following movements:

- Supinate – to rotate the arm and turn the palm upwards.

- Pronate – to rotate the arm and turn the palm downwards.

- Flex – to move the hand towards the lower arm, bending at the wrist joint.

- Extend – to move the hand away from the lower arm, so the wrist and hand are straight at the joint.

- Abduction – moving away from, for example spreading the fingers or moving the arm away from the body.

- Adduction – moving towards, for example bringing the fingers back together or moving the arm towards the body.

When the muscles of the hand and lower arm contract, they pull on the tendons that are attached to the fingers. This creates the movement.

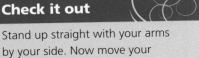

Check it out

Stand up straight with your arms by your side. Now move your arms outwards – this is known as abduction. Next, move your arms back towards your body – this is known as adduction. Make a list of which lower arm muscles you used when you adducted, then abducted, your arms.

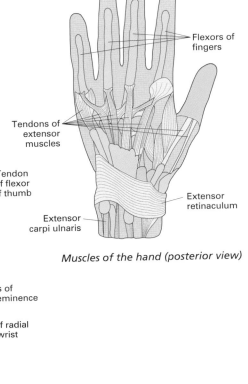

Flexors of fingers

Tendons of extensor muscles

Extensor retinaculum

Extensor carpi ulnaris

Muscles of the hand (posterior view)

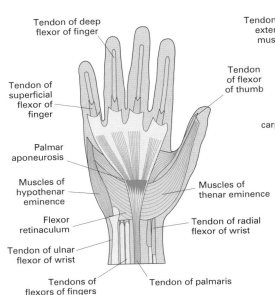

Tendon of deep flexor of finger

Tendon of superficial flexor of finger

Tendon of flexor of thumb

Palmar aponeurosis

Muscles of hypothenar eminence

Muscles of thenar eminence

Flexor retinaculum

Tendon of radial flexor of wrist

Tendon of ulnar flexor of wrist

Tendons of flexors of fingers

Tendon of palmaris

Muscles of the hand (anterior view)

Muscle of hand	Location	Action
Hypothenar muscles	Below little finger on the palm	Flexes, adducts and abducts little finger
Thenar muscles	Below thumb on palm of hand	Flexes, adducts and abducts thumb

Muscles of the hand

Key terms

Anterior – front view.

Ulnar – the same side of the arm as the little finger.

Medial – mid-line, near the middle.

Radial – the same side of the arm as the thumb.

Check it out

Wiggle your fingers and then clench your hands to form a fist; can you see the muscles and tendons in your forearm and hands contract and move? Make a note of the muscles that you are using.

Key terms

Plantar flexes – action to point foot down.

Dorsi flexes – action to position heel downwards and toes pointing upward.

Lateral – at the side of something.

Posterior – located behind, or at the back of something.

Longitudinal arch of foot – runs across the bone, sideways.

Muscle of forearm	Location	Action
Flexor carpi radialis	**Anterior** side of forearm (inside joint across to thumb side)	Flexes and abducts wrist
Flexor carpi ulnaris	Along **ulnar** side of forearm (little finger side)	Flexes and adducts wrist
Palmaris longus	Anterior **medial** side of forearm	Flexes wrist
Flexor digitorum sublimis	Down medial side of forearm	Flexes fingers
Pronator teres	Anterior side of forearm across elbow joint	Pronates forearm, turns wrist down and flexes elbow
Anconeus	Small triangular muscle, which lies on the elbow joint	Abducts the ulna and stabilises the elbow joint
Extensor digitorum	Back of forearm on **radial** side	Extends fingers
Extensor carpi ulnaris	Back of forearm on ulnar side	Extends and adducts wrist
Extensor carpi radialis brevis	Radial side of forearm	Extends and abducts wrist
Extensor carpi radialis longus	Radial side of forearm (thumb side)	Extends and abducts wrist

Muscles of the lower arm

Structure and functions of the muscles of the lower leg and foot

The table below shows the muscles that flex and extend the lower leg and foot. The toes move in the same way as the fingers — the muscles contract, then use the same pulling force to create movement, using the tendons to manipulate the toes. Located at the ankle is a band of tendons that hold the muscles in place, known as the Achilles tendon. This tendon is an extension of the gastrocnemius and soleus muscles and it is the strongest and thickest tendon in the body.

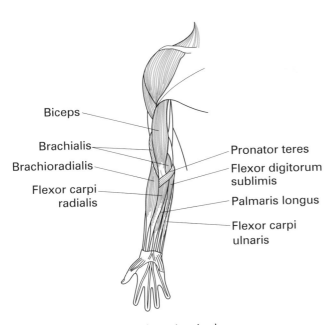

Biceps

Brachialis

Brachioradialis

Flexor carpi radialis

Pronator teres

Flexor digitorum sublimis

Palmaris longus

Flexor carpi ulnaris

Muscles of the lower arm (anterior view)

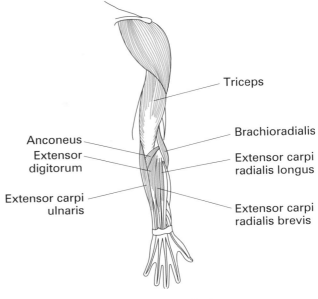

Triceps

Anconeus

Extensor digitorum

Extensor carpi ulnaris

Brachioradialis

Extensor carpi radialis longus

Extensor carpi radialis brevis

Muscles of the lower arm (posterior view)

Muscle of lower leg	Location	Action
Gastrocnemius	Forms calf muscle at back of lower leg	Points toes downward (**plantar flexes**) and propels body when walking or running
Peroneus longus	Lower part of shin bone	Bends ankle to pull foot upwards and turns feet to face outward
Soleus	Below the gastrocnemius, at back of lower leg	Helps posture by steadying leg and pointing toes (plantar flexes)
Tibialis anterior	**Lateral** side of tibia, down shin bone	Bends ankle to pull foot upwards (**dorsi flexes**) and turns feet to face one another
Extensor digitorum longus	Lateral part of shin bone	Bends ankle to pull foot upwards, turns feet to face outward and extends toes
Extensor hallucis longus	Partly behind tibialis muscle, down shin bone	Extends big toe
Flexor digitorum longus	Inside of back of calf	Plantar flexes and inverts foot Flexes toes and supports inner **longitudinal arch of foot**

Muscles of the lower leg

Anatomy and physiology

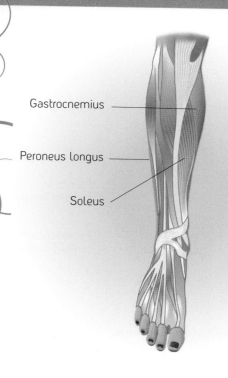

Gastrocnemius

Peroneus longus

Soleus

Gastrocnemius and soleus muscles

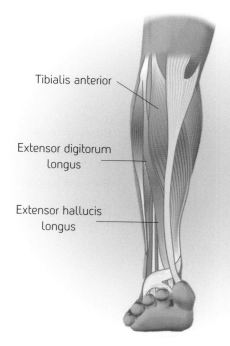

Tibialis anterior

Extensor digitorum
longus

Extensor hallucis
longus

Tibialis anterior muscle

Check it out

In a seated position point your foot downwards – this is known as plantar flex. Straighten your foot and point your toes upwards – this is known as dorsi flex. List the muscles you are using.

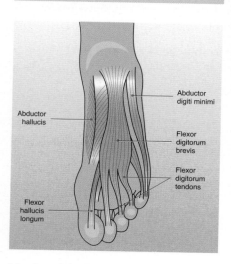

Abductor
digiti minimi

Abductor
hallucis

Flexor
digitorum
brevis

Flexor
digitorum
tendons

Flexor
hallucis
longum

Muscles of the foot

Muscle of foot	Location	Action
Abductor hallucis	Along medial border of the foot	A muscle of the foot that abducts the big toe
Flexor hallucis longus	Begins at the lower posterior surface of the fibula, down to the sole of the feet towards the big toe	Flexes all joints of the big toe, plantar flexion of the ankle joint
Flexor digitorum brevis	In the middle of the sole of the foot	Flexes lateral four toes
Abductors digiti minimi	Down the lateral side of the foot	Flex and abduct the little toe

Muscles of the foot

Bones

Under our skin we have a skeleton made of bones. Our bones are covered by muscles, which are attached to the skeleton by tendons. Our bones are connected to each other with ligaments. The human skeleton consists of 206 bones, from our skull to the tips of our toes and fingers. Larger bones such as the skull, sternum, ribs, pelvis and femur bones all contain **bone marrow**, which produces stem cells, for example erythrocytes (red blood cells) and leucocytes (white blood cells). From birth, our bones continue to grow and usually stop growing during our teenage years.

Structure of bones

There are two main types of bone tissue:

- Compact — this forms the outer shell of bones and is very hard.

- Cancellous — known as spongy, this type is found beneath compact bone. It forms a mesh of bony bars with spaces filled with bone marrow.

Function of bones

Functions of bones:

- Produce blood cells in the bone marrow (including red and white blood cells and platelets)

- Support the soft tissue and provide attachment for muscles

- Protect vital organs

- Assist movement (as muscles contract they move the bones)

- Store minerals (for example, calcium which is then released into the blood)

Bones of the lower arm and hand

The radius and ulna form the bones of the lower arm, with the ulna on the little finger side and the radius on the thumb side. The hand is made up of 27 bones in total: the wrist consists of eight carpal bones, the hand has five metacarpal bones, each finger contains three phalange bones and each thumb contains two phalange bones that total 14 phalanges.

Key term

Bone marrow – soft, fatty, porous connective tissue that fills the cavities of bones. It is made up of living cells, nerves and blood vessels.

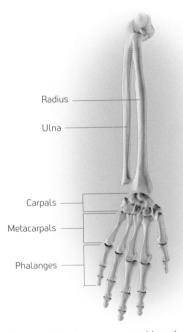

Bones of the lower arm and hand

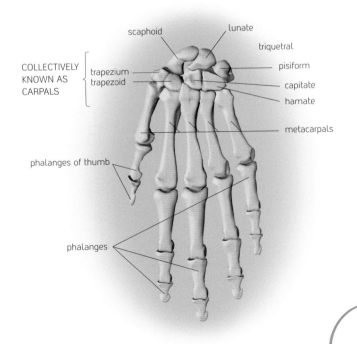

Bones of the hand and wrist

Bones of the lower leg and foot

The legs and feet support the weight of the whole body and the lower leg, which begins below the knee (the patella), consists of the tibia and fibula. The tibia is on the big toe side and the fibula on the little toe side. There are seven tarsals (ankle), five metatarsals (foot) and 14 phalanges (one toe has two phalanges and the others have three each).

The foot has two types of arch that provide support, act as shock absorbers and assist with posture. There are two **transverse arches** and two **longitudinal arches**.

Key terms

Transverse arch – runs across the bone, sideways.

Longitudinal arch – runs across the bone, lengthways.

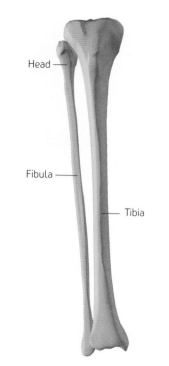

The tibia and fibula (lower leg)

Head

Fibula

Tibia

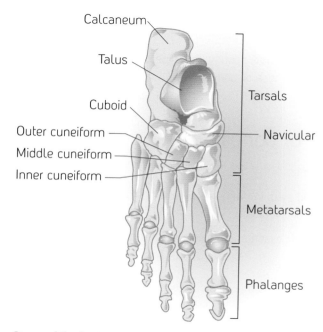

Calcaneum

Talus

Cuboid

Outer cuneiform

Middle cuneiform

Inner cuneiform

Tarsals

Navicular

Metatarsals

Phalanges

Bones of the foot

Blood

The composition of blood

Blood is composed of 55 per cent plasma and 45 per cent blood cells. Blood transports nutrients and removes waste products. The heart pumps blood through the arteries and veins of the body, to transport blood to the vital organs. The blood transports valuable nutrients and removes waste products, as it flows through the vessels. The arteries carry oxygenated blood away from the heart to the organs, and veins carry deoxygenated blood back to the heart. Capillaries are tiny vessels that are connected to the arteries and veins. They have very thin walls to allow nutrients to be transferred easily to the body's organs and waste products from the body's organs, through capillary exchange.

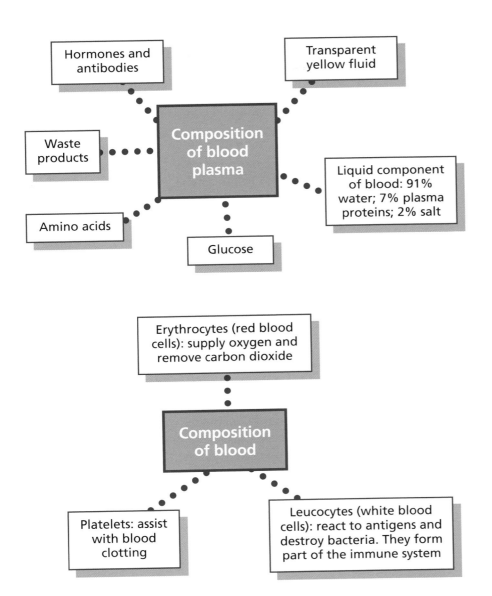

Arteries	• Thick elastic walls
	• Blood pumped out of heart at great force
	• Maintain blood pressure
	• Contain oxygenated blood
Veins	• Thinner walls than arteries
	• Slow blood flow and smooth flow
	• Contain valves to prevent blood flowing in wrong direction
	• Pressure or contraction of muscles helps blood flow, by pushing the blood upwards
	• Contain deoxygenated blood

Differences between arteries and veins

Function of blood

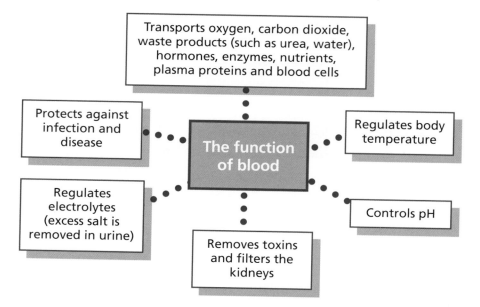

Transports oxygen, carbon dioxide, waste products (such as urea, water), hormones, enzymes, nutrients, plasma proteins and blood cells

Protects against infection and disease

The function of blood

Regulates body temperature

Regulates electrolytes (excess salt is removed in urine)

Controls pH

Removes toxins and filters the kidneys

Arteries and veins of the lower arm and hand

Arteries carry oxygenated blood, bringing oxygen to the cells. Deoxygenated blood, carrying waste products, is carried away in the veins. When massaging the lower arm and hand or using a heat treatment like a thermal mitten, you will warm the circulating blood and increase blood flow to the area. The increased blood flow brings nutrients to the area, removes waste products, produces a healthy skin colour and softens the tissue. This will also apply when working over the lower leg and foot area.

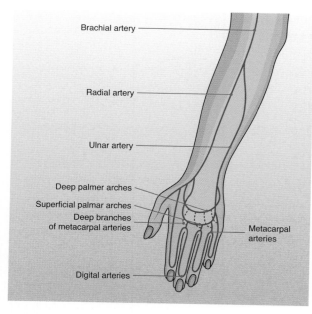

Brachial artery

Radial artery

Ulnar artery

Deep palmer arches
Superficial palmar arches
Deep branches of metacarpal arteries

Metacarpal arteries

Digital arteries

Arteries of the lower arm and hand

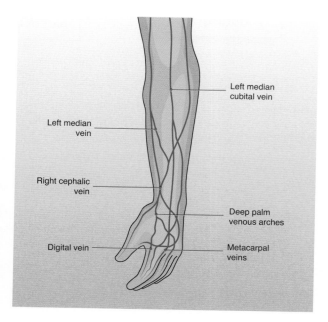

Left median cubital vein

Left median vein

Right cephalic vein

Deep palm venous arches

Digital vein

Metacarpal veins

Veins of the lower arm and hand

The main arteries of the forearm are the ulnar and radial arteries. These arteries continue to the palmar arches, located in the palm of the hand. The arteries then lead on to the metacarpal and digital arteries of the palm and fingers.

The digital veins in the fingers connect to the deep palm venous arches in the palm and then continue to the cephalic and basilica veins of the lower arm.

Arteries and veins of the lower leg and foot

Just below the knee are the anterior and posterior tibial arteries. The peroneal artery branches off from the posterior tibial artery. From the anterior tibial artery, the dorsalis pedis artery forms at the ankle. The posterior tibial artery divides at the ankle to form the medial and laterial plantar arteries. The plantar arteries connect to the dorsalis pedis artery and extend to form the digital arteries.

Top tips

- When feeling for a pulse, place your finger on the radial artery in the wrist (on the thumb side of the wrist).

- If a client has poor circulation it could lead to chilblains (painful, itchy swellings). A massage and heat treatment to the area will help improve circulation.

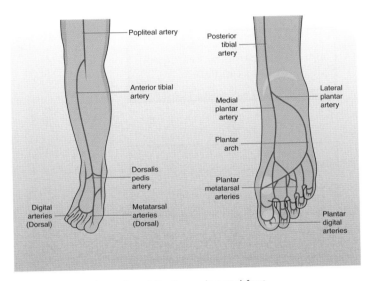

Anterior view of arteries of the lower leg and foot

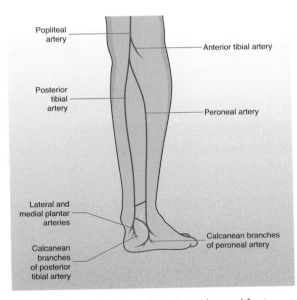

Posterior view of arteries of the lower leg and foot

The digital veins in the toes drain into the plantar and dorsal venous arch. This connects to the dorsal pedis veins and then the superficial veins, known as the saphenous veins, which join the iliac vein. The deep veins are the posterior tibial vein, which joins the peroneal vein, and the anterior tibial vein, connecting to the popliteal vein at the knee.

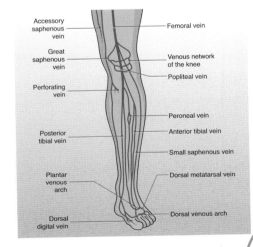

Anterior view of veins of the lower leg and foot

Key terms

Lymphocytes – white blood cells that make up part of the immune system. They identify and destroy foreign bodies, for example bacteria or viruses.

Lymph – a straw-coloured fluid derived from plasma containing small amounts of oxygen and nutrients.

Tissue fluid – (interstitial fluid) occupies the space between the lymph capillaries and blood capillaries.

Think about it

Have you ever had very swollen feet? This happens because of a build-up of excess **tissue fluid** in that area. It can occur if a person has been sitting for too long, during pregnancy or where the lymphatic system is not working properly. A twisted ankle can lead to a build-up of tissue fluid in the area to give added protection.

Top tip

As a nail technician, you can massage the area to speed up the removal of excess tissue fluid, as long as it is not contra-indicated.

The lymphatic system

The lymphatic system is the 'waste disposal unit of the body' – it collects waste products produced by the body and removes them. It also collects any excess fluid from the tissues and absorbs lipids (fats) and gets rid of them. The lymphatic system carries **lymphocytes**, which defend the body from the invasion of viral, bacterial or fungal infection. The lymphatic system is like the blood circulation, although the vessels are much finer than blood vessels. Blood plasma passes from the blood capillaries and bathes the tissues, which passes into the lymphatic vessels and become **lymph**.

Lymph is a straw-coloured fluid derived from plasma and contains small amounts of oxygen, nutrients, proteins, waste products, toxins, lipids, carbon dioxide and urea. Approximately 100 ml of lymph is formed per hour and it is continuously replenished.

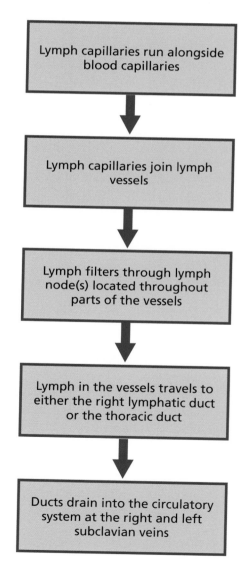

Lymph capillaries run alongside blood capillaries

↓

Lymph capillaries join lymph vessels

↓

Lymph filters through lymph node(s) located throughout parts of the vessels

↓

Lymph in the vessels travels to either the right lymphatic duct or the thoracic duct

↓

Ducts drain into the circulatory system at the right and left subclavian veins

The lymphatic system

Functions of the lymphatic system

The lymphatic system has three main functions:

- It maintains the fluid balance by collecting and returning interstitial fluid and plasma to the blood.

- It absorbs lipids from the intestines and transports them to the blood.

- It supports the immune system by producing lymphocytes to defend the body against disease.

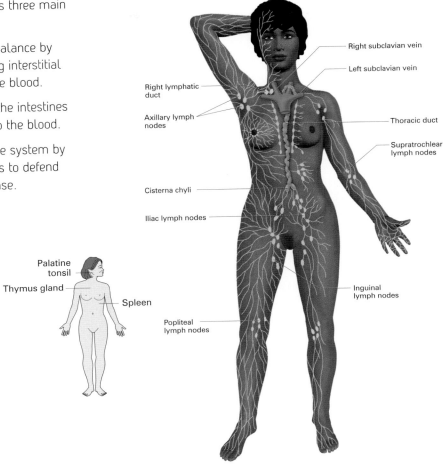

The lymphatic system of the body

Right subclavian vein

Left subclavian vein

Right lymphatic duct

Axillary lymph nodes

Thoracic duct

Supratrochlear lymph nodes

Cisterna chyli

Iliac lymph nodes

Inguinal lymph nodes

Palatine tonsil

Thymus gland

Spleen

Popliteal lymph nodes

Waste products pass from the cells into the tissue fluid, back into the lymph capillaries

Nutrients and oxygen pass from the blood through the capillary walls and into the tissue fluid

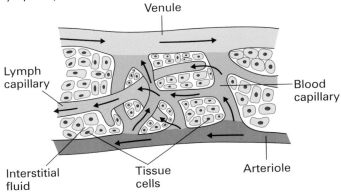

Venule

Lymph capillary

Blood capillary

Interstitial fluid

Tissue cells

Arteriole

The exchange of tissue fluid

Check your knowledge

1. What are the five layers of the epidermis called?

2. What does the subcutaneous layer contain?
   a) Adipose
   b) Collagen
   c) Elastin
   d) Sweat

3. Which sweat gland is found all over the body?
   a) Eccrine
   b) Apocrine

4. What is mitosis?

5. What is the best definition of a cell membrane?
   a) Small structure
   b) Controls all cell functions
   c) The outer cell wall
   d) Powerhouse of a cell

6. What are the three layers of the skin called?
   a) Papillary, reticular, dermis
   b) Epidermis, dermis, subcutaneous
   c) Epidermis, eccrine, apocrine
   d) Epidermis, dermis, adipose

7. What are the functions of the skin? (Remember SHAPES.)

8. What attaches bone to bone?

9. What attaches muscle to bone?

10. What are the three types of muscle called?

11. What is the correct name for the 'waste disposal unit of the body'?
    a) Circulatory system
    b) Muscular system
    c) Skeletal system
    d) Lymphatic system

12. Which is correct? The feet has:
    a) 7 tarsals, 5 metatarsals and 14 phalanges.
    b) 8 carpals, 5 metacarpals and 14 phalanges.

13. Why are the hands and feet very sensitive to touch?

14. How does a hand cream with AHAs affect mature hands?

15. What is the function of fingernails and toenails?
    a) To make the fingers and toes more attractive.
    b) To protect the fingers and toes.
    c) To use tools.

16. What is the lunula?

17. How long does it take for fingernails and toenails to grow back?

Skin and nail analysis

What you will learn

- The importance of carrying out a nail and skin analysis
- How to identify nail and skin conditions
- Diseases and disorders of the nail and skin

Key terms

Analysis – looking at the nails, skin and cuticles and determining their condition.

Contra-indication – skin disorder or disease that prevents or restricts a treatment.

Contagious – a disease that can be passed from one person to another.

Restriction – a limitation or reduction.

Adaptions – changes that are made to a treatment plan to suit the individual client.

Direct cross-infection – when a person is infected by a contagious person by being in direct contact with them, for example through touch.

Indirect cross-infection – when a person is infected because they have been in contact with something, for example a tool, that has been used on a client with a contagious disease.

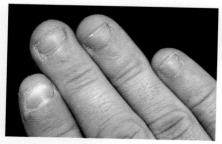

Severely bitten nails

Think about it

If you do not identify a contra-indication, then you and every person you come in contact with could be either **directly** or **indirectly cross-infected**.

Introduction

Having a good understanding of nail and skin **analysis** is vital to the nail technician, and you will need this knowledge and understanding to complete assessments for all the practical skills units.

The importance of carrying out a nail and skin analysis

As a nail technician, you need to understand that there are many **contra-indications** that can prevent a treatment from happening. The client may suffer from a nail or skin condition that could be **contagious**, might be caused pain if worked upon, or the treatment could cause the condition to worsen. If none of these possibilities applies, then the treatment can be performed with **restrictions** or **adaptions**; for example, if a client has a very old bruise on their arm, then either avoid the area or avoid putting pressure on it.

What would you do?

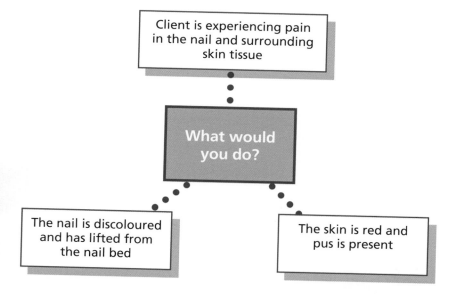

Not every client will have perfect nails and skin, which means that you must understand and be able to recognise every possible contra-indication to enable you to make an informed decision as to whether or not to perform or adapt a treatment. Some conditions such as excessively dry nails are not contagious and would benefit from regular ongoing treatments.

How to identify nail and skin conditions

The consultation process

Before you plan the client's treatment, as part of the **consultation** process, you must first check for contra-indications. This unit identifies the relevant nail and skin diseases and disorders that are applicable to a nail technician and would be contra-indicated. During the consultation, if you recognise a contra-indication, you must not say to the client what you think it is. Nail technicians are not medical professionals and might make a wrong diagnosis. Instead, inform the client that you think there appears to be a problem and advise them to visit their GP.

Secondly, you will need to check the general health of the skin and nails. Do they look healthy? Are there any concerns?

Key term

Consultation – discussion between client and nail technician to determine treatment plan.

Consultation techniques

While performing a skin and nail analysis and checking for contra-indications, you will need to carry out the following procedures:

- visual checks – look at the condition of the skin and nails

- manual checks – feel the skin to determine if it is healthy

- questioning – ask the client if they have had any problems or concerns with their skin and nails

- referring to client's record card – you will need to establish if the client has visited the salon before to find out what treatments they have had. Also check for previous contra-indications, contra-actions and allergies as they will have an impact on your treatment plan.

Look at the flow chart of visual and manual checks to be carried out during analysis.

Think about it

While training to become a nail technician, you might not have the confidence or experience to instantly recognise a problem. To help you, create some flash cards with photographs of the condition and a brief description as a prompt.

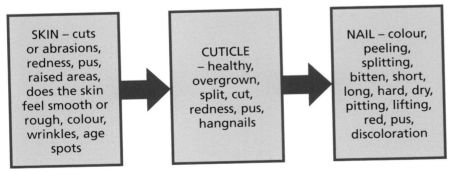

SKIN – cuts or abrasions, redness, pus, raised areas, does the skin feel smooth or rough, colour, wrinkles, age spots

CUTICLE – healthy, overgrown, split, cut, redness, pus, hangnails

NAIL – colour, peeling, splitting, bitten, short, long, hard, dry, pitting, lifting, red, pus, discoloration

Visual and manual checks during analysis

Top tip

When examining the nails and skin for contra-indications, never touch the client's hands or feet. Perform visual checks first and use the hand towel to turn the client's hands or feet over to check both sides. If the client had a condition that could cross-infect, you could become contaminated if you touch the client. Once you are ready to begin the treatment, wipe over the area with a hand or foot sanitiser to cleanse the area.

Top tip

Do not perform a manual check until you are sure there are no contagious conditions present.

Think about it

Examine your own nails, cuticles and skin. What condition are they in?

Think about it

Look at the table summarising contra-indications and decide whether each is a disease or a disorder.

Diseases and disorders of the nails and skin

A disease is a condition that is contagious, such as onychomycosis. A disorder is non-contagious, such as onycholysis.

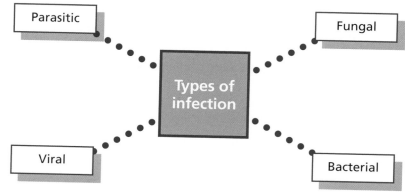

Types of infection

The following table summarises the skin and nail diseases and disorders that you will need to know about. This knowledge will enable you to advise clients before any treatment begins. Some of the conditions will be infectious (can be cross-infected) and others will be non-infectious. There are other conditions that do not relate to a nail or skin disease or disorder but must be taken into consideration when performing a consultation.

Condition	Description	Cause	Treatment (contra-indicated or restricted)
Ridges	**Longitudinal** (vertical) grooves in the nail plate	• Nail naturally grows that way • Part of ageing process, illness or damage to **matrix**	**Buff** the nails and apply **ridge filler base coat**
	Long ridges that run either lengthwise (vertically) or across the nail (horizontally)	• Vertical ridges are normal in adults and increase with age • Can be caused by psoriasis, poor circulation or frostbite • **Horizontal ridges** are caused by high fevers, pregnancy or measles	Buff the nails and apply ridge filler base coat
Corrugations (furrows)			
Beau's lines	**Transverse** lines or furrows on nail plate	During illness, nail cells in matrix stop reproducing. Once reproduction begins again, lines will be evident but will eventually grow out	• Regular manicure or pedicure • Buff the nails and apply ridge filler base coat

Onychorrhexis (on-ee-ko-rex-is)	Split, weak, brittle nails – the dry, brittle nail may peel and split	• Lack of oil in nails • Skin and nails exposed to chemicals or detergents • Change of weather • Unhealthy diet • Illness or medication • Too much buffing or filing	• Nail strengthener • Keep nails short • Wear gloves when using chemicals • Apply hand and nail cream • Regular manicures *Note:* Condition could worsen if nail enhancements applied
Hangnails	Cuticle down the side of the nail plate separates, leaving a long hangnail	Dryness	• Clip away during a manicure • Use a hand and nail cream regularly
Whitlow (panaritium)	• Small abscesses at the side or base of the nail • Swollen, red, infected (pus present)	• Viral (herpes simplex virus) or bacterial • Damage to area with sharp object or having finger in mouth (thumb sucking in children)	Refer client to their GP
Bruised nail	Dark blue/black patch under the nail plate where blood has attached itself	Trauma	Avoid area while painful, then a dark enamel can be applied to disguise the discoloration
Habit or tic	• Damage to the nail as a result of regular picking or biting • Can damage the matrix	Can be related to stress or a nervous condition	Manicure with care

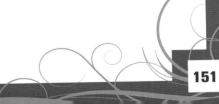

Black streaks	• Usually small black streaks across nail plate, often around the top of the nail near the nail bed • More common in dark-skinned than light-skinned people	• Indicative of heart problems or malignant melanoma • An indication of hormonal changes and imbalance, as in the first stages of pregnancy • A vitamin B12 deficiency • Trauma can also cause black streaks that tend to run the length of the nail, rather than around the top of the nail bed	Seek GP approval before performing any treatments
Splinter haemorrhage	• Tiny streaks of blood running lengthways up the nail plate • Non-contagious	Trauma	• Avoid until the area is pain-free, then use dark varnishes to conceal • Always work carefully in the area
Blue nails	Blood colouring to nail bed	• Bad circulation • Heart problems	Manicure or pedicure with massage to help with circulation
Cuts and abrasions	Red, swollen, possibly infected (pus may be present)	Injury to skin surrounding the nail	• Contra-indicated to the working area: avoid area until fully healed • If cut and abrasion is not directly in the working area then cover and protect while working
Onychia	Inflammation of the matrix with pus present	Tools not **sterilised** correctly; poor sanitisation can cause a bacterial infection	• Contra-indicated to the working area: avoid area until fully healed • Refer client to GP

Redness or inflammation	Red and swollen area	Infection or allergic reaction	Contra-indicated: avoid area until fully healed
Allergy	• Red, swollen, irritated or raised areas • Urticaria (hives)	An allergic reaction to an irritant or ingredient within a product	• Perform **patch tests** (24 hours prior to treatment) • If client has a reaction after or during treatment, then remove products and apply cold compress; see GP if irritation persists • Document the reaction on their record card
Undiagnosed lumps and swellings	Raised and tender area	Infection or trauma	Contra-indicated: avoid area until fully healed
Damaged nails	Split or broken nail plate	Trauma	• If it is only the free edge, then cut the nail • If high up onto the nail plate, it is contra-indicated: trim and avoid area until the nail grows back • If no infection is present, nail repair can be made with silk and resin
Eggshell nails	Very thin and fragile nail plate with a white curved free edge	• Medication • Chronic illness • Systemic disorder • Nervous disorder • Diet	• No nail extensions allowed • Regular manicure (no soaking of nails, as nails change shape when wet and polish will chip off; also they are prone to damage)

Discoloured nails	Nails are stained – often a brownish-yellow colour	• No base coat worn under dark enamels • Smoking	• Use a four-way buffer to remove surface stain and perform a manicure • Advise client to wear base coat before applying enamel
Pterygium (pet-er-ee-gee-um)	• Overgrown cuticles Cuticles grow very low down on to nail plate • If too long, they may split and become infected	Neglect or excessive removal previously	Regular manicures (client can pre-soak for a few days before the manicure to soften for easy removal)
Recent scar tissue	Scar will feel either smooth or bumpy and will be a different colour to the surrounding skin	Injury or surgical procedure	Contra-indicated: avoid area until fully healed (more than 6 months old)
Hyper-keratosis	Thickening of the stratum corneum and the stratum granulosum due to abnormal keratin production; usually affects elbows, knees, palms and soles	Can be caused by vitamin A deficiency or chronic exposure to arsenic	• Do not rub or exfoliate area as it will stimulate skin growth and make condition worse • Refer clients to their GP, who will prescribe topical creams to remove the excess skin if required
Diabetes	• Lack of skin sensation • Thin skin that is slow to heal and prone to damage/infection • Poor condition of skin (cuticles and nails generally show poor health)	Too much glucose in the blood because the body cannot use it properly (pancreas does not produce any or enough insulin to help glucose enter body's cells or insulin does not function correctly)	Need GP approval before performing any treatments

Contact dermatitis	• Red, inflamed skin • Dry, cracked skin • Itchy skin, small blisters	• Similar to eczema, but not hereditary • Caused by external irritants; for example, chemicals	• Avoid contact with skin irritants • Wear personal protective equipment (PPE) when needed, such as powder-free gloves • Ensure all products are removed properly • Wash hands regularly • Moisturise regularly • Use a barrier cream or very oily creams • Refer client to GP
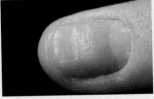 Eczema of the skin	• Underactive sebaceous gland • Red, inflamed skin • Dry, cracked skin • Itchy skin, small blisters	• Inherited condition • Stimulated by irritants such as chemicals, pollen, temperature changes, hormone level changes, stress and certain fabrics	• If not infected, use a very oily cream or a barrier cream • Refer client to GP
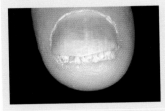 Eczema of the nail	• Inflammation, ridges, horizontal ridges, infection, pitting • Nail plate will lift and become thicker	Internal factors	If the area is not infected or painful, a gentle manicure can be performed
Psoriasis of the nail	• Inflammation, pitting, Beau's lines • Nail plate is thick and curved, and will lift	Internal factors	If the area is not infected or painful, a gentle manicure can be performed
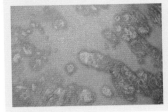 Psoriasis of the skin	• Red and silver scaly patches of skin • Can become infected if skin breaks – with bleeding, pus and inflamed areas	Unknown cause but related to stress	• Can be treated as long as there is no infection • Patch test with products 24 hours prior to treatment

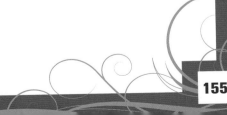

Warts	• Raised areas of skin on the fingers or hands that feel rough and hard • Can be dark or flesh coloured in appearance • Can be one or many grouped together • Very contagious	Human papilloma virus	• Contra-indicated: avoid area until wart has been treated • Refer client to GP
Verruca vulgaris (plantar warts)	• Found on soles of feet • Circular patches on the skin surface with a large black dot or lots of small black dots inside • Vary in size and shape • Appear flat, as they grow inward due to pressure of body weight • Very contagious	Human papilloma virus	• Contra-indicated: avoid area until verruca has been treated • Refer client to GP
Scabies	Animal parasite that burrows under the skin leaving wavy, grey lines	**Parasitic**	• Contra-indicated: avoid area until fully healed • Refer client to GP
Ringworm of the skin	Small, scaly red patches that grow outwards, then heal in the centre, to create rings varying in size	Fungal infection	• Contra-indicated: avoid area until fully healed • Refer client to GP
Nail infections	Red, swollen, infected (pus may be present)	Bacterial, fungal or viral infection	• Contra-indicated: avoid area until fully healed • Refer client to GP

Onychocryptosis (on-ee-co-crip-toe-sis) 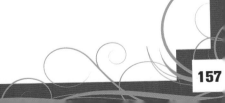	Ingrowing toenails (nail grows into nail wall) – infected (pus may be present), inflamed	• Incorrect filing or cutting • Ill-fitting shoes • Neglect	Refer to chiropodist or GP
Onychoptosis (on-ee-cop-toe-sis)	Shedding of whole or part of nail	May result from certain diseases – for example, syphilis – or as result of fever, trauma, systemic upsets or adverse reaction to drugs	Refer client to GP
Onychophagy (on-ee-co-fa-jee)	• Bitten nails, with little or no free edge (often exposing the hyponychium) • Often the area is red, swollen and infected	Severely bitten nails	• Unpleasant-tasting nail varnishes designed to discourage nail biting, but client has to want to stop • Regular weekly manicures • Can have short artificial nails applied, to prevent nail biting and encourage natural growth
Onycholysis (or onycholisis) (on-ee-co-li-sis)	The nail separates from the nail bed, leaving a large uneven area of free edge	Internal disorders such as psoriasis, eczema or lifting nail plate away with tool; for example, nail file when filing the side of the nail	Contra-indicated: avoid area until fully healed
Onychomycosis (tinea unguium) (on-ee-com-ee-co-sis)	• Ringworm of the nail • Yellow-green patches under nail plate • Nail can be brittle and may start to lift	Fungal infection	• Contra-indicated: avoid area until fully healed • Refer client to GP

Skin and nail analysis

Tinea pedis (athletes foot) 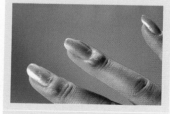	• Ringworm of the feet, usually found in between the toes but can spread over the feet • Dry, scaly with small blisters that burst • Can dry out and reoccur	Fungal infection	• Contra-indicated: avoid area until fully healed • Refer client to GP
Pseudomonas	• Green between nail plate and artificial nail • Bacteria present when artificial nails applied or enter after application • More associated with onycholysis or paronychia, where damage already exists • Pus and pain present around nail surrounding tissue	• Bacterial infection between natural nail plate and nail bed or between an artificial nail and natural nail plate, leaving a green by-product of the infection	• To help prevent this infection individually cleanse each nail plate, sanitise client's skin and wash your hands before each treatment • Not easily cross-infected • If client has the infection then remove nails, lightly buff, remove moisture and surface oils • Client must keep nail plate clean and dry until it hardens again • Wear gloves and refer client to GP • Don't use nail file on infected nail then on healthy nail – throw all disposable tools away and sterilise and sanitise all tools and the working area
Paronychia (pa-ro-nic-ee-ah)	Redness and pus present at the nail wall	Bacterial or fungal infection	• Contra-indicated: avoid area until fully healed • Refer client to GP
Onychatrophia (atrophy) (on-ee-cat-row-fee-ah)	• Nail becomes smaller – may waste away • Opaque and ridged	• Damage to matrix • Nervous disorder or disease	• Contra-indicated: avoid area until fully healed • Refer client to GP

Onychauxis (hypertrophy) (on-ee-cork-sis)	Thickening of nail plate – may change colour	• Irritant; for example, ill-fitting shoe or rubbing nail • Internal disorders, infections or neglect	If no infection present, can perform regular treatments
Onychogryphosis (on-ee-co-gri-fo-sis)	Thickening and curving of nail	• Internal factors – increased production of nail • Ill-fitting shoes • May be part of ageing process	• Contra-indicated: avoid area until fully healed • Refer client to GP
Leuconychia (lu-co-nic-ee-ah)	White patches on nail plate	Air pockets form on nail from trauma or damage to matrix	• Will grow out • Can use a dark varnish to disguise • Regular manicures
Koilonychia (coy-lo-nic-ee-ah)	Nail curves upwards in a spoon shape	Inherited or side-effect of anaemia (iron deficiency) or overactive thyroid gland	• Contra-indicated: avoid area until fully healed • Refer client to GP
Hallux valgus	• Bunions – swelling of big toe joint pushes the toe close to the second toe so they look distorted • Painful and inflamed	• Often hereditary • Injury • Arthritis or muscular imbalance	If not infected then perform treatment carefully

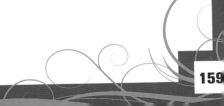

Corns and calluses	• Pressure to skin on or between toes causes areas of thick skin to form • Corns press on to deeper layers, causing pain	Friction from ill-fitting shoes or too much running	• Remove with **rasp**, exfoliate, foot mask, paraffin wax or bootees and moisturise • Regular pedicures
	• Calluses are larger and wider than corns • Found on bony areas of soles of feet – may be painful	Friction from ill-fitting shoes or too much running	• Remove with rasp, exfoliate, foot mask, paraffin wax or bootees and moisturise • Regular pedicures
Varicose veins	• Protruding veins in legs • Bluish/purple in colour – may be painful	• Damaged or weak valves in veins cause blood to pool in that area • Occurs in mature, overweight or pregnant people (hormonal changes); worse if person stands for excessive period of time	• Refer client to GP • Do not massage affected area
Chilblains	• Can affect hands or feet • Skin appears red, purple and blue in patches – painful and itchy	• Poor circulation • Aggravated by cold weather	• Regular massage and heat treatments • Refer client to GP
Phlebitis	• Inflammation of superficial vein • Red, tender, long thin veins appear on surface – area is warm, itchy, swollen, hard and tender • If infected, additional symptoms may include fever, pain and breakdown of skin	Can occur without cause or through injury or medical procedure	GP approval required before treating

Epilepsy	• Abnormal electrical discharge in the brain interrupting normal functions • Epileptic seizure symptoms include muscle twitching, abnormal sensations, emotional symptoms and loss of consciousness	Possible causes include: • abnormalities in the development of the brain • lack of oxygen during birth • infections (meningitis or encephalitis) • brain tumour • cerebral thrombosis or haemorrhage (stroke)	Check with GP before treatment
Recent broken bones, fractures and sprains	• Client should inform nail technician but always ask them during the consultation • Observe any visible casts, post-surgery scars, dressings or discomfort	Injury or brittle bones	• Be aware of health and safety considerations • Ensure client is comfortable sitting for a period of time • Do not perform treatment directly on an area where a broken bone, fracture or sprain is present
Muscular aches and pains	Pain, muscular nodules and inflammation present in area to be treated	• Strain • **RSI** • Injury • Accident	Massage can alleviate aches and pains but if they are related to an accident do not work upon this client without a GP letter

How to identify contra-indications which prevent or restrict treatments

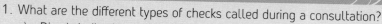

Key terms

Beau's lines – lines that form on the nail from side to side

Buff – using either a leather buffer or four-way buffer that produces a shine on the nail plate

Horizontal ridges – lines or ridges that form on the nail plate from side to side

Longitudinal – lines that run from the cuticle to free edge

Matrix – where new nail cells are formed

Patch test – if concerned that a client may have an allergy to a product then test a small amount on the skin and observe for 24 hours

Parasitic – caused by animal parasite that lives in the skin

Rasp – tool to remove hard, dead skin from feet

Ridge filler base coat – used on ridged nail to give a smoother finish when enamelling

RSI – repetitive strain injury, from poor posture or incorrect lifting and carrying

Sterilise – to destroy all living organisms

Transverse – lines that run from side to side

Top tip

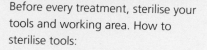

Before every treatment, sterilise your tools and working area. How to sterilise tools:

- Wash in hot, soapy water (detergent) to remove debris.

- Choose an appropriate method:
  ○ Autoclave – for metal tools
  ○ UV cabinet – all types of tools (metal, plastic, nail files, etc.)
  ○ Chemical baths – for disinfection and storage of metal tools.

Check your knowledge

1. What are the different types of checks called during a consultation?
   a) Direct, indirect and questioning
   b) Visual, manual and questioning

2. What is the medical term for bitten nails?
   a) Pterygium
   b) Onychophagy
   c) Onychatrophia

3. What is an infection of the nail wall called?
   a) Onychauxis
   b) Leuconychia
   c) Paronychia

4. What is the nail shaped like a spoon called?
   a) Koilonychia
   b) Onychogryposis
   c) Leuconychia

5. What is a bunion called?
   a) Hallux valgus
   b) Onychatrophia
   c) Onychocryptosis

6. What is ringworm of the nail?
   a) Onychoptosis
   b) Onychomycosis
   c) Onycholysis

7. What is direct cross-infection?
   a) When an infected person touches another person
   b) When an infected person comes in contact with a tool that is used on another person

8. What are the four different types of infections?

9. What type of infection is ringworm?
   a) Bacterial
   b) Viral
   c) Fungal
   d) Parasitic
   e) Can be bacterial or viral

10. What type of infection is paronychia?
    a) Bacterial
    b) Viral
    c) Fungal
    d) Parasitic
    e) Can be bacterial or fungal

Provide manicure and pedicure treatments

What you will learn

- Prepare for manicure and pedicure treatments
- Provide manicure and pedicure treatments

Key terms

Manicure – treatment performed on the hands and lower arm, working on improving the condition of the nails, skin and cuticle.

Pedicure – treatment performed on the feet and lower leg, working on improving the condition of the nails, skin and cuticle.

Top tip

When a client books in for nail extensions, either ask them about the condition of their nails, cuticle and skin or, if in person, make a visual analysis. If they are in poor condition, recommend a manicure treatment or series of treatments. This will improve the condition of the nails before having nail extensions, creating a better finish and generating more profit for the salon.

Key term

Cross-infection – when someone who has a contagious condition passes it to another person.

Introduction

Together, **manicures** and **pedicures** are the foundation of the professional nail technician's skills, on which they can build more advanced techniques. Both treatments are very popular in nail bars, spas and salons, for both male and female clients, as they can be performed to improve the condition of the nails, cuticle and skin or purely as a relaxation treatment. Also, for clients who intend to have nail enhancements such as fibreglass nail extensions or nail art, nails in good condition, with healthy cuticles, are a perfect base for the nail technician to work upon.

There are other reasons why a client will choose to have a manicure or pedicure – for example they may want to stop biting their fingernails or prevent the occurrence of ingrowing toenails. It is the responsibility of the nail technician to perform a thorough consultation and analysis to determine the client's needs, then design an individual treatment plan. This unit also looks at how to turn a basic treatment into a luxury treatment by incorporating additional products and equipment that enhance the effects of a manicure or pedicure.

Manicures and pedicures offer the client a range of benefits.

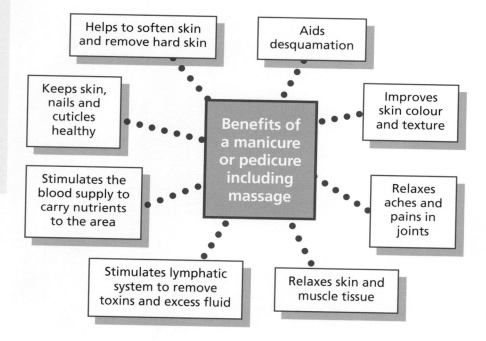

Helps to soften skin and remove hard skin

Aids desquamation

Keeps skin, nails and cuticles healthy

Improves skin colour and texture

Benefits of a manicure or pedicure including massage

Stimulates the blood supply to carry nutrients to the area

Relaxes aches and pains in joints

Stimulates lymphatic system to remove toxins and excess fluid

Relaxes skin and muscle tissue

Prepare for manicure and pedicure treatments

In this section, you will find out about the preparation required to perform a manicure or pedicure treatment, including yourself as the nail technician, the client and the working area. It is just as important to prepare yourself as it is to prepare for the treatment, since this will ensure good time management, prevent **cross-infection** and allow you to deliver a competent treatment.

Salon requirements for preparing yourself, the client and the work area

Preparing yourself

Before a client arrives at the salon to have a manicure or pedicure treatment, the working area and technician must be prepared fully to ensure the treatment runs smoothly. As a nail technician, you have a professional image to maintain and this is vital to your success and that of the business. When training to become a technician, you are assessed on your personal presentation and hygiene. These standards are set by the awarding bodies that your assessors must follow during your assessment. You will be expected to continue these high standards throughout your career.

To learn more about professional presentation, see Follow health and safety practice in the salon, page 17.

Preparing the client

When a client has a manicure and/or pedicure treatment they need to be positioned correctly. This will depend upon the size of the nail studio, salon or spa and if the client is having additional treatments at the same time. When a client has a pedicure, always remember to provide a towel for their lap to protect their modesty and their clothing from the products used. To learn more about the importance of health and safety as part of client preparation, see Follow health and safety practice in the salon, page 19.

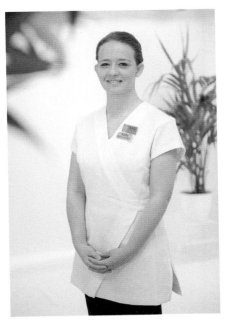

Maintain a professional image

> ### Top tip
>
> Before leaving for work, have a look at your appearance in a full-length mirror and ask yourself, do I look professional? If you do not follow the designated dress code, you instantly create a poor image of your workplace, your colleagues and yourself. These basic guidelines are vital to the success of any business.

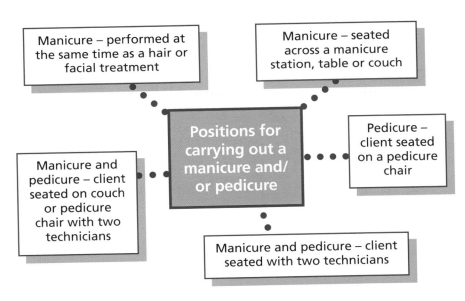

- Manicure – performed at the same time as a hair or facial treatment
- Manicure – seated across a manicure station, table or couch
- Manicure and pedicure – client seated on couch or pedicure chair with two technicians
- **Positions for carrying out a manicure and/or pedicure**
- Pedicure – client seated on a pedicure chair
- Manicure and pedicure – client seated with two technicians

Preparing the working area

The location of the treatment will influence how you set up the work area. However, always begin by sterilising all your tools and sanitising the working area — to learn more, see Follow health and safety practice in the salon, page 23.

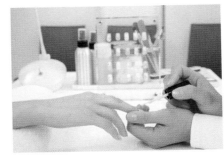

Good preparation helps to ensure a successful treatment

When performing a manicure it is ideal to perform the treatment across a manicure station, where all your products and tools can be neatly and safely stored. However, if you are working across a table or alongside another treatment, then a trolley can be used as an alternative. Remember, if the manicure is being performed alongside another treatment, you will need to support the client's arm and wrist, either on the arm of a pedicure chair or use a rolled-up towel on your lap (make sure the client is comfortable). When setting up your station or trolley ensure you have all your products and equipment; then you will be prepared for every eventuality.

Environmental conditions suitable for manicure and pedicure treatments

It is important to create a perfect environment for the client's treatment so that they feel totally relaxed and to enable you to perform the treatment effectively.

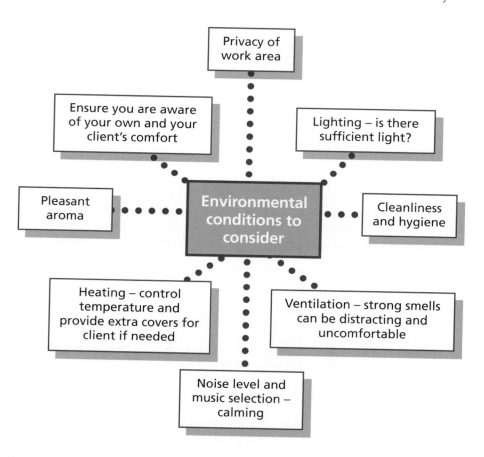

To learn more about suitable environmental conditions in the workplace, see Follow health and safety practice in the salon, page 26, and Provide and maintain nail enhancement, page 227; and for information on the Performing Rights Regulations, see Working in the beauty-related industries, page 111.

Provide manicure and pedicure treatments

Salon life

My story

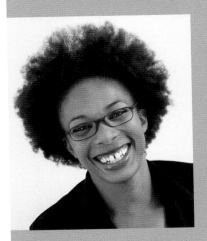

My name is Alex and I work as a nail technician in a busy city-centre nail studio. I have 15 years' experience and have worked on many different clients, some with very specific needs. I am passionate about my line of work and have had many happy clients over the years.

Unfortunately, because I have had a really successful career, I recently let down my professional guard and my attitude became a little too relaxed. A client came in for a pedicure treatment during a very busy Saturday morning and I was too busy to perform a full consultation. The client, who had never had a salon treatment before and had never worn enamels, had her toenails painted. Shortly afterwards, she had a mild allergic reaction to the enamel and after I talked with her she disclosed that she had very sensitive skin. Usually she would avoid most products, including enamels, make-up and perfume. If I had completed a full consultation I would have discovered this earlier and performed a skin test with certain products like mask and creams. I would have also chosen alternative enamels, as I could have used solvent-free, water-based products that are free of ingredients like toluene or formaldehyde. This was a very difficult lesson to learn and thankfully the client gave me a second chance. I learned to always remain professional and put the needs of the client first in order to uphold the reputation of the salon and the quality of the services we provide.

Ask the experts

Q How do you perform a skin test?

A Select the products that might be a possible allergen, like creams for instance, and apply a small amount on the inside of the arm or near the wrist and leave for 24 hours. The client must monitor the area; if it feels warm and itchy, or if there is redness or blistering, then they have had a reaction.

Q Is there anything else that I can do to minimise the chances of a client having a reaction?

A Yes, choose products that do not contain known allergens, like lanolin or formaldehyde, and try to have a range of products for a more sensitive skin.

Benefits of offering the service for the nail technician

- Excellent retail opportunity for recommending products: cream, scrub, enamel remover, nail files
- Repeat business, recommending and booking in clients for their follow-up treatments and promoting additional services
- Can be a promotional offer where a manicure and pedicure treatment could include nail art or as a course of treatments to prepare nails in poor condition to be ready for artificial nails
- Can be promoted with additional treatments like paraffin wax or electrical heat treatments

Benefits of the treatment/service for the client

- Softens and nourishes the skin, cuticles and nails
- Improves the colour and condition of the skin and nails
- Relaxes tired muscles and achy joints
- Visually improves appearance of hands and feet, showing latest enamelling techniques
- Provides individual treatment plans

Frequently asked questions:

Q How short should I cut toenails if the client wants a French polish?

A Leave a slightly longer free edge. This will produce a nice effect, but if you leave the nails too long they could press against the skin and cause discomfort.

Q What if a client wants a really short free edge?

A Do not cut or file below the flesh line or you will expose the hyponychium and the area will be prone to an infection.

Q Should I buff toenails?

A If the nails are not ridged or stained and are a healthy length then do not buff as it will stimulate nail growth and clients do not want to keep cutting their toenails.

Q Why should I recommend aftercare products to every client?

A They maintain the effects of the treatment and will increase the salon's profits.

Q Why do I need to learn about the ingredients of manicure and pedicure products?

A If you recognise an ingredient and learn about its effects, you can understand how a product works. Also you need to understand the side-effects, to prevent damage. For example, most chemicals are harsh and if they are left on too long they could cause dryness to the nail and skin area.

Top tip

It is important to perform an allergy test, just remember to ask your clients when they book an appointment whether they have any known allergies or very sensitive skin. It takes less time to perform a skin test than the time it will take to deal with an unhappy client who has had a reaction.

Consultation techniques used to identify treatment objectives

During the consultation process, perform visual and manual checks of the area and ask questions to determine if there are any contra-indications with the client's skin, cuticle or nails. Performing a good consultation will help you to decide if the treatment needs to be adapted and what the client's expectations are, which will enable you to create an individual plan. You will also need to discuss whether the nails need cutting and the required shape of the nail.

To learn more about consultation techniques, see Client care and communication in beauty-related industries, page 39, and Provide and maintain nail enhancement, page 228.

The importance of carrying out a nail and skin analysis

To learn more about the importance of nail and skin analysis, see the unit on Skin analysis on page 147.

How to select products, tools and equipment for manicure and pedicure treatments

There is a vast range of manicure and pedicure products, tools and equipment available to suit a variety of needs. Whether you are in industry or education, you will be trained to use these items and you will need to understand how, when and why to use them so you have the necessary knowledge to create suitable treatment plans for individual clients.

Manicure and pedicure tools and equipment

Some of the following tools, which are usually made of metal, plastic or rubber, can be washed, sterilised and reused. There are also disposable items made of wood or plastic.

Trolley or manicure station

A manicure treatment is usually performed on a manicure station, which should be of the correct height and width for safe use. A trolley or manicure station can be used to store products and tools ready for use — it usually has drawers for storage and a wrist support for the client.

Manicure or pedicure soaking bowl

Nail soak or pedi soak with warm water is added to the bowl. The nail bowl has specially designed finger holes, so that the client can comfortably and effectively soak their nails in the bowl. Pedicure bowls are much larger in size in order to fit both feet in comfortably. They usually have a flat bottom so they are safe and secure while the client's feet are soaking. Soaking their nails will cleanse the area and prepare the nails for further work.

Nail brush

Nail brushes are used when soaking the client's nails in a manicure bowl, either to remove dirt and debris from under the free edge or to remove oil from the nails before enamelling.

Rubber hoof stick

A plastic or wooden tool, with a flat rubber end that is used to gently push back overgrown cuticles, to aid removal of excess cuticle.

Nail buffers

There are three different types of buffer, which are used to stimulate the blood

Top tip

Between clients, sterilise and wash your tools and refresh and sanitise the working area. Aim to keep the area tidy during treatments. This will prevent cross-infection and present a professional environment, which will give your clients confidence in your performance.

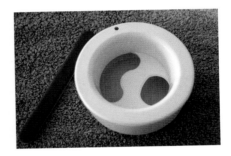
Manicure bowl

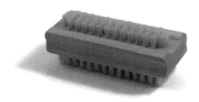
Nail brush

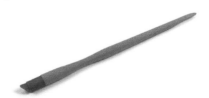
Hoof stick

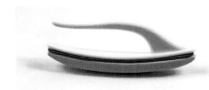
Nail buffer

Provide manicure and pedicure treatments

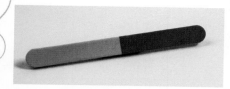

Three-way buffer

supply to improve nail growth, create a healthy colour, produce a shine and smooth out any surface lines or ridges.

- A chamois leather-covered pad with a plastic handle is used with buffing paste but does not create a high-shine finish.

- Three- or four-way buffers or buffer blocks do not require a buffing paste. They create a high shine and are more effective at producing a smooth nail than the leather pad.

- Electric nail buffers are used as a quicker option. They create the same effects as the manual buffers but again the leather pad creates the least shine.

Cuticle knife

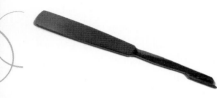

Cuticle knife

A metal tool, used to remove the eponychium and lift overgrown cuticle ready for removal with the nippers.

Cuticle nippers

A metal tool, used to remove excess cuticle and any hangnails.

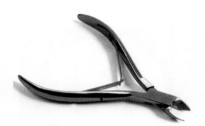

Cuticle nipper

Manicure scissors

Designed to cut fingernails, they can be straight or curved in shape.

Pedicure toenail clippers

Designed to cut strong toenails, they are much more effective at cutting than scissors.

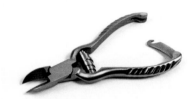

Toenail clippers

Callus shaver, foot rasp, foot file, ceramic foot file or pumice stone

These are all used to remove hard skin from the feet by gently grating it away. They can be used on either dry or pre-soaked feet but are more effective when the skin is dry.

Orange sticks

Orange sticks are multi-purposed and can be used either as they are or tipped with cotton wool. They can be used to apply cuticle products to the nail or when tipped with cotton wool they can remove enamel that has accidently been applied to the skin. They are made of wood and, for hygiene reasons, are disposable.

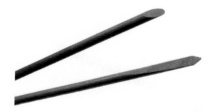

Orange stick

Emery board

An emery board has two sides: a fine side to file fingernails into shape and a coarse side to file toenails. It can also be used to file fingernails to shorten them. However, it is advisable to cut the nails with scissors, as too much filing using the coarse side can create friction, which produces heat that can dry out the nails.

The grit quantity determines how coarse or fine a file will be:

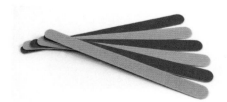

Emery boards

- 80 grit — extra-coarse
- 100 grit — coarse
- 180 grit — medium
- 240 grit — fine.

Emery boards can only be cleaned using special cleaners and then sterilised in the UV cabinet, but ideally they should be disposed of after use, as it is difficult to clean them fully.

Spatulas
These can be made of wood (disposable) or plastic (reusable) and are used to remove products from their container, either to be dispensed or as a palette/surface to work from.

Barbicide jars
These contain a **disinfectant** solution and are placed on the workstation to store pre-sterilised metal tools, including scissors, cuticle knife, nippers and clippers.

Wrist support cushion
A cushion or a rolled-up small towel is used to support the client's wrist during a manicure.

Waste bin or rubbish bowl
A lined, pedal waste bin or a lined waste bowl is placed next to the nail technician to maintain hygiene standards.

Lined dishes or bowls
Dishes or bowls containing consumables such as cotton wool are placed on the workstation. A further bowl can be used for the client's jewellery if applicable. Bowls can also be used to warm oil for cuticle treatments.

Towels and couch roll
These can be used to protect trolleys from damage that can occur from manicure or pedicure products such as enamel remover. They can also be used to protect the client's clothing, the working area and nail technician. Towels or face cloths can either be dampened with hot water or dampened with cold water and warmed in a towel heater, and then used to remove products such as exfoliators or massage oil.

Cotton wool or tissues
Cotton wool is used to apply or remove products, for example nail varnish remover and antiseptic. Both can be used as an alternative method for separating the toes when enamelling.

Gown
A gown can be worn by the client to protect their clothing.

Protective arm tissue
Protective arm tissues are used to protect the client's clothing.

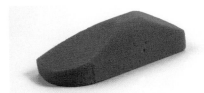

Pumice stone

Top tip

There are other more durable and easy-to-clean nail files on the market, including glass, crystal and ceramic stone files. These files can be washed to ensure complete removal of nail particles and can be used on natural or artificial nails, creating a smoother, damage-free nail. Invest in better quality tools and you will benefit financially and professionally.

Key term

Disinfectant – a chemical solution that will destroy most micro-organisms.

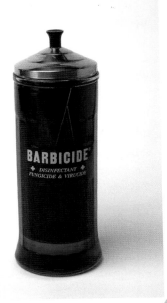

Barbicide®

Top tip

To reduce the salon's outgoings, always be aware of ways to be cost-effective. Here are some suggestions:

- Split tissues, cotton wool pads and couch roll.

- Use reusable tools that can be washed and sterilised, instead of disposable tools, for example plastic spatulas and glass nail files.

- Use the correct amount of product.

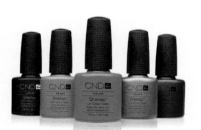

Key terms

Oil-in-water mixture – a product that has more oil in it than water.

Beeswax – wax produced by bees in a hive.

Lanolin – oil found on sheep's wool.

Cocoa butter – a yellow-white fat from cocoa beans.

Liquid paraffin – mineral oil.

Emulsifying agent – allows hand to glide/slip along skin during massage

Emollients – moisturisers that contain oil and water to nourish skin and prevent water loss. Contain either an oil-in-water solution or water-in-oil solution. More oil makes it a heavier product (cream). More water makes it a lighter product (lotion).

Clingfilm or foil

Clingfilm or foil can be used with a paraffin wax treatment. Once the wax has been applied, the area is wrapped in clingfilm or foil to retain the heat and enhance the effects of the treatment. They are also used to prevent the wax breaking up and making the working area untidy.

Thermal mittens and bootees

Thermal mittens, used during a manicure treatment, and thermal bootees, used during a pedicure treatment, are electrical heat treatments. Heat enhances the effects of products applied to the skin, allowing them to penetrate deeper. Heat is also relaxing for sore muscles and joints.

Paraffin wax

Paraffin wax can be used during a manicure or pedicure treatment to soften the skin, nourish the nails and relax the muscles and joints. The wax can be heated to an average temperature of 49°C in a paraffin wax bath. It is applied to the skin by a brush from the wax heated in a bath or from a cartridge containing the wax that is warmed in a heater, and is sprayed onto the skin's surface.

Manicure and pedicure products

Remember, never waste products. Be cost-effective and always use the correct amount, or it will affect your salon's profits.

Cuticle massage cream

The cream is applied to the cuticles and then the nails are placed in the manicure or pedicure bowl containing warm water and nail or pedi soak, to soften the cuticles for easy removal.

Ingredients: **oil-in-water mixture** – **lanolin**, **cocoa butter**, **liquid paraffin** (**emollients**); **beeswax** (**emulsifying agent**)

Cuticle oil

Cuticle oil, or massage oil that has been warmed over a bowl of hot water, can be used as a cuticle treatment to nourish and soften dry cuticles.

Cuticle remover

The main purpose of a cuticle remover is to loosen and release the cuticle for further cuticle work. The remover may contain harsh chemicals such as potassium hydroxide or sodium hydroxides which are **alkaline** and also **caustic**. When the cuticle remover is applied to the cuticles it softens and breaks down the cuticle. If left on too long, it will irritate and dry out the cuticle. There are milder formulations that contain **AHAs**, derived from plants that break down the skin cells.

Ingredients: 2.5% solution of potassium hydroxide or sodium hydroxide and glycerine (emollient)

Buffing paste

Used with a chamois leather buffer to remove surface ridges and produce a shiny nail plate, creating a smoother nail for enamelling.

Ingredients: **talc**, **kaolin**, **stannic oxide**

Lotions and creams

Lotions and creams are emollients that soften the skin and cuticles and can be used to perform the massage during a treatment. They may contain other benefits, including anti-ageing properties such as sunscreen to prevent age spots, AHAs to minimise wrinkle depth, collagen to make the skin plump or, for the feet, peppermint to cool the skin.

Massage cream or oil

Oil or cream media have a high oil content so that they remain on the skin surface during massage. They help the hands to glide over the area, and are especially good for very dry skin.

Nail varnish remover or enamel remover

The remover is a **solvent** that dissolves enamel. It is applied to cotton wool and then wiped over the nails. It usually contains acetone, but acetone-free removers can be purchased for clients who wear artificial nails. Acetone is also used to remove artificial nails, as it is a strong and effective chemical, but it can be very drying to the nail plate.

Ingredients: solvents (acetone, ethyl, butyl acetate), glycerol, mineral oil

Nail enamel thinners or solvents

Thinners are used to dilute old enamel that has become too thick to use.

Ingredient: ethyl acetate

Nail varnishes or enamel

Enamels carry colour within them and are applied to the nail to add colour, either in a matt or shiny finish.

Ingredients: nitrocellulose and resin (**film formers**), ethyl acetate, butyl acetate (solvent), isopropyl myristate (**plasticiser**)

Base coat

This protects the nail plate, as it is applied before enamel to prevent the enamel staining the nail plate. It also provides a smooth base to apply enamel on to and helps the enamel last longer.

Ingredients: **resins**, nitrocellulose, plasticisers

Ridge filler

This has a thicker consistency than base coat and is used to fill ridges so as to create a smoother finish when enamelling.

Ingredients: nitrocellulose, plasticisers, resin, **fibres**

Key terms

Alkaline – measure of alkalinity on a pH (potential of hydrogen) scale

Caustic – a chemical substance that destroys living tissue

AHAs – alpha hydroxy acids, from sources such as fruit. They cause the skin to produce new cells faster, exfoliating the skin.

Talc – a fine-grained white, greenish, or grey mineral.

Kaolin – a fine clay.

Stannic oxide – a white powder that is insoluble in water.

Key terms

Solvent – a liquid that dissolves other substances such as enamel. When added to enamel it helps the enamel to dry and to keep the correct consistency (not too thick or thin).

Film formers – hold the colour of the enamel.

Plasticiser – provides flexibility to reduce chipping of enamel.

Resin – gives enamel its flexibility and helps it adhere to the nail plate.

Fibres – make the ridge filler thicker in consistency.

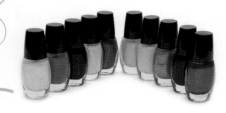

Nail enamels

Top coat

This protects the nail plate and is applied over the top of an enamel to give a shiny finish and to help prevent the enamel from chipping.

Ingredients: nitrocellulose, plasticisers, resin

Nail strengtheners and hardeners

Applied like a base coat, these strengthen/harden weak nails.

Ingredients: aluminium potassium sulphate (film-forming plastic resin), formaldehyde (film-forming plastic resin), resins, glycerols

Quick-dry spray

This is spayed over the enamel to reduce drying time and harden the enamel.

Ingredients: mineral oils, silicone (**lubricant**), natural oils, alcohol

Hand or foot cleansers

Antiseptic cleansers are used on cotton wool to wipe over the skin to remove dirt, sebum, sweat and body products.

Hygiene spray

An antiseptic that is sprayed over the area to sanitise it.

Nail bleach

This is used to whiten the nail plate and surrounding skin.

Ingredients: **hydrogen peroxide**

White pencils

Used under the free edge to create a whiter tip and reduce staining of the free edge.

Ingredients: aluminium potassium sulphate, formaldehyde, resins

Hand/nail soak

Hand/nail soak is added to warm water in a manicure bowl to cleanse and nourish the area. It also enhances the effects of the cuticle massage cream and aids removal of excess cuticle.

Ingredients: vary between manufacturers — may include essential oils such as lavender, chamomile or peppermint (soothing aroma and antiseptic)

Foot soak (pedi soak)

Foot soak is added to warm water in a foot bowl to cleanse, sooth, cool and revitalise the feet.

Ingredients: vary between manufacturers — may include herbs such as peppermint oil extracts (cooling, reduce odour and revitalising) or green tea (an anti-oxidant to cleanse body of toxins), avocado oil (moisturising), essential oils like lavender, vanilla or jasmine (soothing aroma), Epsom or Dead Sea salts

Key terms

Lubricant – provides a smooth or slippery surface

Hydrogen peroxide – a chemical that bleaches the nail.

Top tip

Foot soaks containing magnesium-rich salts are extremely effective at relieving tired and aching muscles.

Check it out

Look at the ingredients labels of the products you use. Do you recognise them? If not, revise the ingredients above – this could be a question in your next test.

(contain mineral magnesium to soothe aching muscles, reduce inflammation and swelling)

Manicure and pedicure specialist treatments

To turn a basic treatment into a luxury manicure or pedicure, a nail technician can use any of the following equipment.

Thermal mittens and bootees

To use mittens or bootees:

1 Apply either a cream, lotion, oil or mask to the hands or feet.

2 Wrap the hands/feet in plastic liners or clingfilm before inserting into the mitts or bootees for 10–15 minutes.

3 Remove the hands/feet and remove the plastic liners.

4 As the massage is performed, the tissues are softened and the joints are relaxed, which will enhance the effects of the massage and the cuticle work.

Warm oil treatments

Warm oil will soften and nourish dry nails, cuticle and skin. Various types of vegetable-based oils can be used, for example olive oil. Pour a small amount of oil into a small bowl, then place the bowl into a larger bowl of hot water to warm the oil. Remove the small bowl and place the fingertips into the oil for five minutes, then continue with the treatment.

Exfoliators (foot/hand scrubs)

Exfoliators contain abrasive particles, which are either synthetic or natural, such as salt scrubs. They exfoliate the skin's surface by removing dead skin cells, especially hard patches found on the soles and palms. Use a large circular movement, as small movements will cause skin irritation and damage.

Hand mask

Usually applied after exfoliating to soften, nourish and revitalise the skin, a hand mask may also have anti-ageing benefits.

Ingredients: vary between manufacturers — may include AHAs (to thin the skin to minimise wrinkle depth), collagen (to plump the skin), plant extracts (to lighten age spots), rosemary (to moisturise and protect), vitamin A (aiding cell renewal), aloe vera and chamomile (to soothe), nut oils (to soften), vitamin E (to moisturise)

Foot mask

Usually applied after exfoliating to soften, nourish, cool and revitalise the skin.

Ingredients: vary between manufacturers — may include peppermint oil (reduces odour, revitalises and cools), kaolin clay (to deep cleanse), cocoa butter (to soften)

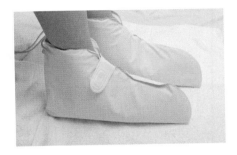

Thermal bootees

Top tip

If a client has very dry or overgrown cuticles, use the mittens or bootees before the cuticle work. If the client suffers from arthritis, use them before massaging. This is when the individual treatment plan that suits the client is most relevant, and being aware of these details will make you an outstanding nail technician.

Key term

Exfoliator – a product that contains abrasive particles that remove surface skin cells.

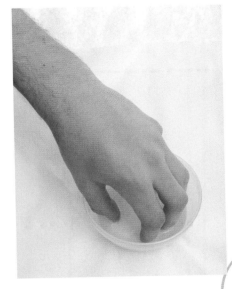

Warm oil treatment

Paraffin wax

To use a paraffin bath:

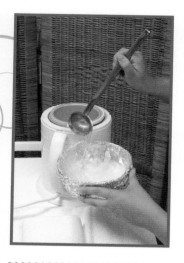

1. Line a plastic bowl with foil and use the ladle to dispense the melted wax into the bowl.

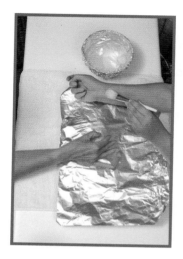

2. Quickly distribute a rich cream over the skin and place the client's hand, palm up, over a large piece of foil that has a small towel underneath. Then test the wax on your wrist to check the temperature first and next on the client's wrist, as they could be more sensitive to the heat than you are.

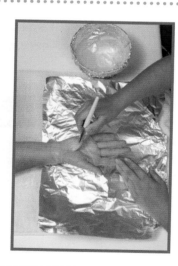

3. Quickly apply the wax to the client's hand and wrist area – do not use too many brush strokes, as the wax will now begin setting. Turn the client's hand over and apply to the opposite side.

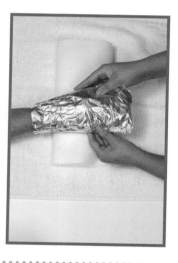

4. Wrap the hand in the foil to retain the heat and maximise the effects of the wax.

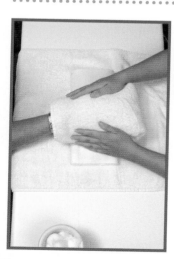

5. Now wrap the hand in a towel to slow down the cooling of the wax.

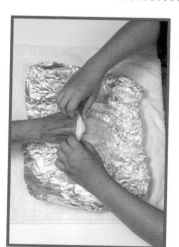

6. Once the wax has set, uncover the area and peel off the wax to reveal soft, smooth skin and relaxed muscle tissue and joints.

Nail and skin conditions and contra-indications

To learn more about:

- nail and skin conditions

- diseases and disorders of the nail and skin that prevent or restrict manicure and pedicure treatments

see the Skin analysis unit on page 147.

Structure and functions of the nail and skin and muscles, bones, arteries and veins and lymphatic vessels of the lower arm, hand, lower leg and foot

To learn more about the anatomy and physiology of the lower arm, hand, lower leg and foot and their relevance to manicure and pedicure treatments, see the Anatomy and physiology unit, page 121.

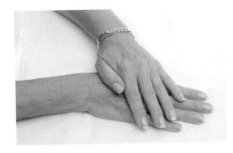

Provide manicure and pedicure treatments

A good knowledge of products, tools and equipment will allow you to design the correct treatment plan to suit the individual client. Once you understand the basics and the effects of certain products, you can perform an effective manicure or pedicure treatment.

How to communicate and behave in a professional manner

To learn more about the importance of communication and professional ethical conduct, see Client care and communication, page 35.

Health and safety working practices

To learn more about health and safety in the workplace and legislation that affects working practices, see Follow health and safety practice in the salon, page 1, and Provide and maintain nail enhancement, page 223.

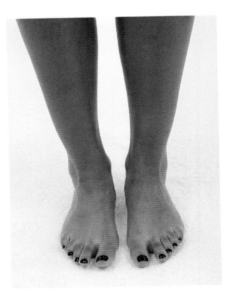

> **Top tip**
>
> Promote additional treatments, such as paraffin wax, warm oil and thermal mittens and bootees, to enhance the effects of your treatments, improve the client's satisfaction and to make more profit for the salon.

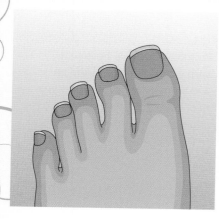

A square nail with curved corners

Provide manicure and pedicure treatments

Top tip

Never presume to know what fingernail shape a client wants. During the consultation, discuss shapes. You can recommend a shape that would best suit them, but if a client specifies a different shape, you will have to do want the client wants, to ensure a happy outcome.

The importance of positioning yourself and the client correctly

We looked briefly at the importance of correctly positioning yourself and the client in Salon requirements for preparing yourself, the client and the work area (see page 165). To find out more, see Follow health and safety practice in the salon, page 19, and Provide and maintain nail enhancement, page 225.

The importance of using products, tools, equipment and techniques to suit the client's treatment needs, nail and skin conditions

First, you must understand how to perform a basic manicure or pedicure treatment — either of these treatments will take 45 minutes. A luxury treatment with extras such as an exfoliator and paraffin wax will take an hour.

Toenail shapes

To prevent ingrowing toenails, cut the nails straight with clippers, then file them straight with curved corners just above the flesh line to leave a short free edge. If the nails are incorrectly cut and filed, they will begin to grow into the skin and an infection may occur. In this case, the client should see their GP for treatment.

Fingernail shapes

Round

A short and neat shape that is ideal for professionals such as nurses or cooks, who need a strong short nail.

Squoval

This is the strongest nail shape, incorporating a square shape with curved corners. It is very popular, especially for those who have long nails or artificial nails.

Square

The shape produces very straight sides and a blunt straight line at the free edge. This is a strong shape but looks so blunt that it can make fingers look short and wide and is not very flattering.

Oval

The nail is filed into an egg shape (oval), producing a slightly weaker nail, although it is more flattering to short fingers with wide nails and gives a more feminine appearance.

Pointed (tapered)

This is a very old-fashioned shape that is weak and prone to damage — it is best not to recommend it.

Claw (or hook)

The nail naturally curves and becomes very thick – this condition is known as onychogryphosis (see Skin analysis, page 159). The nail should be kept short to minimise the appearance of a claw shape.

Fan

The nail is much wider at the free edge than the nail attached to the nail bed and creates a fan shape. Correction work is required – the nail should be filed to create an oval shape.

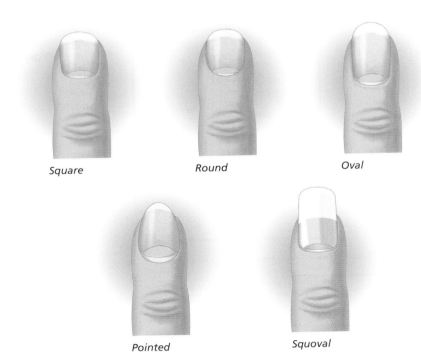

Square   Round   Oval

Pointed   Squoval

Provide manicure and pedicure treatments

Think about it

Before you perform a manicure or pedicure treatment, revise the unit on Skin analysis (see page 147), as you will need to check for contra-indications.

Basic manicure procedure

Once your treatment plan has been created and you have sterilised your tools, prepared your working area and the client is positioned comfortably, then you can begin.

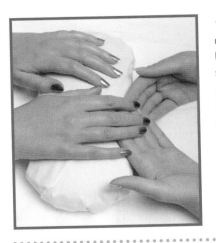

1. During the consultation, discuss the client's needs. You should include the preferred nail length, shape, type of varnish, etc. If there are no contra-indications, you can begin the service.

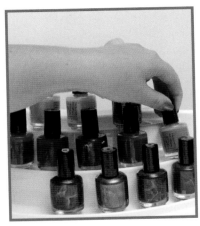

2. Ask the client to choose the varnish she would like. Provide a wide range of colours for the client to choose from including clear, light, dark, matt, frosted and French polishes.

You should recommend a varnish that is suitable for the client.

3. Remove any existing nail enamel from both hands and check the condition of the nails and cuticle in their natural state. Sanitise the hand to prevent cross-infection while you carry out a manual contra-indication check.

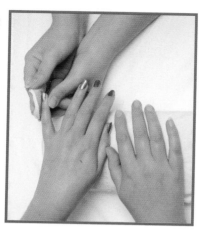

4. If the nails require cutting to shape, use the nail scissors and dispose of the nail cuttings from both hands.

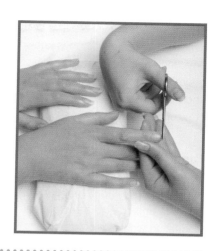

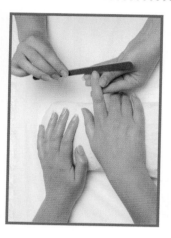

5. Use an emery board to file the nails into the desired shape, using the correct movements at a 45° angle and holding the end of the file. File from the outside in, then change sides and repeat — do not use a sawing action (going back and forth would create friction, which produces heat and dries out the nail, causing it to split and peel). File only the nails on the right hand.

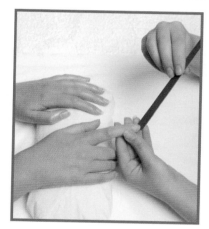

6. After filing the nails into the correct shape, perform upward strokes with the emery board to seal the free edge layers and prevent dehydration of the nail. This technique is known as bevelling.

7. Using a spatula, remove a small amount of cuticle cream from the pot and then use an orange stick to distribute to each nail of the right hand.

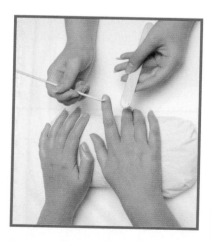

8. Massage the cream into the nails and cuticles of the right hand, two fingers at a time. This will aid absorption of the product.

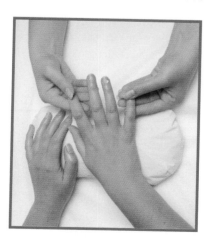

9. Dispense nail soak into a manicure bowl and add warm water. Now soak the right hand to soften the cuticles further and repeat steps 5–8 on the left hand.

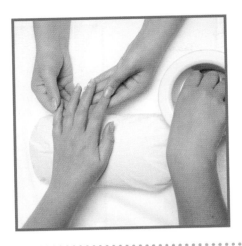

10. Remove the right hand and dry thoroughly with a towel.

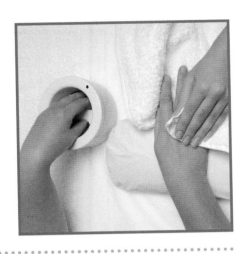

11. Using either a cotton bud or a cotton wool tipped orange stick, apply cuticle remover to the cuticle area. Do not re-dip the cotton bud or orange stick, as this will contaminate the product.

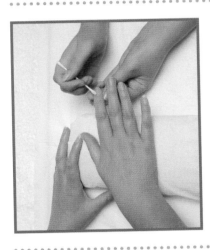

12. Using a hoof stick, perform small circular movements and gently ease back the cuticle.

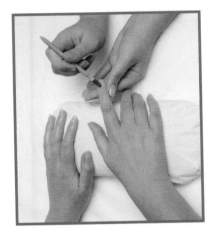

13. Use the cuticle knife flat at a 45° angle and perform circular movements from the outside in to ease the excess cuticle away from the nail plate. Then flip over the knife and repeat on opposite side of nail plate. Also keep the knife damp, so it glides along the nail plate without scratching the nail.

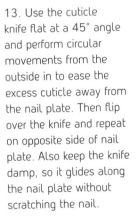
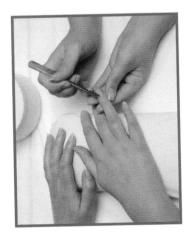

14. Use the cuticle nippers to trim any excess cuticle. Do not pull or you will damage the cuticles.

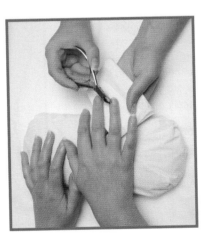

Top tip

To produce more effective results, when working on each nail, support each finger securely to prevent damage and enhance stability.

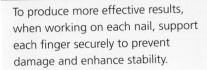

Top tip

Remember do not take too much cuticle or it will bleed and it will create access for infection.

15. Repeat the bevelling movement again and repeat steps 9–15 on the left hand.

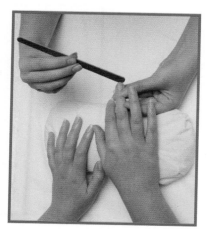

16. Choose the appropriate massage medium – this could be oil, cream, hand lotion or talc – and begin the massage (see Different massage techniques and their benefits, page 189).

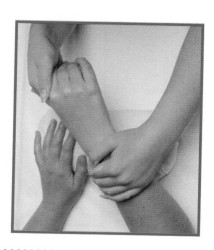

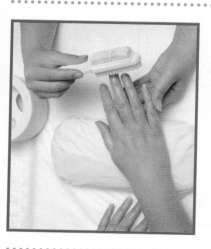

17. Use soapy water and a nail brush to remove the oil from the nail plate. If you do not, this will act as a barrier when enamelling.

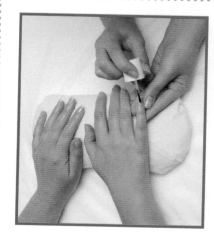

18. If the client chooses to have enamelling, first apply a base coat, nail strengthener or ridge filler.

19. Apply two coats of coloured enamel, with minimal brush strokes and without flooding the cuticle or staining the skin. If you apply enamel to the skin, use either a cotton bud or orange stick tipped with cotton wool soaked in enamel remover and carefully remove enamel. Apply a top coat to prolong the life of the enamel and quick-drying spray.

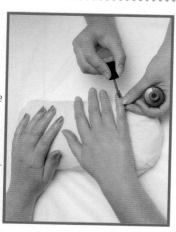

20. Check your client is happy with the results.

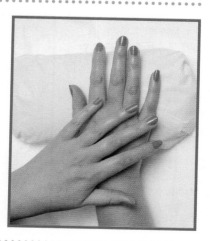

Top tip

Buffing the nails – this can be done either after filing (step 5) or at the end of the treatment (step 17) if the client does not want enamelling but a natural sheen. Use either the chamois buffer (with or without paste) or the four-way buffer, depending upon the desired effect.

Basic pedicure procedure

The procedure for a pedicure treatment is essentially the same as a manicure treatment, so what has been performed on the hands is repeated on the feet with some minor differences. Buffing would not be performed on the feet unless there were ridges, discoloration, problems with nail growth or the client did not want enamelling but did want a natural sheen to their nails. Buffing stimulates nail growth and clients do not want their toenails to grow as fast as their fingernails. Also, feet tend to have more hard skin, known as calluses, so the technician would work more on the problem areas.

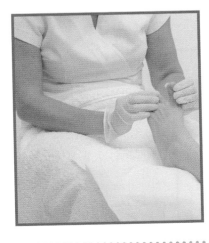

1. During the consultation, discuss the client's needs and check for contra-indications. Once you are ready to begin, wipe over the area with a sanitiser or antiseptic lotion and remove old enamel, if present, with enamel remover on a cotton pad.

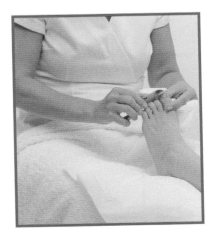

2. Cut the toenails on the left foot straight across if they are too long.

3. File the toenails on the left foot straight with curved corners, to prevent ingrowing toenails.

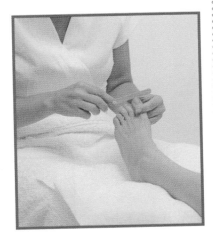

4. Using a spatula, remove a small amount of cuticle cream from the pot and then use an orange stick to distribute to each nail of the left foot. Massage the cream into the nail and cuticle of the left foot, two fingers at a time. This will aid absorption of the product.

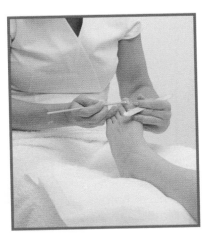

5. Dispense foot soak into a pedicure bowl and add warm water. Now soak the left foot to soften the cuticles further and repeat steps 1–5 on the right foot.

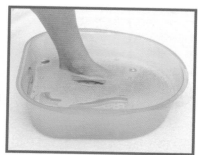

6. Remove the left foot and dry thoroughly with a towel. Then, using either a cotton bud or a cotton wool tipped orange stick, apply cuticle remover to the cuticle area. Do not re-dip the cotton bud or orange stick, as it will contaminate the product.

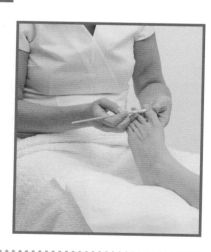

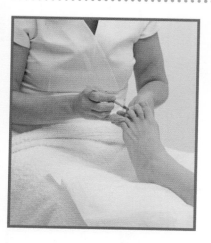

7. Using a hoof stick, perform small circular movements and gently ease back the cuticle.

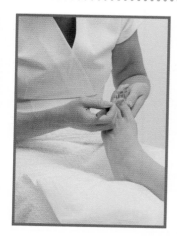

8. Next, use the cuticle knife flat at a 45° angle and perform circular movements from the outside in to ease excess away from the nail plate. Then flip over the knife and repeat on the opposite side of nail plate. Keep the knife damp so it glides along the nail plate without scratching the nail. If the cuticles are very overgrown then use the cuticle nippers to trim any excess cuticle but do not pull or you will damage the cuticles. Do not remove too much as the toenails do not require it.

9. A foot scrub can be used to help remove any calluses. Remove the product from the tub with a spatula then apply to the skin using large circular movements to lift away the dead skin cells. A rasp can be used if the calluses are very hard and require further work.

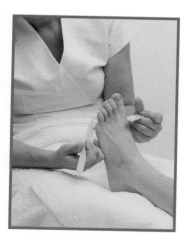

10. Choose the appropriate massage medium – this can be either oil, cream, lotion or talc – and begin the massage (see Different massage techniques and their benefits, page 189).

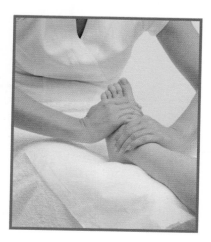

11. If enamelling is required, use soapy water and a nail brush to remove any oil from the nail plate (as oil will act as a barrier). Place cotton wool or tissue between the client's toenails. Before enamelling, apply a base coat, nail strengthener or ridge filler. Apply two coats of coloured enamel, with minimal brush strokes and without flooding the cuticle or staining the skin. If you apply enamel to the skin, use either a cotton bud or orange stick tipped with cotton wool soaked in enamel remover and carefully remove enamel. Lastly, apply the top coat to prolong the life of the enamel and quick-drying spray.

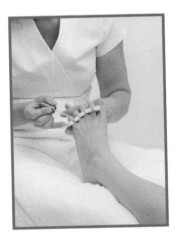

12. Check your client is happy with the results.

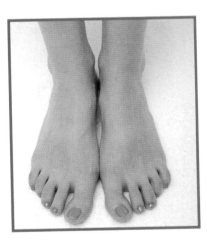

Nail finishes and techniques

Application of enamel

There are many tips that can help to produce a smooth application of enamel, with long-lasting results that will not chip, peel or look streaky.

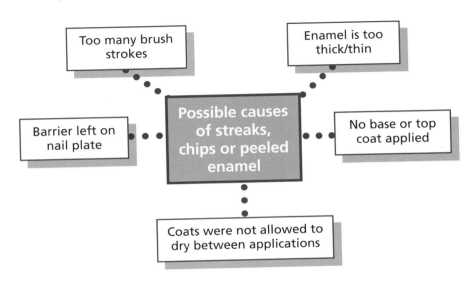

Too many brush strokes

Enamel is too thick/thin

Barrier left on nail plate

Possible causes of streaks, chips or peeled enamel

No base or top coat applied

Coats were not allowed to dry between applications

> **Top tip**
>
> A rasp can also be used before soaking the feet, which is often more effective as the skin is dry.

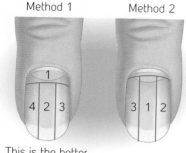

Method 1   Method 2

This is the better method for wide nails

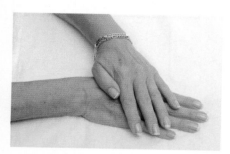

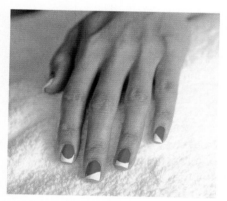

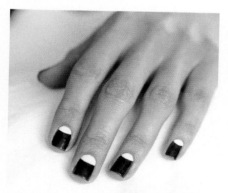

Variations on the traditional French polish – the top image shows an American French polish, which uses more natural bases

Clear or coloured enamelling

There are two methods of applying clear or coloured enamel either with three or four strokes that must not be too close to the cuticle or too close to the sides of the nail. Method 1 with four strokes is better for clients with a larger nail plate.

French polish enamelling

There are different methods of application and colour intensities with French polish kits, from very natural tones, including beige, pink or peach bases, and from natural whites to bright whites for the free edge.

To carry out a general application:

1 Apply a base coat.

2 Apply the white enamel to the free edge, either free-hand or by using special guide strips.

3 Peel off the guide strips (if used), then apply the flesh-coloured enamel.

4 Lastly apply the top coat.

There are also new versions of the original French polish design, as originally the French polish had very white tips with a flesh-toned sheer base.

American French polish

A more natural effect is created with a more natural white and flesh-toned bases.

Reverse French

A dark colour like black is applied to the whole nail and then a light colour like white or silver is applied to the free edge.

Reverse French with double French

This is the same as a reverse French but the lunula is also painted the same colour as the free edge.

Funky French

This is where a clear or natural base is applied with glitter, metallic or holographic polish on the free edge.

Chevron French polish

White tip is applied from the left-hand side downwards and across on an angle, then repeated from the right-hand side.

Using the correct products, tools, equipment and techniques to avoid adverse effects

With everything you do, it is important to have excellent knowledge of the treatment procedure and understand what the effects are. This includes the correct use of tools, equipment and products, as what you decide to do during a treatment can either have positive or adverse effects. If the desired effects are not achieved, a number of issues can arise.

Check it out

Once you have mastered a basic French enamel, why not try out a funky French? To maximise on your assessment you could incorporate a manicure or pedicure assessment with a nail art assessment.

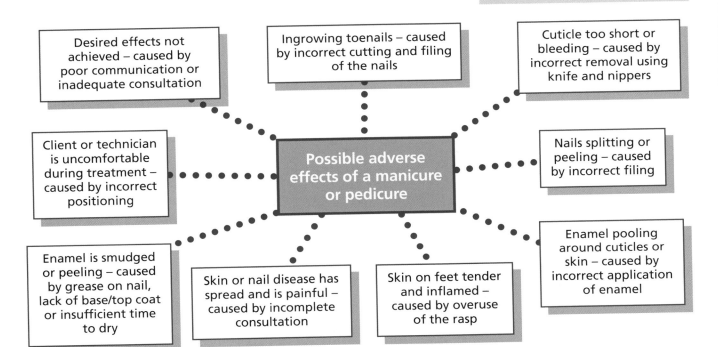

Desired effects not achieved – caused by poor communication or inadequate consultation

Ingrowing toenails – caused by incorrect cutting and filing of the nails

Cuticle too short or bleeding – caused by incorrect removal using knife and nippers

Client or technician is uncomfortable during treatment – caused by incorrect positioning

Possible adverse effects of a manicure or pedicure

Nails splitting or peeling – caused by incorrect filing

Enamel is smudged or peeling – caused by grease on nail, lack of base/top coat or insufficient time to dry

Skin or nail disease has spread and is painful – caused by incomplete consultation

Skin on feet tender and inflamed – caused by overuse of the rasp

Enamel pooling around cuticles or skin – caused by incorrect application of enamel

How treatments can be adapted to suit the client's needs

When performing a manicure or pedicure, you will need to assess which products, tools and equipment to use, depending upon the client's individual requirements. This is where you need to learn how to adapt a basic treatment.

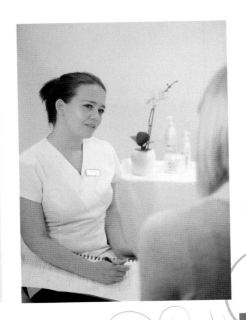

Considerations	How to adapt
The cuticles are healthy and not overgrown	Do not use the cuticle nippers – use the cuticle knife instead
Male client	No enamel Buff the nails Firmer massage Extra work on overgrown cuticles
Clients who are very thin and bony	Perform lighter massage movement or the client will feel uncomfortable

Provide manicure and pedicure treatments

Considerations	How to adapt
Larger clients with more adipose or muscle bulk	Perform deeper massage movement or the client will not feel the benefits of the massage
Bruised nail	If it is not tender, then a manicure can be performed with the application of a dark enamel to disguise the bruise
Severe eczema of the skin	If area is not infected but excessively dry, perform a nourishing treatment, e.g. paraffin wax or an intensive mask. Exfoliators will irritate the skin which is already very thin. Usually the cuticles will be dry and short, so no cuticle work should be performed
Split nail	Will require a nail mend, using a fibreglass or silk wrap (see Provide and maintain nail enhancement, page 255)
Old false tan	If it is a patchy tan, it can be removed with coarse exfoliators
Arthritis	Be gentle when massaging and use paraffin wax or mittens/bootees to help relieve aches and pains. Make sure the client has sufficient support when performing a treatment
Very short nails	Gently file any uneven areas to prevent further damage
Overgrown cuticles	Spend extra time working on the cuticles with the knife and nippers
Very dry skin and cuticles	Use products that contain more oil to nourish the skin and nails, e.g. rich hand cream or cuticle oil
Mature skin	Use more nourishing products with anti-ageing properties
Poor circulation	Spend more time massaging to increase circulation and any of the heat treatments
Nails with an old set of artificial nails or damaged nails from wearing artificial nails	Time must be added to remove the old set effectively before the manicure can begin. Also the nails will probably be damaged and thin, so no buffing (nails already too thin) or enamelling (would highlight nails)
Calluses	Extra time needed to remove hard skin and a heat treatment, e.g. paraffin wax, would soften area
Ridges on the nails	Buff to remove them and produce a smooth shiny nail
Thin and weak nails	Cut the nails short, massage with a rich cream to nourish the nails and increase blood supply
Discoloured nails and skin	Either bleach the nail, use white pencil or use a four-way buffer to remove the stain

Assess your client's needs and adapt the treatment

Top tip

Never provide the same treatment for every client, as they will all have different needs and requirements. You must maximise the effects produced, while making the client feel extra special.

Check it out

Use the guidance given in the table (Assess your client's needs) to practise creating individual treatment plans. Then imagine a client with several of the considerations listed in the table and create a treatment plan for them: for example a thin, bony client with arthritis, very dry weak nails and cuticles. What would you do? Try a few more combinations to help you prepare for your next practical assessment.

Different massage techniques and their benefits

Massage is one of the most important parts of any treatment, as it induces relaxation and enhances the effects of the treatment. There are different massage media that can be used, including cream, oil and talc (talc is used more on a lower leg and foot massage, if the client has very hairy legs and feet).

Massage classification

There are different types of massage movements, but the three main types that can be used during a manicure or pedicure treatment are effleurage, petrissage and tapotement.

Effleurage

This is a stroking movement, where the hands glide smoothly over the area; it can be performed either with light or deeper (but not very deep) pressure. Effleurage is used at the beginning and end of a massage and also to link movements together, to prevent the technician from breaking contact with the skin. The movement introduces the technician's touch to the skin, helping to induce relaxation, and also helps the technician to end the massage without a sudden stop. Effleurage is so versatile that it is even used to distribute the massage medium over the area.

Petrissage

Petrissage can consist of kneading, friction, knuckling, pinching, rolling and scissor movements, where the skin and muscle tissues are lifted then compressed away from underlying structures. The movements work at a much deeper level than effleurage, aiding relaxation of tense tissue fibres and improving muscle tone.

Tapotement or percussion

This movement consists of hacking and cupping, which produce a quick, stimulating, rhythmic effect, where the fingers break contact with the skin. This movement will improve muscle and skin tone, as it stimulates the area.

Manicure massage routine

Begin with an effleurage movement and start with light movements getting deeper each time. Use a wrist support for the client and support the area.

1 Effleurage from the hand up the right arm, over the elbow and back down towards the hand, repeat six times.

2 Perform circular thumb movements up the inside of the right forearm and slide back down, repeat four times.

3 Perform circular friction movements over the back of the hand, up and down each metacarpal.

> **Top tip**
>
> Once you have learned the basic massage routine, you can adapt it to suit your client. If a client wants a longer massage with no enamelling then this is acceptable, as the treatment will not take any longer and will not affect your timings or profit.

4 Move the fingers and thumbs in a circular movement to the right and then left, while supporting the hand.

5 Support the client's hand and place the client's finger between your first and middle finger, then gently pull and twist the client's finger.

6 Support the client's forearm with one hand and interlock your fingers with the client's fingers and move the wrist back and forth.

7 Perform circular thumb movements on the client's palm.

8 Repeat step 1 but begin with a deep effleurage movement and finish with a light movement.

9 Finally, with one hand on top of the client's forearm and the other directly below, slide your hands down the arm over the hands until you slowly remove your hands from the client's fingertips.

10 Repeat the massage to the left hand and forearm.

Pedicure massage routine

Begin with an effleurage movement and start with light movements getting deeper each time:

1 Effleurage the whole foot and lower leg. Repeat four times.

2 Hold the foot with one hand and with the other hand perform petrissage movement from the foot up the calf, slide back down. Repeat four times.

3 Place the hands on top of each other and place on the calf, with thumbs positioned on the front of the leg. Using both thumbs perform thumb kneading up the front of the leg and slide back down. Repeat four times.

4 Perform thumb frictions to the upper foot by criss-crossing thumbs from the toes to the ankle. Slide back down and work from one side to the other.

5 Thumb friction to sole of foot

6 Thumb friction to the heel of the foot

7 Support the ankle with one hand and rotate the foot one way then the other way.

8 Rotate each toe one way then the other.

9 Support each toe individually between the thumb and 1st finger then pull downwards. Repeat on each toe.

10 Massage the whole foot and lower leg with deeper movements, finishing with light pressure. Repeat four times.

11 Finally, with one hand on top of the client's lower leg and the other directly below, slide your hands down the leg over the foot until you slowly remove your hands from the client's toes.

12 Repeat the massage to the left foot and lower leg.

Contra-actions that may occur during and following treatment and how to respond

A **contra-action** is a reaction that has occurred from a treatment being performed and affected the area that has been treated. It could include an adverse reaction, known as an allergic reaction, where the skin and nail become red, swollen and itchy, with blisters.

During the consultation, you must ask the client if they have an allergy, then use this information to make any necessary changes to the treatment plan. If the client has very sensitive skin but is unaware of an allergy, then a skin test can be performed 24 hours before the treatment. The client may react to a number of products, such as enamel or hand cream, so when aftercare advice is given, you must inform the client of what they must do.

A contra-action could also occur if a treatment was not correctly performed and health and safety procedures were not followed, for example:

- infection in the cuticle or nail area from excessive removal of the cuticle or cutting and filing the nail too short
- faulty equipment — not checking whether the thermal bootees or mittens were working correctly; if they are too hot this could cause deep **erythema** burns to occur
- paraffin wax too hot could cause deep erythema burns
- incorrect product choices, such as exfoliating a client with eczema (skin already very thin).

Key term

Contra-action – an allergic reaction to any aspect of the treatment. The skin may appear red, swollen and itchy.

Key term

Erythema – where blood circulation is stimulated by an increase in temperature, resulting in blood capillaries rising to the skin's surface to expel excess heat, causing the skin to redden.

The importance of completing the treatment to the satisfaction of the client

To learn more the importance of client feedback, see Client care and communication in beauty-related industries, page 47.

The importance of completing treatment records

To learn more about record cards, see Client care and communication in beauty-related industries, page 42.

Provide suitable aftercare advice

Providing the correct aftercare advice is essential so that the client can maintain the effects of the treatment and knows what to do in the event of a contra-action. It will also encourage the client to make any necessary changes to how they look after their hands and feet, especially if they have any concerns such as bitten nails or calluses. The client will also need to know what to do if something happens for the first time, for example a hangnail.

It is important that you inform the client of what to do should they suffer from a contra-action after the treatment. They must:

- remove products immediately and apply a cold compress
- remove any enamel applied with enamel remover on a cotton pad – not pick it off with their nails
- if irritation persists, see their GP
- inform the nail technician so it can be documented on the record card.

You should also advise the client:

- when to return for their next treatment
- to wear protective groves when using any household or industrial cleaners at home or at work or when gardening or performing any outside work such as cleaning the car
- to use nail scissors to remove damaged nails and file correctly with an emery board
- not to bite nails or surrounding skin
- not to use nails as tools, for example to pick off old enamel
- not to use sharp objects to clean under the nails – instead use a nail brush with hot soapy water
- not to wear ill-fitting shoes
- for those who suffer from feet odour, wash feet regularly, change socks or tights daily and apply a deodorising foot powder or foot spray
- to ensure feet are completely dry after bathing, to prevent the skin becoming inflamed and split
- to avoid wearing high-heeled shoes, as this can cause calluses and will also affect posture, causing joint and muscular pains.

The client can maintain the effects of the treatment and improve the condition of the skin, nails and cuticle by:

- using hand cream or lotions throughout the day
- using cuticle cream
- applying a foot and body cream every day after bathing
- using a foot scrub or hand scrub weekly
- applying base coat and top coat when using enamel at home
- for those with weak nails, using a nail strengthener
- using a buffer.

To learn more about providing the client with clear advice and recommendations, see Client care and communication in beauty-related industries, page 43.

Check it out

Use the computer to create an aftercare leaflet that incorporates all different kinds of aftercare advice that you can provide at the end of your treatment to ensure you have covered all areas. This could act as a prompt to gain further assessment, when selling and promoting products and services.

Check your knowledge

1. What are the benefits of a manicure or pedicure?

2. What are possible contra-actions to a manicure or pedicure treatment?
    a) Direct cross-infection
    b) Indirect cross-infection
    c) A reaction that happens as a result of the treatment or an allergen

3. What type of movement is effleurage?
    a) A kneading movement
    b) A stroking movement
    c) A tapping movement

4. By what other name is the tapotement movement also known?
    a) Percussion
    b) Psoriasis
    c) Paraffin

5. What shape should toenails have?
    a) Round
    b) Oval
    c) Pointed
    d) Straight with curved corners

6. What is the strongest fingernail shape?
    a) Squoval
    b) Round
    c) Oval
    d) Pointed

7. What is the average temperature of paraffin wax?
    a) 23°C
    b) 44°C
    c) 49°C

8. Name an ingredient in cuticle remover.
    a) Potassium hydroxide
    b) Hydrogen peroxide
    c) Alpha hydroxy acids

9. What is the effect of a solvent?
    a) Thins very thick enamel
    b) Provides flexibility
    c) Nourishes the nail plate

10. What is the effect of plasticiser?
    a) Lubricates
    b) Provides flexibility
    c) Acts as an emollient

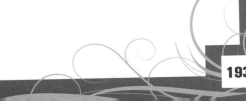

Getting ready for assessment

The manicure and pedicure units are differently assessed in VRQs and NVQs, using a combination of assessment methods, as specified below. You cannot simulate any practical assessment but you must be aware of the criteria and be proactive during practical sessions to cluster assessments for more than one unit at a time.

City & Guilds		VTCT	
NVQ	VRQ	NVQ	VRQ

Service times: 45mins for a manicure/pedicure and 1hr for a luxury manicure/pedicure
 	
Evidence :
• Should be gathered in a realistic working environment, and simulation avoided
• You must demonstrate that you have met the required standard for all the outcomes, assessment criteria/ skills and ranges
 	
Knowledge and understanding will be assessed by:
• a mandatory written question paper
• oral questioning
• written and oral questions can also be done as a GOLA online test
• practical assessment
• completion of an assessment book/ portfolio
	Service times: Not applicable to this qualification
	
	Evidence:
	• You can take either the online test or complete knowledge tasks in the assignments
	• There is no particular time limit set for the completion of an assignment (tasks)
	• Assignment is graded pass, merit or distinction
	• GOLA online tests are pass or fail
	• Practical tasks are graded pass, merit or distinction
	• 3 pre-observations must be completed (each with a treatment plan), before the final observation and should include a combination of:
	  • use of heat
	  • hand or foot mask
	  • exfoliation
	  • dark enamel
	  • French enamel
	• Final observation must include one of the following manicure finishes:
	  • dark enamel
	  • French enamel
	
	Knowledge and understanding will be assessed by knowledge tasks or an online GOLA test
		Service times: Pedicure 50mins and a standard manicure 45mins
		
		Evidence:
		• It is strongly recommended that the evidence for this unit be gathered in a realistic working environment
		• Simulation should be avoided where possible
		• You must practically demonstrate that you have met the required standard for this unit
		• All outcomes, assessment criteria and range statements must be achieved
		• Your performance will be observed on at least three occasions for each assessment criteria
		
		Knowledge and understanding will be assessed by:
		• internally-assessed workplace performance using a variety of methods
		• a mandatory written question paper – these questions are set and marked by VTCT
			Service times: Pedicure 50mins and a standard manicure 45mins
			
			Evidence:
			• It is strongly recommended that the evidence for this unit be gathered in a realistic working environment
			• Simulation should be avoided where possible
			• You must practically demonstrate that you have met the required standard for this unit
			• All outcomes, assessment criteria and range statements must be achieved
			• Your performance will be observed on at least three occasions for each assessment criteria
			
			Knowledge and understanding will be assessed by:
			• a mandatory written question paper
			• oral questioning
			• portfolio of evidence

Provide nail art

What you will learn

- Prepare for nail art service
- Provide nail art service

Top tip

Use a training hand with nail tips to practise new designs, as this can be a good way to help clients choose their own designs and can be used as a visual aid, especially for clients who are hearing impaired.

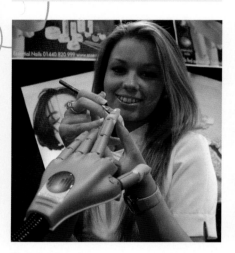

Training hand

Think about it

Before the client arrives, make sure you have sanitised the working area, washed, sterilised and stored your tools correctly, checked the client's record card and washed your hands. To learn more about disorders and diseases that can be cross-infected through poor hygiene, see Skin analysis, page 147.

Top tip

It is the employer's responsibility to provide the correct working environment and it is your responsibility, as an employee, to maintain it. To ensure a safe and healthy working environment, you need to understand what the legal responsibilities of the employer and employees are.

Introduction

Nail art can begin with just painting a colour onto either natural or artificial nails. As a nail technician, you will need to master and develop this skill. Nail art has become a very popular extension to a regular nail service such as a manicure or pedicure treatment. It takes a lot of practice, and you will need a very good eye for detail and a lot of patience. Remember that not all clients will be devotees of nail art – some may only indulge in nail art for a special occasion and require only a basic design, while others may want the most elaborate and extravagant design to fit their nail enhancements. It takes careful discussion and a detailed client consultation to determine which method of nail art to carry out and it is a good idea to make a display of your own designs to give the client an idea of what is available.

There are many different nail art techniques. This unit will look at the different types and effects to be achieved. All you need to achieve these designs is a little imagination and the correct equipment.

Prepare for nail art service

Preparation is vital to ensure you are ready to perform any type of nail art design that a client might ask you to create. It also demonstrates a professional attitude and promotes good time management. A nail technician also needs to be aware of the importance of sterilisation and sanitisation of all tools, the working area and themselves, as this is part of the preparation process.

Salon requirements for preparing yourself, the client and the work area

Before a client arrives at the salon to have a nail art treatment, the working area and technician must be prepared fully, to ensure the treatment runs smoothly.

As a nail technician, you have a professional image to maintain which is vital to your success and that of the business. When you are training to become a technician, you are assessed on your personal presentation and hygiene. The standards for these assessments are set by the awarding bodies that your assessors must follow when you are being assessed. Throughout your career you will be expected by employers, clients and colleagues to continue the high standards that you had to maintain throughout your studies. The basic salon requirements are the same as when you prepare

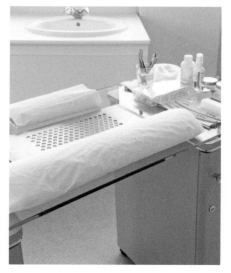

A station set up for a nails service

for a manicure or pedicure treatment – see Provide manicure and pedicure treatments, page 165, and Follow health and safety practice in the salon, page 19.

Environmental conditions suitable for nail art services

It is important to have and maintain the correct environmental conditions to ensure a safe, healthy and effective treatment is performed. Good environmental conditions include adequate lighting, ventilation, temperature and comfort, which enable the technician to perform the treatment correctly and ensure the safety, health and comfort of the client and yourself. To learn more about environmental conditions, see Provide manicure and pedicure treatments, page 166, and Provide and maintain nail enhancement, page 227, and for the legislation that enforces these conditions, see Follow health and safety practice in the salon, page 5.

Consultation techniques used to identify service objectives

To identify the service objectives required to create an individual treatment plan, good communication skills, such as what we say or our body language, are vital. Consultation techniques include being an active listener, demonstrating good questioning techniques, ensuring understanding between the technician and the client, the location of the consultation, demonstrating good body language and having legible written communication. To learn more, see Client care and communication in beauty-related industries, page 41.

The importance of carrying out a nail and skin analysis

As a nail technician, you must understand the importance of carrying out a nail and skin analysis during the consultation. There are many contra-indications that can prevent a treatment from happening – the client might suffer from a nail or skin condition that could be contagious, it could be painful to work on or the treatment may make the condition worse. If none of these possibilities applies, then the treatment could be performed with restrictions or **adaptations**, for example if a client had a very old bruise on their arm, then either avoid the area or apply minimal light pressure. To understand in depth what a nail technician must know to perform a competent and thorough analysis, see the Skin analysis unit, page 149.

Top tip

Ensure the salon has appropriate music playing in the background at the correct volume to create a pleasant environment. Because there will be strong-smelling odours from the types of treatments being performed, think about the aroma of the salon. Essential oils on pot pourri or in oil burners will help create a soothing environment.

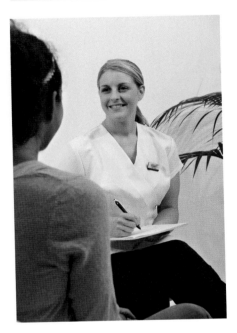

Use all types of communication to perform an effective consultation

Key term

Adaptation – changes to a normal procedure because of a contra-indication.

Top tip

Successful businesses understand the importance of good communication skills, so practise your skills at every opportunity and observe senior colleagues for ideas and inspiration that you can use.

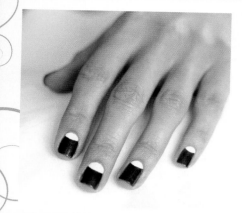

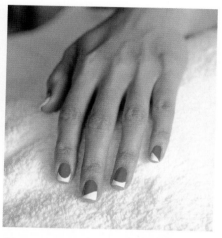

An unusual and reverse French manicure

How to select products, tools and equipment to suit client's service needs and nail conditions

It is important to select the correct products, tools and equipment for the nail art treatment you will provide, and this can only be achieved if you understand what is available to you. For information about the following products, tools and equipment that you will need to perform a nail art treatment, see Provide manicure and pedicure treatments, page 169:

- Top coat and base coat
- Enamels
- Enamel removers
- Cuticle oils
- Orange sticks (see also page 201)
- Workstations.

How to choose a nail art design

It is important to display your nail artwork so clients can see what types of designs are available. This can be done by creating designs on nail tips or taking photographs of nail art designs, which can be put on to display boards in the salon. Start your display board with easier designs, progressing to more elaborate creations that require more intricate work. Remember to price the nail art designs accordingly, as the more intricate the work, the more time-consuming and costly it will be for the client. Often the most elaborate nail art designs are the ones that really attract the clients.

Change your display boards every season, so in summer ensure that you are displaying designs consisting of warm colours such as reds, yellows and oranges. In nature, warm colours represent the changing of the seasons. They also energise us, preparing us for summer sunshine, although these colours may be too bold for some clients who prefer more subtle colours. Therefore, display the lighter side of a warm palette with pinks, pale yellow and peach colours. Summer colours are used in spring, but are much more muted. In winter, you will find that clients are attracted to the cooler colours — blues, greens and purples — as the days shorten and clothing becomes darker in preparation for the winter months. In autumn, choose more neutral shades such as greys, soft browns/beige, pale pink and soft brown tones.

Most salons that offer a nail art service will have themed display boards showing a range of designs reflecting the time of year, for example Halloween, Valentine's Day and religious celebrations such as the Chinese new year, Diwali and Christmas.

Colours and trends in nail art

Every season, there is an ever-growing range of nail varnishes, with new and more innovative colours being designed to help create the masterpiece design your client is looking for. Colours can be mixed together to match any outfit, theme or occasion, although the majority of clients will want a look that they can wear on their nails every day. Clients consider nail art to be a statement personifying who they are.

If your client shows an interest in nail art, begin by looking at their personality and clothing. Show them your designs and if they appear to be conservative (traditional) in taste, suggest subtle designs and colours for their nails, such as a neat French polish with some delicate nail art or sheer striping flicks. Alternatively, a client who likes to follow fashion trends and has an extrovert (outgoing) personality may be open to more dramatic designs with rhinestones and bolder colours. All your clients are individuals and it is a good idea to ask the client to bring in a picture of what they want.

A talented nail technician can flatter any client's nails by suggesting suitable designs and colours, but if the client chooses to have nail extensions you will have the opportunity to use your artistic flair to the full. Public perception of nail art has also changed over the past few years, with many clients no longer choosing glitzy designs just for special occasions. Red, the colour of sophistication, has been joined by deep purple, blue, green, black, even yellows and neon colours, as nail art has become a part of everyday life. While nail technicians have kept abreast of new techniques, nail companies have continued to develop new and innovative methods of nail art.

Choosing your nail art brushes

For anyone aspiring to become an outstanding nail technician, with the ability to perform creative nail art designs, a professional set of nail art brushes is a necessity. These types of brushes are designed to be used only for the purpose of nail art and the effects they can create can be breathtaking.

As nail art designs become more and more popular, clients' requests are likely to become more creatively demanding. To carry out the more complex designs you will need to use a variety of nail art brushes. It is advisable to pay a reasonable amount for brushes to ensure you achieve the best results. With good care, brushes can last throughout your career. Cheaper varieties will fall apart quite quickly. A good-quality nail art brush must have sable hair, as this will ensure accuracy and precision in your designs and will withstand constant cleaning.

Below we look at the types of brushes available and the effects that can be achieved.

Nail art brush

This brush can be used to paint pictures and designs **free-hand** using acrylic paints, but try to buy the best-quality, fine-tip brush you can afford. Brushes come in a variety of sizes from very small to large and can be made from sable, nylon or synthetic hair, which can vary from flexible to stiff. The type of brush you need will depend upon the design you are creating and the effect you wish to achieve.

Liner brush

This is a wider but much shorter brush, and it is used to paint nail art with thicker lines or to cover larger areas, as in enamelling the nail.

Top tip

Nail art designs that are advertised are normally displayed on large plastic tips and will look very different on a natural nail. Also, some aspects of nail art are much easier to do on a nail tip than a small natural nail, so keep both of these points in mind when recommending designs for clients.

Check it out

To learn the effects of each of the brushes, practise designs on nail tips using all the brushes to master your nail art skills, ready for your practical assessments.

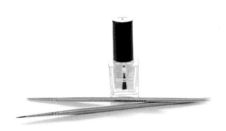

Different sized striping brushes

Key term

Free-hand – creating a design without using stencils.

Striping brush

This is a very thin, narrow brush that is available in different sizes with varying lengths and thicknesses, and is used to produce long, straight lines. Shorter striping brushes are good for detail as they produce lines that are thicker, allowing you to create flowers and spots. The longer and thinner the brush, the finer and longer the lines it produces, so they are good for zigzag and straight strokes on the nails. Once you have mastered the basics, you can use this brush to produce flicks and curves. Striping brushes are also available with a crooked neck, making the brush easy to use when held in an upright position.

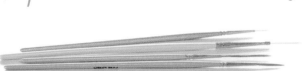

Fine detail brush

This is the smallest nail art brush and is used for hand-painting details or placing dots on the nail plate. The brush is short and tapered into a fine point. It can be used for creating very detailed designs.

A selection of nail art brushes

Flat/flat-angled brush (shading brush)

This brush comes with flat square or angled sides, making it the brush of choice if you are creating an intricate nail art design. It can also be used for creating large flower designs, shading the inside of a larger design or filling in a design. By using different colours on each side of the brush, you can create a swirl effect. Both flat and flat-angled brushes are also referred to as 'shading' or 'angular' brushes.

Fan brush

This type of brush creates texture and blends colours together – it is perfect for striping and layering multiple colours onto nails. As opposed to the striping brush that creates straight lines, the fan brush is more versatile, as it gives the nail colour more of an airbrush effect. This brush can also be used to smooth over a gold- or silver-leaf application.

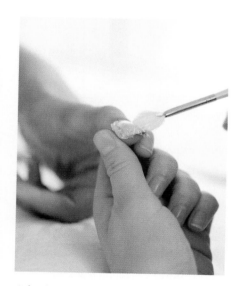

Dotting brush

The dotting brush has the smallest tip of all the nail art brushes – it is often referred to as the 'marbler'. It is ideal for creating small dots and designs and for swirling colours to create a marbling effect.

Glitter dust brush

This brush is designed to be used with glitter dust powder and liquid mixer. Simply dip the nail art glitter brush into the dust mixer, making sure that a ball of mixer forms at the end of the brush. Next, select your chosen glitter colour and dip the loaded brush into the dust with a rolling movement. Then apply the fluid to the nail, creating the design of your choice. Remember to apply two coats of sealer to the nails to maintain the life of the design, and to clean the brush in acetone or enamel remover after use.

A fan brush in use

Choosing your tools

Just as brushes are an important aspect of nail art, there are various other tools that are equally important in helping to create elaborate designs and making you a master of nail art.

Brush cleaning/storage jar

Maintenance of your brushes is very important and a storage and cleaning jar is required in your kit. It is made from a durable plastic with a screw-on lid and interior brush holders to prevent the brushes from becoming misshapen.

Dappen dish

A Dappen dish can hold enamel remover to clean brushes during a treatment, for example to clean a glitter dust brush when re-dipping the brush to obtain more glitter.

Dotting and marbling tools

A dotting or marbling tool resembles a pencil (a wooden dowel) with a metal ball head of a small and/or medium size (some have a two-sided head). It can be used to blend layers of wet paint to create a marbling effect or for fine paint application to create lines, swirls and dots, for example when creating flowers. It is also ideal for picking up gems and securing them in place on the nail. The tool can vary in size from very small to large, depending upon the effect required.

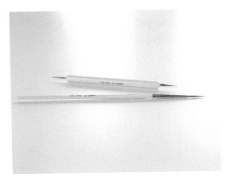

A dotting or marbling tool

Orange stick

You can never have too many of these, as they can be used in almost every nail art application or nail care treatment. They can be used to pick up rhinestones and secure them into varnish. Orange sticks are very inexpensive and can be bought in bulk, so never be without them.

Embossing tool

This tool is used to create raised designs (a **3D effect**) on the nail plate. It is a syringe-like tool that is filled with acrylic paint. When the plunger is depressed, the paint is pushed out of the tip to create patterns and lines. The designs incorporate dots, lines and commas to create the 3D effects. Remember to seal the design once the paint has completely dried.

Nail adhesive/glue

This is used both to adhere artificial nails to natural nails and decorations such as rhinestones or beads to the nails. It is sometimes advisable to use nail glue for extra security if you are placing a stone that stands proud on the nail and might otherwise fall off.

Stencils

Nail art stencils are similar to the ones that children use to create pictures, only they are much smaller and have a sticky back to keep them in place. Stencils are an excellent way of creating great designs if you are not good at hand-painting and can be purchased with particular themes such as flowers, butterflies, shapes and patterns. They can also be used if a themed nail art design is needed, such as holly or Christmas trees. Stencils are applied to a dry nail and painted over. When the paint has dried the stencil is removed, leaving the chosen design behind on the nail.

Key term

3D effect – a raised design that protrudes outwards

Top tips

- If you smudge your application of enamel or nail art, use a cotton wool tipped orange stick with enamel remover to clean the area.

- Remember that nail glue will bond in seconds and is extremely strong, so take extra care when using it and always follow the manufacturer's instructions.

Top tips

- If the guide tapes are pressed down too firmly, when they are removed they could peel away the base coat and damage the enamel finish.

- Advise the client to reapply the sealer every couple of days to maintain the life of the nail art and avoid any chips. This is also a good way to promote the sale of products and increase the salon's profits.

Guide tapes

These are self-adhesive tapes, which are placed over the smile line of the nail and make it easy to paint a French manicure. Once the white tip is dried, they are removed, leaving a perfect line.

Sealer

With all nail art designs it is important to 'seal' your designs on completion, when the nail is completely dry. It is advisable to use a sealer to fix the paint and bring out the depth of colour. The sealer will also maintain the nail art's shine whereas a regular top coat may react with the paint or cause it to perish.

Palette/paint mixing tray

It is a good idea to invest in a palette, preferably plastic, that you can wipe clean after use. You can place your paints on it ready for use or it can be used to mix paints or glitter together to create additional colours or effects. Palettes are available in a range of sizes, but for nail art a small or medium palette is advisable.

Craft knife

This tool is used for cutting and making personal stencils from masking tape or 'frisket film'.

Rhinestone picker-up

This tool will do exactly what it says, as it picks up and secures gems in place on the nail.

Stork scissors

These are an essential item to have in your nail art tool kit. They are normally gold in colour and are small, sharp scissors used in all aspects of nail art, including the cutting of striping tape or foil.

Tweezers

Tweezers are an integral part of your nail art kit. They can be used for picking up stickers, water decals (transfers) and rhinestones. Angled, pointed or flat-headed (straight-nose) tweezers are available – choose whichever ones make your nail art design a little easier to do.

Nail art 5-gram/10-gram empty storage pots

These clear pots, with screw-on lids, are perfect for storing all your nail art bits and pieces such as confetti, beads, charms, rhinestones and dangles.

Compartment storage case

Storage cases with compartments are available in many different sizes and are perfect for keeping all your nail art products neat and tidy, such as rhinestones, beads, stickers and transfers. The case looks professional and will allow the client to choose a colour and design.

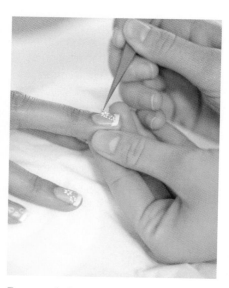

Tweezers being used

Varnish carry case

Mobile nail technicians find this case handy for carrying nail enamels and paints.

Carry case

A nail technician's carry case is available in a range of colours and sizes, although they should all have the same basic structure or layout to ensure that the products and tools stored inside are protected from damage. An ideal carry case should be aluminium-framed, with internal trays to store tools securely. It should be strong yet lightweight, and built for longevity and, depending upon the size and amount of stock you have, may usefully have wheels on the base with a detachable top section, which can be used as a vanity case.

Training hand

A training hand is an artificial hand that can be used to practise nail art designs on. Replaceable plastic nail tips are used on the hand.

Nail art products and techniques

There are a range of nail art products that will enable you to create a wide variety of designs. It is a good idea to practise using all the different types to create your own unique designs.

Nail enamels

Selecting a nail enamel involves more than just choosing the colour. There are many different types of varnish available, from matt to metallic, as shown in the table below.

> **Top tip**
>
> Cutter punch tools are used to cut shapes into a plastic tip before it is applied and these are mainly used for competition work or advanced nail art designs.

> **Check it out**
>
> Paint nail tips to experiment with different enamel finishes and learn visually what effects each enamel creates.

Type of nail enamel	Uses
Cream	The polish we associate with reds. It is creamy and rich, glossy and shiny, but not shimmery or glittery; some have extra shine, so that nails look wet.
Matt	Matt shades are the opposite of glossy; they look 'flat' – more like the nails have been polished with a felt-tip pen.
Pearlescent or frosted	These are shimmery shades and they sparkle instead of just shining, but contain no glitter. Some pearlescent varnishes contain fish scales, which gives them a shimmering appearance. To maintain that effect, use a sealer on the nails, as a normal top coat will flatten the scales and dull the appearance of the varnish.
Opalescent	Shades have a distinctive 'mother-of-pearl' effect, as they glisten and reflect other colours in different lights.
Glitter	Shades come in a variety of colours and contain glitter pieces. Some glitter varnishes are more subtle and contain tiny specks of glitter, while others are more dramatic and contain noticeable chunks for a dramatic and bold effect.
Metallic	A finish that makes the nails appear like metal. The most popular shades are gold, silver and copper.

Types of nail enamel

Top tip

Do not try to thin old, thick enamel with nail varnish removers or paint thinner as it will damage the enamel's ability to work effectively.

There is also a big difference in the quality of the enamels you can purchase and the difference is not necessarily in the price. A good polish is easy to apply with no streaking, has good colour depth and good adherence, resisting chipping. With poorer quality enamel, no matter how many layers you apply, it still feels uneven in application, does not look smooth and will begin to chip immediately after application. To ensure the life of an enamel, always store it away from sunlight and heat. Purchase small bottles rather than large ones, because trends are constantly changing and nail enamel has a limited shelf life. If you have not used a bottle of enamel for a while and the bottle will not open, simply run the neck of the bottle under warm water until it softens and the top will come off easily. Another way to extend the life of an enamel that has begun to thicken is to add a little nail varnish thinner.

Nail art painting

Nail art paints are used to create a free-hand design and are water-based. They give a very dense colour and are designed to be used over an enamel: first, paint your desired shade onto the natural or artificial nail, then use the correct size of brush or marbling tool to apply your design.

- To achieve fine stripes and a sophisticated look, use a very long, thin brush.

- To create a design of flowers or dots of colour, use a dotting tool.

- For the nail technician with slightly limited artistic capabilities, stencils can be used to create a dramatic effect: simply put the stencil over the nail and then paint over. When the paint is completely dry, remove the stencil and the chosen design will be imprinted on the nail.

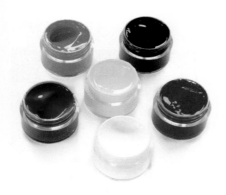

Nail paints in pots

There is a vast selection of acrylic paints available and they come in a range of colours — you are only limited by your imagination for the designs you want to create. Nail paints are also easy to remove if you make a mistake — simply wipe the nail over with a wet nail wipe or cotton wool bud and the paint will come off.

Marbling

This technique mixes two or more colours together to create a dramatic effect on the nails. It is advisable to use contrasting colours over a clear base coat. To ensure the effect is dramatic, first use the larger round end of the marbling tool and apply blobs of the chosen colours down the centre of the nail. Then, using the smaller end of the marbling tool or fine brush, begin to make quick 'S' strokes or flicking movements to swirl the colours together. Continue with this technique until the nail is covered. Once the marbling has dried, apply two coats of top coat to ensure its sheen and seal the design.

Top tip

Paints available in containers that come with a brush, ready for use, are called nail art stripers.

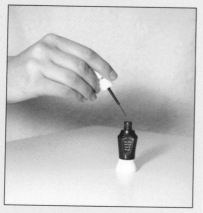

Nail art striper

Foiling

This is another very easy and highly effective method of nail art, giving you the ability to create different designs by using a variety of foils applied over a painted nail. The nail can have either a base coat alone or, for added dramatic effect, foiling can be applied over coloured enamel

The application of foil is a quick process. As the foil is purchased on a roll, there is no need to start cutting the foil in the shape of the nail — merely place the foil over the nail plate. First, a white adhesive is applied in a very thin layer to the nail plate. The adhesive will turn clear in colour and then the foil (pattern-side up) can be applied straight over the nail. The foil is pressed into place with a rubbing action of the thumb or with a cotton wool bud; the foil will stick into place only where the adhesive has been applied. Pull off the foil backing and the foil will remain on the nail.

Foil will add a whole new look to the nail, whether it covers the whole nail, to create stripes, or is just applied to the tips. Foils look amazing and make the nails shimmer and shine. Once the application is complete, a special sealer is applied in numerous layers to maintain the life of the foil. It is advisable not to use a top coat, as it can destroy the delicate layer of the foil.

Gold or silver leaf

For something a little different, gold or silver leaf is the perfect choice — it will give the nails an antique look. Be very careful when applying the leaf, as it is very fragile and crumbles easily. Apply foil adhesive to the area of the nail where you want the design to be and allow it to become tacky before you apply a small amount of the leaf. Alternatively, enamel can be used instead of the adhesive. Once applied, gently rub over the area with a fan brush and then seal to ensure longevity of the design. The leaf can be applied to the whole nail, free edge or torn into small pieces and placed randomly.

Polish secure

This term applies to all nail techniques that require varnish or enamel to secure the chosen design, including rhinestones, pearls, foil shapes, flatstones and beads. Polish secure refers to the application of small stones that are placed into wet nail enamel, which acts as a bonding agent to hold accessories in place.

Rhinestones

These stones come in a variety of sizes and colours and resemble precious or semi-precious stones. They can be made of glass or plastic and reflect the light, giving an illuminating effect. There are many shapes available, including round, oval, triangle and square. Depending upon the effect to be achieved or client preference, rhinestones can be placed upon the nail to achieve a dramatic but refined effect or, by simply applying a single stone, enhance an already manicured nail. Once the rhinestone is secured in place, seal with a top coat to ensure it stays on and advise the client to reapply top coat again at home because although rhinestones are small, they will stand proud on the nail (a 3D effect). Rhinestones are widely available on the Internet — prices vary, as does the quality; a good-quality rhinestone will be made of either glass or crystal and will not become dull or lose its lustre, so buy wisely.

Flatstones

Flatstones are available in different sizes, shapes and colours. They are flatter in structure than rhinestones and are a less expensive alternative. They tend to stay on longer than rhinestones because they do not protrude. However, they have a tendency to lose their sparkle, especially once a layer of top coat has been

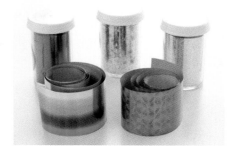

Foil

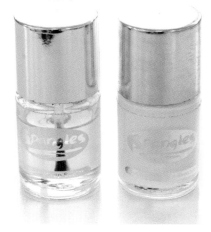

Base coat and nail adhesive

Top tip

Applying gold or silver leaf to the whole nail is not advisable as the leaf creases easily. There are foils that look like gold leaf that could be used over the whole nail, as an alternative to avoid the possibility of the leaf creasing.

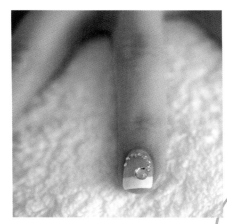

Rhinestones

applied. It is a good idea to apply a thicker layer of top coat to the wet enamel and push the stones in using a rhinestone picker-up or orange stick — this will give the nail its shiny finish and hold the stones in place without the need to seal them.

Pearls

These are flat-backed plastic beads that resemble pearls and they are the perfect complement for a bridal party. They are very pretty and popular, as they are available in different sizes.

Stone shapes

A wide range of glass shapes, of all sizes and colours, are available to enhance any nail art design.

Foil shapes

These are little pieces of shiny or metallic-looking plastic that are cut into different shapes, including stars, hexagons, circles and animals such as rabbits or cats.

Metal studs or leaves

These are a polish secure method of applying glitzy jewellery to the nails without having to put a hole into the nail plate. The studs are available in different shapes and are gold or silver in colour. They are placed into wet enamel and, because they are usually hollow, adhere well to the nails.

Glitter

The use of glitter varnishes or dust can enhance or create a unique nail art design. Glitter can be applied to the whole nail or used to make patterns to highlight a particular section of the nail.

Glitter varnishes are painted straight onto the nail, using either the brush supplied in the varnish or a fine nail art brush to create lines and patterns.

Glitter dust creates a more dramatic and specific effect. The dust is picked up with a glitter dust brush that has been dipped in sealer mixer. The effect created on the nail plate is solid and dense in appearance. Like all nail art, glitter dust will need to be sealed — gently apply a thick layer of sealer to ensure the glitter dust does not move. The sealer can also be applied directly to the nail, so if you want glitter on the nail tips, then paint the sealer in that area and dip the tip into the dust — this will ensure a dramatic and perfect finish.

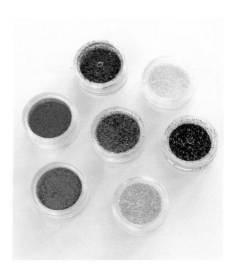

Glitter dust pots

Transfers

A transfer (also known as a decal) is usually formatted on a background of white gloss paper which, when it comes into contact with water, releases the design onto the nail surface. The design you choose may depend on whether the nail is natural or painted. Transfers can be removed easily by wiping over the nails with an acetone-free varnish remover.

There are two different types of transfer:

- Self-adhesive – this is an extremely quick and very effective method, where the transfer is peeled off a protective backing and stuck directly onto the nail.

- Water-release – this method is more complicated and time-consuming. The transfer requires soaking off its backing sheet. Place the transfer face-down in a small container of water until it slides off. If you are going to adopt this method it is always advisable to invest in good-quality transfers, to ensure they do not disintegrate when they are placed in water.

Transfers are a fantastic way of providing good-quality nail art within minutes and designs include seasonal themes, characters and flowers.

Nail tape

Striping nail tape is available in many different colours and patterns and can be used for simple or more complex designs. It has a sticky back that is placed on the nail and pressed down. The first step is to enamel the nails as this is the backdrop for the nail art design. Then place the tape onto the nail in the chosen design and press down firmly with an orange stick to ensure the tape is stuck. Trim the edges with a pair of small, sharp scissors and apply a top coat over the tape.

Laser strands (very fine, twisted metal strands) catch the light at all angles and produce an attractive effect. They are available in lots of different colours, or you could use two-tone laser strands to give a great finished effect to the nails.

Nail stickers

Nail stickers can be used to create elaborate, unique designs and are one of the easiest, quickest and simplest forms of nail art products on the market today. Simply peel off your chosen design with tweezers and position it on the nail plate. The stickers are very versatile as they can be positioned anywhere and at any angle. They can be themed for parties such as Halloween or Christmas. The designs are sometimes bold with striking colours, which can be combined with other nail art designs, or they may be subtle with rhinestones for a wedding celebration or holiday. Many nail companies supply nail stickers even for the smallest nails, which can be used for a children's birthday party.

Embossed designs

Before you start nail painting with the **embossing** tool, it is advisable to practise basic techniques so you get the feel of the tool and the flow of the acrylic paint that you are using. Embossed nail designs are created using a syringe-like tool that is filled with acrylic nail paint to create raised designs on the nails. When pressure is applied to the plunger, the paint is forced out of the nozzle, similar to decorating a cake. So the slower you go, the more accurate you will be and the more confident your technique will become. This is a technique that you will need to master to ensure your design looks effective, but it is easy to do, as only three strokes are used, including a dot, a line and a comma shape. Almost any design can be achieved, from a flower to a strawberry sundae.

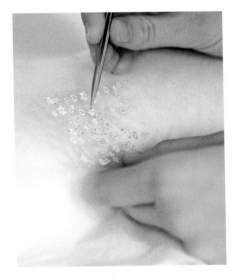

Self-adhesive transfers

Top tip

If the edge of the striping tape starts to lift a little after the top coat has been applied, use an orange stick to hold it in place until it sticks.

Key term

Embossing – decorating the nail with a design.

Think about it

Why not have a nail art treatment yourself, using a variety of methods, and follow the aftercare advice you would give a client? Experience working and living while wearing nail art. This will give you an idea of any problems the client may have in maintaining and removing the nail art.

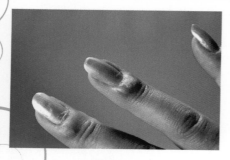

Paronychia – a contagious nail condition that is contra-indicated for all treatments

Key term

Skin and nail diseases and disorders – conditions that could be contagious or made worse by performing a nail art treatment.

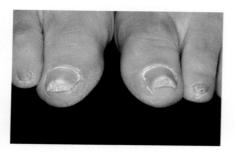

Onychomycosis – a contagious nail condition that is contra-indicated for all treatments

Check it out

Create skin and nail diseases/ disorder flashcards with images and text, to help you revise the knowledge you will need for your assessments.

Remember that acrylic paint does not have a lustre or sheen when it dries, so always finish with two coats of top coat or sealer and when you want to change the design it can quickly be removed with a nail varnish remover.

Everything that you will need to carry out these designs is available in an embossed nail art kit. It contains syringes, various shades of acrylic paint, a container to store the tools and a sponge, which must be kept damp as this will help keep the acrylic paint moist and ready for use. Maintain your kit by washing out the syringes in warm water and if the nozzle becomes blocked or the flow of paint becomes uneven, remove the nozzle and clean with a fine wire.

Nail conditions and contra-indications that prevent or restrict nail art

There are many nail conditions and contra-indications that will either restrict or prevent you from performing a nail art treatment. You must be able to recognise these, and either not perform the treatment, asking the client to seek medical advice, or adapt the treatment plan to suit the individual client. To learn more about **skin and nail diseases and disorders** and contra-indications, see the Skin analysis unit, page 150.

Structure and functions of the nail

To learn more about the anatomy and physiology of the nail and skin, to understand their relevance to nail art treatments, see the Anatomy and physiology unit, page 132.

Provide a nail art service

How to communicate and behave in a professional manner

It is not enough just to be able to perform an outstanding treatment, as clients want to receive the full package, which includes the nail technician demonstrating excellent verbal, written and non-verbal communication skills, and demonstrating a professional manner and attitude. By using good communication skills, you can create a professional environment for all. To learn more about communication and professional ethical conduct, see Client care and communication in beauty-related industries, page 35.

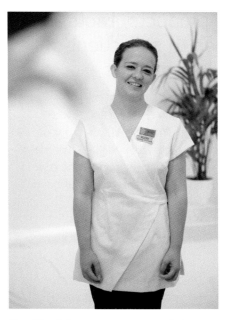

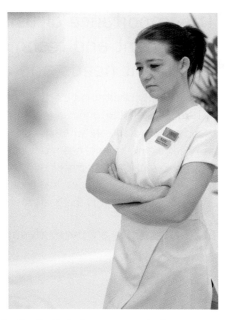

Good body language or non-verbal communication is vital when communicating with clients

Think about it

When practising treatments on your peers, perform a role play activity to practise communication skills. This will help you to become more relaxed and confident in your approach when working on real clients.

Health and safety working practices

When a technician demonstrates the correct health and safety working practices, it is observed by their employer, colleagues and clients. This will create a professional image not only for the technician but also for the business, as clients will have confidence in the technician's abilities, and this will help to develop the salon's reputation. To learn more about health and safety in the workplace and legislation that affects working practices, see Follow health and safety practice in the salon, page 5, and Provide and maintain nail enhancement, page 225.

The importance of positioning yourself and the client correctly

It is essential that the technician and client are correctly positioned during the treatment, to ensure both are comfortable. For the technician, this will prevent muscular and skeletal aches and pains, including repetitive strain injury (RSI), from occurring. The treatment can also be performed safely, to avoid damage to the client, technician and working area. To find out more, see Follow health and safety practice in the salon, page 19, and Provide and maintain nail enhancement, page 237.

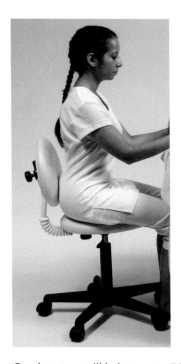

Good posture will help prevent RSI

Top tip

Always be aware of your posture when you are working. Before the client arrives, check your stool is at the correct height and position, as this is one way to ensure you avoid RSI.

Top tip

Having a manicure before a nail art treatment will improve the condition of the skin and nails and form a healthier area to create more effective nail art.

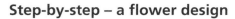

The importance of using products, tools, equipment and techniques to suit client's treatment needs and nail conditions

Once you fully understand the types of products, tools, equipment and techniques available, you can begin to create a range of designs that will become more elaborate with time and experience. The unit Provide manicure and pedicure treatments has many products and techniques that you will need to perform a nail art treatment – for information on how to enamel and how to file the different nail shapes, see pages 178 and 179. Remember that good application of enamel is the basis for nail art.

Step-by-step – a flower design

Equipment required:

- Base coat
- Pink enamel
- White and yellow paints
- Dotting tool
- Top coat

Application:

1 Apply base coat to all nails.

2 Apply pink enamel to all nails, with two applications.

3 Using the dotting tool, first apply the yellow dot for the centre of the flower, then use the dotting tool and apply the white dots for the petals.

4 Allow the paint to dry and apply top coat.

Step-by-step – self-adhesive transfers with French polish

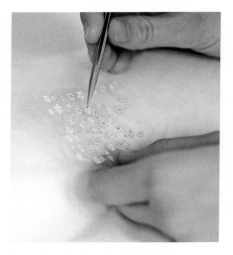

Removing the transfer carefully

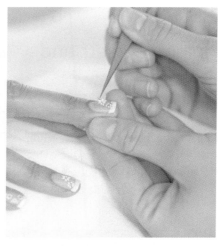

Carefully choosing the location of the transfer

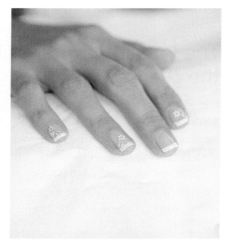

The finished result

Equipment required:

- Self-adhesive transfers
- Flat-headed tweezers
- Base coat
- French polish base and white enamels
- Top coat

Application:

1 Apply base coat.

2 Apply French polish.

3 Use tweezers to remove transfer from the backing sheet.

4 Place transfer on the nail.

5 Apply top coat once.

Step-by-step: simple striping

Equipment required:

- Base coat
- Dark enamel (black)
- Top coat
- Silver glitter paint
- White paint
- Striping brush

Application:

1 Apply base coat to all nails.

2 Apply black enamel to all nails, with two applications.

3 Use the striping brush with the silver glitter paint. Start at the left-hand side and move the brush vertically across the nail, with a quick and smooth sweeping movement, to create the middle line. Then create another two lines using the same method, one above and one below the middle line.

4 Apply two stripes of white in between the silver stripes, using the same method.

5 Once dry, apply top coat once.

Top tip

When applying water-release transfers, follow the steps for self-adhesive transfers but pre-soak the transfer in water or use a damp cotton wool bud and rub the reverse of the transfer to release it.

Water-release transfers work best on wet or tacky enamel.

Step-by-step – marbling

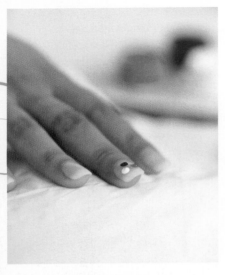

Three drops of coloured paint before marbling

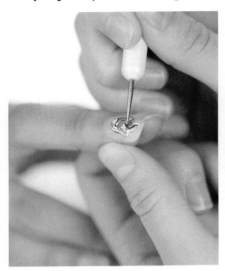

Swirling the colours together

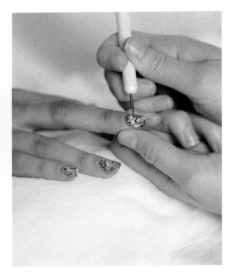

Continue swirling until final result achieved

Top tip

Coloured enamel can be used, especially if the whole nail is not having marbling, as this will create a new effect.

Top tip

The two-ended marbling tool has a large and a small ball to create different effects.

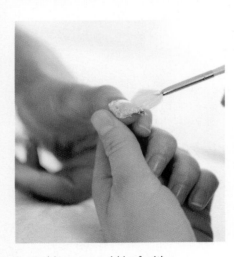

Smoothing over gold leaf with a fan brush

Equipment required:

- Base coat
- Red, white and blue paint
- Marbling tool/dotting tool
- Top coat

Application:

1 Apply base coat to all nails.

2 Using the dotting tool, apply three drops of the three coloured paints.

3 Swirl the red paint into the other colours to create a marbling effect.

4 Once the paint is dry, apply top coat once.

Step-by-step – gold leaf

Equipment required:

- Base coat
- Red enamel
- Adhesive
- Top coat
- Gold leaf
- Fan brush
- Tweezers and/or cocktail stick

Application:

1 Apply base coat to all nails.

2 Apply two coats of red enamel to all nails (leave to dry).

3 Ensure gold leaf is the correct size. Use the tweezers and a cocktail stick to pull apart.

4 Apply top coat or adhesive to the areas that require gold leaf, place the gold leaf onto the nail and smooth over with the fan brush.

5 Apply top coat once.

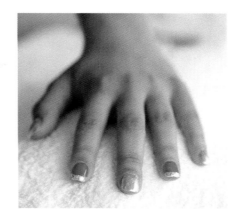

Step-by-step – a cherry design

Equipment required:

- Base coat
- White enamel
- Black paint and fine detail brush
- Green rhinestone
- Red glitter dust

- Glitter dust brush
- Dappen dish with enamel remover
- Top coat
- Orange stick

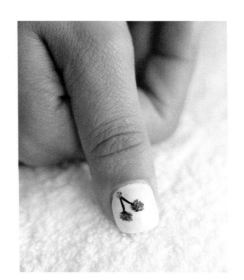

Application:

1 Apply base coat to all nails.

2 Apply two coats of white enamel to all nails (leave to dry).

3 Apply black paint with the fine detail brush to create the stalks (leave to dry).

4 Using the glitter brush, dip into the mixer and ensure a ball of the mixer forms at the tip of the brush. Load the glitter dust on the tip of the brush using a rolling action.

5 Apply the glitter to the area and then use the brush to flatten down the glitter so it does not protrude.

6 Remember to clean the glitter brush in the Dappen dish before dipping back into the mixer or glitter.

7 Apply a dot of top coat, pick up the green rhinestone with a damp orange stick and place onto the nail (see picture for location).

8 Leave to dry and apply top coat.

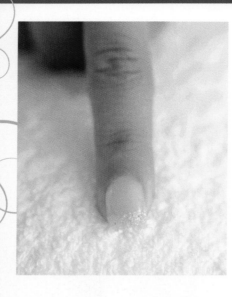

Step-by-step – a glitter-tipped free edge (funky French)

Equipment required:

- Base coat
- Top coat
- Pale pink enamel
- Pale pink glitter
- Glitter dust brush
- Dappen dish with enamel remover

Application:

1 Apply base coat to all nails.

2 Apply two coats of pale pink enamel to all nails and allow to dry.

3 Apply top coat to the free edge.

4 Using the glitter brush, dip into the mixer and ensure a ball of the mixer forms at the tip of the brush. Load the glitter dust on the tip of the brush using a rolling action.

5 Apply the glitter to the area and then use the brush to flatten down the glitter so it does not protrude.

6 Remember to clean the glitter brush in the Dappen dish before dipping back into the mixer or glitter.

7 Once the glitter is dry, apply a top coat.

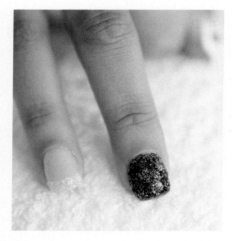

Step-by-step – a three-colour glitter effect (stained glass effect)

Equipment required:

- Base coat
- Top coat
- Green, pink and blue glitter
- Glitter dust brush
- Dappen dish with enamel remover

Application:

1 Apply base coat to all nails (allow to dry).

2 Apply dots of top coat where the green glitter will go.

3 Using the glitter brush, dip into the mixer and ensure a ball of the mixer forms at the tip of the brush. Load the green glitter dust on the tip of the brush using a rolling action.

4 Apply the green glitter to the area and then use the brush to flatten down the glitter so it does not protrude.

5 Remember to clean the glitter brush in the Dappen dish before dipping back into the mixer or glitter.

Top tip

When applying three glitter colours to the whole nail, try to keep the applications the same size and shape for a more professional effect.

6 Repeat the process with the pink glitter dust, then the blue glitter dust. This design can be enhanced by using a thin brush to paint black lines between the colours.

7 Once dry, apply a top coat.

Top tip

Use the Dappen dish with enamel remover to clean the brush if you need more glitter, to minimise cross-infection and contamination of the product.

Step-by-step – French polish with a rhinestone flower

Equipment required:

- Base coat
- French polish enamels
- Clear rhinestones
- 1 pink rhinestone
- Top coat
- Orange stick

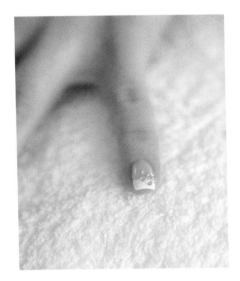

Application:

1 Apply base coat to all nails (allow to dry).

2 Apply a French polish to all nails.

3 While the polish is wet, use a damp orange stick to apply each rhinestone. Start with the pink rhinestone for the centre of the flower. Then apply clear rhinestones around to resemble the petals.

4 Apply top coat.

Step-by-step – French polish with a rhinestone curve

Equipment required:

- Base coat
- French polish enamels
- Small pink rhinestones
- 1 large clear rhinestone
- Top coat
- Orange stick

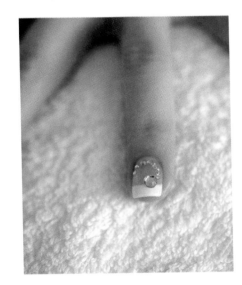

Application:

1 Apply base coat to all nails (allow to dry).

2 Apply a French polish to all nails

3 While the polish is wet, use a damp orange stick to apply each rhinestone. Start with the first pink rhinestone and create a curved line and finish with the large clear rhinestone.

4 Apply top coat.

Step-by-step – French polish with a rhinestone swirl

Equipment required:

- Base coat
- French polish enamels
- 12 small clear rhinestones
- Top coat
- Orange stick

Application:

1 Apply base coat to all nails (allow to dry).

2 Apply a French polish to all nails.

3 While the polish is wet, use a damp orange stick to apply each rhinestone. Start with the centre rhinestone and apply in a swirl finishing at the free edge.

4 Apply top coat.

Step-by-step – French polish with a line of rhinestones

Equipment required:

- Base coat
- French polish enamels
- Small clear rhinestones
- Top coat
- Orange stick

Application:

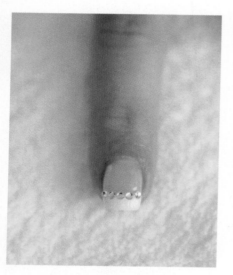

1 Apply base coat to all nails (allow to dry).

2 Apply a French polish to all nails.

3 While the polish is wet, use a damp orange stick to apply each rhinestone. Start on one side and work along the line between the free edge and the nail plate.

4 Apply top coat.

Step-by-step – French polish with rhinestones

Equipment required:

- Base coat
- French polish enamels
- Small clear rhinestones
- Small pink rhinestones
- 1 large pink rhinestone
- Top coat
- Orange stick

Application:

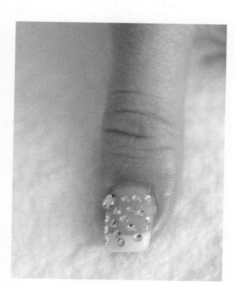

1 Apply base coat to all nails (allow to dry).

2 Apply a French polish to all nails.

3 While the polish is wet, use a damp orange stick to apply each rhinestone. Start with the large pink rhinestone.

4 Apply three lines of clear rhinestones.

5 Apply two lines of pink rhinestones.

6 Apply top coat.

How treatments can be adapted to suit the client's treatment needs and nail conditions

During a consultation you will need to establish if the client has any specific nail conditions that either prevent or restrict a nail art treatment. As long as the nail condition is not contagious and having a nail art treatment will not cause the client any discomfort or cause the condition to worsen, then an adaptation can be done. Nail art can help to disguise certain conditions, such as a bruised nail, as long as a dark polish is applied first.

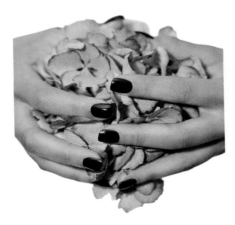

Dark enamel will disguise bruised or discoloured nails

Top tip

Try pearls as an alternative to normal rhinestones. Usually pearls protrude, which is not flattering to clients with large hands. However, there are flat-sided pearls which are more flattering and easier to apply. For a bride, pearls look especially nice with a French polish and are applied to the nail like rhinestones.

Think about it

To learn more about conditions that would not be contra-indicated completely but would have restrictions and how you could adapt a nail art treatment for each of them, see Skin analysis, page 150. This will make you more proficient when designing a treatment plan with a client.

Salon life

My story

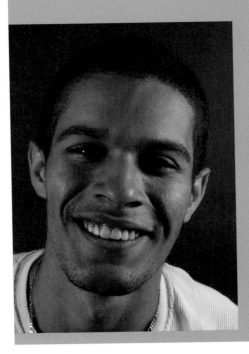

My name is Michael. I am an experienced nail technician and I work in a busy nail bar. My main area of expertise is nail art and I have created many designs, from very basic to competition work. I am especially busy with nail art at the weekend for all kinds of special occasions. One particular weekend I was to perform a luxury manicure for a bride on her wedding day, and she wanted to have a French polish finish. Unfortunately she had an accident early on in the week, trapping her finger in a piano. This had resulted in the majority of her nails being bruised. She was very upset and worried that I wouldn't be able to create the look she wanted. As some of her nails where very dark, I had to discuss her options. I decided to incorporate nail art into the treatment plan to help disguise the bruising. With a darker base coat, rhinestones and paints, I created a more modern version of the traditional French polish – it was still elegant for a bride but disguised the bruised nails.

Experiences like this make me aware that it is important to be able to be flexible and creative as you never know what problems you will need to solve to make a client happy or feel more confident about themselves.

Ask the experts

Q   What else can nail art disguise?

A   Leuconychia, onycholysis, discoloured nails, blue nails.

Q   What about ridged nails, can they have nail art?

A   Yes, but you will need to use a four-way buffer to reduce the ridges' depth first and use a ridge filler base coat.

Top Tip

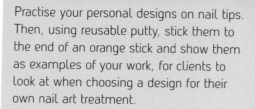

Practise your personal designs on nail tips. Then, using reusable putty, stick them to the end of an orange stick and show them as examples of your work, for clients to look at when choosing a design for their own nail art treatment.

Benefits of offering the service for the nail technician

- Excellent retail opportunity for recommending products like enamel remover, nail files, transfers, glitter and rhinestones.
- Repeat business, recommending and booking in clients for their follow-up treatments and promoting additional services.
- Can be a promotional offer alongside other treatments such as manicure, pedicure or extensions.
- Can be promoted for special events like parties, weddings, school leavers' proms, children's parties.

Benefits of the treatment/service for the client

- Hides any nail imperfections.
- Adds colour, texture and style.
- Improves the appearance of the nails, feet and hands.
- Demonstrates the latest enamelling techniques – for example the funky French enamel.
- Provides individual treatment plans.

Frequently asked questions

Q   During a manicure or pedicure treatment when would I apply nail art?

A   At the end of the treatment when you would normally enamel, just apply the chosen nail art.

Q   When starting out, what nail art should I buy?

A   Usually you can purchase a nail art starter kit from your place of study or your local wholesaler.

Q   How do I get rhinestones to stick to the nail?

A   Use dots of top coat or gel bond on the nail plate to fix them into place.

Q   How do I create a dramatic effect when marbling?

A   Use contrasting colours and do not overblend colours.

Contra-actions that may occur during and following services and how to respond

A **contra-action** is a reaction that has occurred from a treatment being performed and affected the area that has been treated. It could include an adverse reaction, known as an allergic reaction, where the skin and nail become red, swollen and itchy, with blisters. A contra-action could also occur if a treatment was not correctly performed and health and safety procedures were not followed, for example if a nail technician removed too much cuticle or incorrectly removed the client's cuticle, tearing/cutting the skin and causing the area to bleed (see also Provide manicure and pedicure treatments, page 191).

It is important that you inform the client of what to do should they suffer from a contra-action after the treatment. They must:

- remove products immediately and apply a cold compress
- remove any enamel applied with enamel remover on a cotton pad – they should not pick it off with their nails
- if irritation persists, see their GP
- inform the nail technician so it can be documented on the record card.

The importance of completing the treatment to the satisfaction of the client

The way to ensure a client is completely satisfied with a nail treatment is to make sure that when performing the treatment you demonstrate excellent subject knowledge and experience. You will need to have first-rate verbal and non-verbal communication skills to find out all the information needed to create a detailed and individual treatment plan and to ensure the client feels comfortable during the treatment and confident of your abilities. To learn more about the importance of client feedback, see Client care and communication in beauty-related industries, page 47.

The importance of completing treatment records

By law, a nail technician must complete detailed record cards for each client and follow the Data Protection Act 1998, which sets out eight principles that businesses must follow when handling information. To learn more about maintaining confidentiality in line with the act, see Client care and communication in beauty-related industries, page 44.

Aftercare advice

Aftercare and maintenance

After time spent preparing the nails and designing beautiful works of art, it is important to emphasise aftercare advice to the client and ensure they understand

Key term

Contra-action – an allergic reaction to any aspect of the treatment. The skin may appear red, swollen and itchy.

Top tip

When you are discussing aftercare advice always remember to inform the client of what to do in the event of a contra-action occurring after they have left the salon, as they could have a severe allergic reaction and require medical attention.

Think about it

Create a short survey or questionnaire that your clients can complete (anonymously) after a treatment to provide you with honest and constructive feedback on your performance. This will help you to perfect your treatments and support successful assessments in the future.

Top tip

What might feel like harmless chatter with others about a client's personal information is actually against the Data Protection Act and subject to the law's penalties.

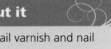

how to protect and prolong the life of the nail art. Advise the client how to care for their nails but not how to do nail art — there is a difference, as you will want the client to return for further treatments. By offering good aftercare advice, your work will last longer and you will have a satisfied client.

Below are some basic aftercare and homecare rules that the client must adhere to so as to preserve the life of the nail art.

- Protect your nails by wearing gloves whenever possible, for example when gardening, doing housework or having your hands exposed to water for prolonged periods of time.

- Apply a sealer every two days to prevent chipping of the nail art or top coat and to prevent yellowing if you have a French manicure. Always recommend the client purchases a sealer to use at home.

- Apply cuticle oil daily to keep the cuticles supple and nourish the natural nails.

- Do not use the nails as tools.

- Avoid picking at the nail art.

- Attend the salon for regular appointments to ensure nails stay looking at their best. Advise the client to return to the salon every two weeks to maintain the designs, but keep in mind the client's occupation because that could determine how quickly the nails will chip and therefore the client may need to return to the salon for maintenance more often than every two weeks.

For basic care of the nails, refer to Provide manicure and pedicure treatments, page 191.

Removal of nail art

It is always advisable to visit the salon every couple of weeks to maintain the nail art and keep it at its best, but if the client discovers the nail designs are beginning to chip and look untidy it may need to be removed at home. Where the designs include varnish, foiling, gold/silver leaf, glitter or transfers, wipe the nails over with a non-acetone varnish remover to remove all products. Where the design consists of marbling or paints, wipe over the nail with a wet wipe or damp cotton wool bud to remove all traces. On occasion, the nail technician might have secured rhinestones to the nail with a minute amount of glue, so if that is the case, remove the polish with non-acetone remover. Then soak the nails in warm water for a few minutes to soften the glue and wipe over again to ensure all is removed. If the nail design consists of foils or tape, remove any polish and peel off the foils/tape with tweezers.

Top tip

If the client follows all the aftercare and maintenance advice given, accidental damage should be limited. Unfortunately, accidents do happen, so it is advisable for the client to contact the nail technician to repair any damage to the nail art designs rather than attempting to repair any damage themselves, which could make it worse.

Think about it

To remove all nail varnish and nail art, the client should use a non-acetone nail varnish remover to prevent dehydration to the nails and damage to nail extensions. A poor-quality nail varnish remover is simply a paint stripper that will remove the micro-organisms that are present on healthy nails.

Check your knowledge

1. What are the different ways glitter can be applied to the nails?

2. How do you clean a glitter dust brush?

3. What tool or brush can create dots or a marbling effect?

4. What enamel creates a flat-looking finish?
   a) Cream
   b) Frosted
   c) Matt
   d) Opalescent

5. What can you use to practise nail art designs on?

6. What brush creates thin lines?
   a) Liner brush
   b) Striping brush
   c) Flat brush
   d) Fan brush

7. What effect is created when two or more paints are mixed together on the nail plate?
   a) Marbling
   b) Striping
   c) Embossing

8. What is glitter dust applied with?
   a) Mixer
   b) Enamel
   c) Base coat

9. What effects are created by a syringe-like tool?

10. They are various sizes, shapes and colours. They can be made of glass, crystal or plastic. They have a 3D effect, are light-reflective and shiny. What is being described?
    a) Flatstones
    b) Pearls
    c) Rhinestones

Getting ready for assessment

Nail art is differently assessed in VRQs and NVQs, using a combination of assessment methods, as specified below. You cannot simulate any practical assessment but you must be aware of the criteria and be proactive during practical sessions to cluster assessments for more than one unit at a time.

City & Guilds		VTCT	
NVQ	**VRQ**	**NVQ**	**VRQ**
Service times: No service times for this unit	Service times: Not applicable to this qualification	Service times: Nail art 30mins	Service times: There are no maximum service times that apply to this unit
Evidence: • should be gathered in a realistic working environment, and simulation avoided • You must demonstrate that you have met the required standard for all the outcomes, assessment criteria/skills and ranges	Evidence: • You can take either the online test or complete knowledge tasks in the assignments • There is no particular time limit set for the completion of an assignment (tasks) • Assignment is graded pass, merit or distinction • GOLA online tests are pass or fail • Practical tasks are graded pass, merit or distinction • 2 Pre observation must be completed (each with a treatment plan), before the final observation • Final observation – the nail art design must be carried out on a minimum of one nail on each hand/foot	Evidence: • It is strongly recommended that the evidence for this unit be gathered in a realistic working environment • Simulation should be avoided where possible. • You must practically demonstrate that you have met the required standard for this unit • All outcomes, assessment criteria and range statements must be achieved • Your performance will be observed on at least four occasions for each assessment criteria	Evidence: • It is strongly recommended that the evidence for this unit be gathered in a realistic working environment • Simulation should be avoided where possible • You must practically demonstrate that you have met the required standard for this unit • All outcomes, assessment criteria and range statements must be achieved • Your performance will be observed on at least three occasions for each assessment criteria
Knowledge and understanding will be assessed by: • a mandatory written question paper • oral questioning Written and oral questions can also be done as a GOLA online test. • Practical assessment • Completion of an assessment book/portfolio	Knowledge and understanding will be assessed by: • knowledge tasks or an online GOLA test	Knowledge and understanding will be assessed by: • internally assessed workplace performance using a variety of methods • a mandatory written question paper. These questions are set and marked by VTCT	Knowledge and understanding will be assessed by: • mandatory written question paper • oral questioning • portfolio of evidence

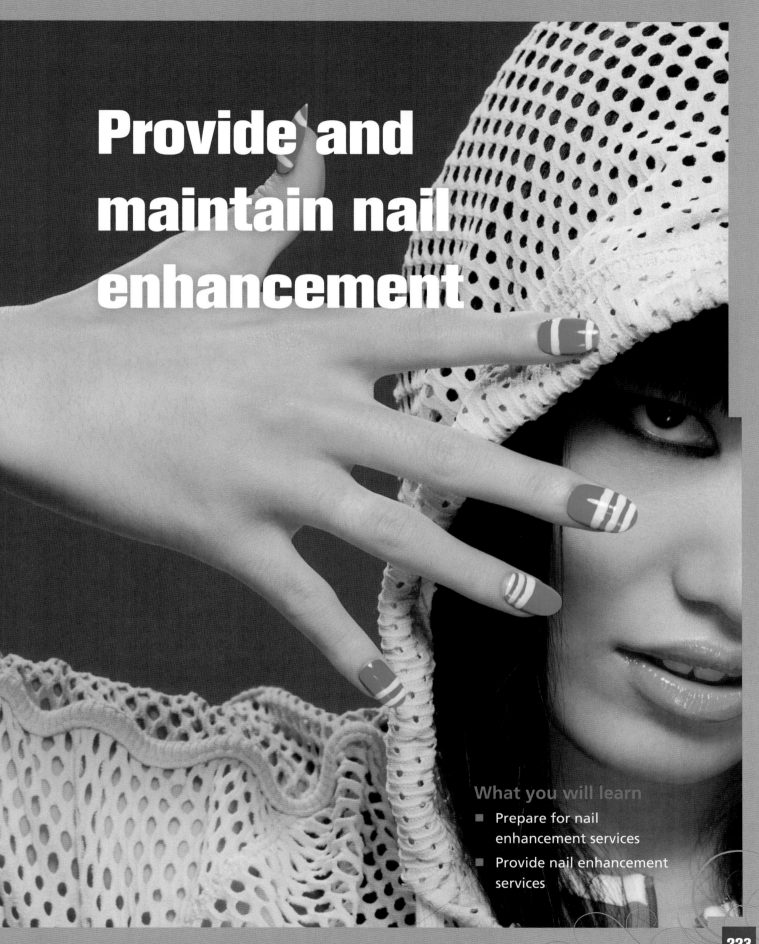

Provide and maintain nail enhancement

Introduction

Artificial nail enhancements are now well-established and popular treatments within the beauty industry. The demand for skilled and qualified nail technicians able to offer this service is increasing, with many nail bars and salons specialising in these treatments alone.

Nail enhancements have an instant visual effect, improving the appearance of the client's hands and allowing them to create the perfect look to finish off a well-groomed image. They are no longer seen as the luxury treatment that they once were. Clients can feel confident about their hands rather than hiding bitten or broken fingernails. The treatment allows the nail technician to increase the length and shape of the natural nail.

In this unit, you will learn how to prepare for nail enhancement services and the application of many methods used within nail technology such as tip and **overlay**, natural nail overlay and sculpt application. It also covers the knowledge and skills you will need in order to be able to apply all nail enhancement systems, including **liquid and powder**, **UV gel** and **fibreglass and silk** wraps. This will enable you, through consultation, to identify the most suitable treatment and nail enhancement system for each client.

Nail enhancements will grow out along with the natural nail situated below. It is therefore important that clients have regular maintenance treatments to ensure their nail enhancements continue to look perfect. If applied and removed correctly and safely, nail enhancements will give the client the desired look without causing damage to their natural nails. The aftercare advice and recommendations that you give the client will also support this.

Key terms

Overlay – a thin coating applied to the natural nail or application over the natural nail tip.

Liquid and powder – the two products that are mixed together to form a strong and durable enhancement system. (For more information, see page 232.)

UV gel – thick gel that is cured into a hard, durable, flexible enhancement using a UV (ultraviolet) curing lamp.

Fibreglass and silk – the strong durable fabrics used in the wrap system.

Think about it

MMA is a big problem in the nails industry. You should educate your clients on the implications of using 'cheap' nail enhancements.

Ban on MMA

Methyl methacrylate (MMA) used with acrylic systems has been banned in the USA, where it was declared to be a poisonous and harmful substance when used on fingernails. Many local authorities within the UK have also banned its use. Responsible manufacturers and salons have switched their clients over to ethyl methacrylate (EMA), a more expensive and safer bonding liquid.

Before you can give a client a nail enhancement treatment, you must be familiar with the Code of Practice for Nail Services produced by Habia, the body that sets the standards for the UK nail industry. These guidelines are designed to protect both the nail technician and the client during and after treatment.

Nail enhancement offers benefits for the client:

- It improves the appearance of the client's hands.
- It enhances the nail appearance with a longer length and an even shape.

- It has an instant visual effect – beautiful, perfect nails.
- It can improve the client's confidence and sense of well-being.

Nail enhancement also offers benefits for the salon:

- It is a regular salon service, ensuring return trips for maintenance.
- It offers an opportunity to sell new products to the client.
- It enhances the reputation of the salon.

Prepare for nail enhancement services

In this section, you will learn about how to prepare yourself, the client and work area for nail enhancement services. This will involve carrying out a consultation and a nail and skin analysis so that you can identify treatment objectives and make recommendations to the client. You will learn which products, tools and equipment to select to suit your client's needs, skin type and nail condition.

Salon requirements for preparing yourself, the client and the work area

It is important to fully prepare for each treatment. This will allow you to concentrate on delivering the best service to each client.

Preparing yourself

You will need to ensure that your personal appearance meets the Code of Practice for Nail Services and your salon's requirements. (To learn more about personal presentation, see Follow health and safety practice in the salon, page 17.)

Both you and the client should also wear suitable personal protective equipment (PPE), as shown below.

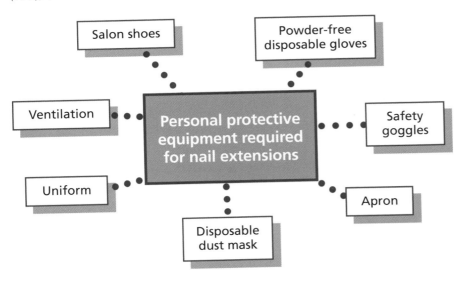

Top tip

Always **sanitise** your hands prior to providing a nail service. Use antibacterial soaps, washes, gels or wipes to disinfect your hands regularly. This will minimise the risk of cross-infection and contamination.

Key term

Sanitise – remove dirt and germs.

Think about it

PPE is there to protect both the nail technician and client. Be sure to choose the relevant PPE for each treatment.

Top tips

- When using liquids and powders always keep the products in **Dappen dishes** with metal lids – this will reduce the odour in the salon. Replace the lids on the pots as soon as you have finished using the product.

- Dispose of liquid-drenched paper roll in a sealed bin liner which is placed in a metal bin with a lid.

Key term

Dappen dish – a small container used to hold liquid products while working.

Top tip

To prevent cross-infection, spray files and buffers and autoclave all metal tools between clients. Where possible, you can bag up a client's files and buffers in a bag with their name on it and this can be kept in a drawer for their use only.

Key term

Cut-out technique – only taking the amount of product required for the treatment using a pump, spatula or spray.

Use of PPE will help to maintain hygiene practices within the salon and minimise cross-infection. The Code of Practice for Nail Services stipulates that certain PPE must be used during treatment. This includes the use of safely goggles while cutting artificial tips and dust masks when filing nail enhancements. To learn more about PPE, see Follow health and safety practice in the salon, pages 7 and 16.

Preparing the client

Once in the treatment area, ask the client to wash their hands and place the client's jewellery in a lined bowl on the desk so that it can be seen. Ensure the client is positioned correctly and comfortably in a chair without wheels. To learn more about the importance of health and safety as part of client preparation, see Follow health and safety practice in the salon, page 19.

Preparing equipment, tools and the work area

Preparing the work area before each treatment will eliminate distractions, prevent the service from overrunning and ensure that it is cost-effective. You will need to place equipment within reach so that you can work at a constant, steady pace.

Set everything up neatly on the nail station. Place clean, sterilised tools and equipment into a sterile bowl or jar containing surgical spirit. Once these have been used, return them to the bowl so that they can be sterilised at the end of the treatment ready for the next client.

Plan ahead where possible for each client by arranging the required products. Use a covered, lined bin for all rubbish, which should be disposed of safely and correctly after the treatment. This will ensure that you follow health and safety regulations. Remember to keep any chemical fumes covered.

Clean and sterilise tools

Disinfect and sterilise tools and the work area prior to and after treatment. This will eliminate the possibility of cross-infection. It is important to be aware of the possible consequences if cross-infection occurs within the salon. Infecting a client through the use of dirty, unsterilised tools or equipment will lead to an unhappy, dissatisfied customer. As word of mouth of their bad experience spreads, other clients may seek treatment elsewhere, the salon's reputation will be damaged and its revenue will be affected. In extreme cases, the salon may be forced to close and could be prosecuted.

There are many types of sterilisation that can be used to maintain equipment. For example, the autoclave is an excellent method that can be used to sterilise metal tools. To learn more about sterilisation equipment and how to use an autoclave, see Following health and safety practice in the salon, page 23.

Provide clean towels and prepare products

Clean towels, which have been freshly laundered at 60°C, should be supplied for each client.

When preparing products for treatment, ensure that you minimise waste by using the **cut-out technique**. It will be cost-effective and with little or no product left over, it will be quicker and easier to clean away at the end of the treatment.

Environmental conditions suitable for nail enhancement services

Lighting

Good lighting is very important as it will enable you to carry out an effective treatment. It will ensure that the area for treatment can be seen clearly. Nail preparation and intricate nail work can cause eye strain for the technician, resulting in long-term problems. Poor lighting may cause you to squint in order to see the treatment area. Daylight will allow colours to be seen clearly. This is vital when working with coloured products or for camouflage work on damaged and bitten nails. To learn more about suitable environmental conditions, see *Provide manicure and pedicure treatments, page 166.*

Overexposure to chemicals – symptoms and prevention

As a nail technician, you will work with chemicals. Many people associate chemicals with something that is bad for them, but the chemicals used and worked with in the nail industry are safe if they are understood and treated with respect. It is important to follow strict guidelines and rules when using, storing and transporting nail products.

You will need to be aware of the dangers of overexposure to products and chemicals and must ensure that every precaution is taken to prevent this from occurring. Every chemical has safe and unsafe levels of exposure – exceeding the safe level will result in overexposure. Overexposure can occur at any time and with any chemical. The most common symptoms of overexposure are skin irritation, headaches, sickness, dizziness, fainting and itchy, watery eyes.

There are three ways a chemical can enter the body:

- Ingestion – accidentally consuming chemicals via the mouth. This can easily happen if the client is allowed to eat and drink at the nail station. Hot drinks attract the vapours from nail products and dust can easily be transferred on to food from hands.

- Inhalation – breathing in fine dust and vapours. The quality of air in the salon must be maintained through using ventilation both in the salon and at the nail station. Face masks may be worn to prevent unnecessary inhalation.

- Absorption – through the skin or cuts and abrasions. Avoid contact with the skin when using nail products and cover any open cuts on both the nail technician and the client.

Material Safety Data Sheets (**MSDS**) provide chemical information on each product, including:

- all potentially hazardous ingredients in the product

- information to help you avoid potential hazards

- how to correctly handle and store products

- how to prevent fires, falls, burns and other accidents

- warning signs of overexposure.

Key term

MSDS – stands for Material Safety Data Sheets.

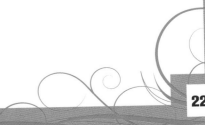

Top tips

Before the treatment, check that:

- the nail station is clean

- all products on the nail station are correctly labelled, with lids on

- required products are within easy reach

- tools are sterilised and placed in surgical spirit during service

- the nail station is on a stable surface

- clean towels are covered by paper roll to catch dust filings.

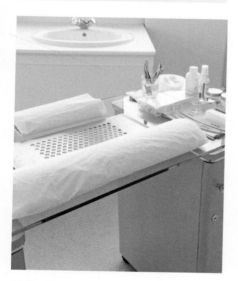

Nail station set-up

Top tip

Always complete a client record card during a consultation. This will ensure you have the client's details at hand and you can record important information; i.e. items bought or colour of polish used. It will also mean another nail technician can service the client if you are ill.

You can acquire these sheets by requesting them from the product supplier. They will be needed when carrying out risk assessments for the salon.

Ventilation

Ventilation is extremely important for your safety. Where ventilation is supplied, it is essential to use it and not to cover it with equipment at the nail station. Ventilation filters must be changed regularly, following the manufacturer's guidelines. A dust extractor can be fitted to the nail desk. These units act like extractor fans, creating a light suction that draws dust from filing through a grille in the top of the desk and into a collection bag or unit. This can then be disposed of regularly. An efficient unit can remove almost all the dust before it disperses into the air.

If ventilation is not used, you may become susceptible to respiratory problems such as asthma and bronchitis, which can be caused by continual exposure to hazardous dust and vapours. Correct ventilation will also protect technicians and clients who wear contact lenses by removing dust from the atmosphere.

Consultation techniques used to identify treatment objectives

The client's needs, including their expectations, preference and the occasion, will ultimately influence their choice of service when booking an appointment. The consultation with the nail technician will determine the system to be used and enable the client to understand the reasons for the system chosen.

Cleansing the treatment area

As part of the consultation, you will need to cleanse the treatment area, removing any existing nail polish or nail enhancements, to restore the nails to a natural condition. This will help you to identify the condition of the nails and skin.

Identifying the condition of skin and nails

The condition of the treatment area must be identified and recorded as part of the consultation. The nails and skin should be analysed by questioning the client. Identifying their occupation, lifestyle and nail and skincare routine will enable you to begin to put together an understanding of the client's requirements. By visually analysing and manually examining the treatment area, you will be able to recommend the correct nail enhancement system for the client at the time of treatment and explain to them the reasons for your choice. As the client returns for further treatment, the condition of the nails and skin may alter and so the treatment may need to be changed, depending on the conclusions you come to during the consultation. For this reason, it is important that a consultation is carried out each time the client returns to the salon, as the treatment requirements will vary.

Preparing the client's service plan

When preparing a service plan, you will need to take into consideration the following factors:

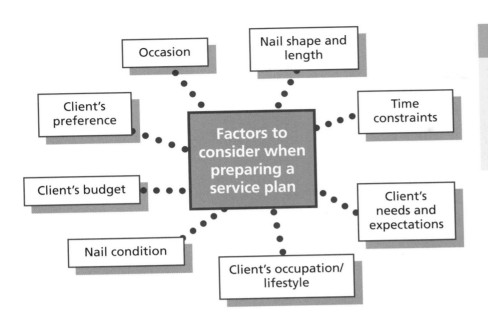

Occasion

Nail shape and length

Client's preference

Time constraints

Factors to consider when preparing a service plan

Client's budget

Client's needs and expectations

Nail condition

Client's occupation/ lifestyle

Top tip

Use a friendly and polite manner when questioning the client. Keep eye contact and show positive body language. Remember to accurately record their responses to your questions.

Obtaining written consent

To complete the consultation, it is vital that you obtain signed, written consent from the client prior to the service. This will confirm the agreement between the client and salon that the service plan outlined will be carried out. It shows that the client understands and consents to the service. Signed consent is required for legal reasons and demonstrates a **duty of care** on the part of the salon and nail technician. As the technician, you will also need to sign the form. Some insurance cover may become invalid if consent is not agreed and signed.

Minors should not be given any nail services without informed or signed parental or guardian consent. If you carry out a treatment on a minor without consent, both the salon and nail technician can be prosecuted as it is illegal. You will also need to have a parent or guardian present during a nail service on a minor. Insurance to carry out the service may be invalidated without the parent or guardian present.

Key terms

Duty of care – a responsibility to ensure that someone does not suffer harm or loss.

Minors – in Scotland a minor is classed as under the age of 16. In England, Wales and Northern Ireland a minor is someone under the age of 18. All minors require parental consent.

How to select products, tools and equipment to suit client treatment needs, and skin and nail conditions

Each of the three systems available – liquid and powder, UV gel and wraps – has their own advantages and disadvantages, as shown in the following table. It is important that the correct product and application is chosen, and you will need to explain clearly to the client why a particular system should be used. Clients will come to the salon with their own ideas and preferences. A product such as liquid and powder (acrylic) is very popular, as it is a well-known system. However, this does not always mean that it is the correct one for the client. For example, length will not be achieved if a natural nail overlay is recommended and carried out. The nail technician makes a professional recommendation for a service and it is up to the client whether or not they agree to have it done.

Top tip

Encourage clients to ask questions so that you can clarify anything they may not understand. This will help to avoid the client having unrealistic expectations.

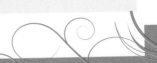

Nail enhancement product	Advantages	Disadvantages
Liquid and powder (acrylic)	• Best-known system and popular choice • Sculpting and tip application is possible • Strongest overlay available • Excellent product for nail-biters • Many colours available with a variety of finishes • Permanent French finish is available • A creative product, enabling many nail art techniques including 3D and embedding • Product can be soaked off rather than buffed off • Can correct irregular natural nail shapes	• Very strong odour • Difficult system to master • Natural nail overlays not commonly applied using this system • The product sets quickly, not allowing much time to perfect application • Some brands require a primer • Completely cured after 48 hours • Some liquid and powder overlays may discolour
UV gel	• Has a high gloss finish • Many colours available with a variety of finishes • Permanent French finish is available • Low odour system • Sculpting application is possible as well as tip application and natural nail overlays • Creates a more flexible artificial nail with medium strength • A natural look can be achieved • Easier system to apply	• Not as strong as acrylic • Leaves a sticky residue – but this can be wiped away • Requires a UV lamp to cure • Difficult to remove with buffing required, although some gels are now removable with acetone • Overexposure can occur if not fully cured • Some gels create a heat sensation when curing under the UV lamp – this may cause client discomfort on the nail plate
Wraps (fibreglass and silk)	• Excellent system for repairing natural nails • Creates very natural-looking, thin and flexible nails with low strength • Minimum odour system • Most gentle system on the natural nail • Quick and easy system to remove, with little damage to the natural nail	• No colour choice available • Sculpting is not generally carried out • Cannot correct irregular nail shapes • Cyanoacrylate resin vapours may cause eye problems • Spray activators may cause problems on sensitive skins • Cannot build structure

Nail enhancement products – advantages and disadvantages

Nail shape, length and condition

The client's nail shape, length and condition will determine the product used. Recommending the most suitable nail enhancements to suit the client's nail shape and condition is vital to finding a system that will give the client the best results possible. To be able to competently recommend a system, you must have knowledge and an understanding of the three systems available. These are shown in the table below.

Nail enhancement product	Nail enhancement application
Liquid and powder	Tip and overlay Sculpt artificial nails
UV gel	Natural nail overlays Tip and overlay Sculpt artificial nails
Wraps (fibreglass and silk)	Natural nail overlays Tip and overlay Natural nail repair

Nail enhancement applications

Salon Life

My Story

My name is Madeleine and I have been a nail technician for six years. A few months ago a woman came into the salon and told me she had been turned away from two other salons because her nails were too short. These salons advised her to go away and grow her nails. She did indeed have severely bitten nails, but I rose to the challenge. The first thing I did was carry out a full consultation. I discovered my client was due to get married in six months and was desperate to have beautiful nails. Together we put together a treatment plan. It began with a luxury manicure including some cuticle work.

Two weeks later, I created some false nail beds using a masque powder, which gave her instant length on her nail beds. This makes the nail beds a very natural pink colour. Then I was able to apply a lovely set of short tips with a fibreglass overlay. My client was ecstatic! For the first time in her life she had beautiful nails.

She returned every two weeks for maintenance and in no time her nails grew to a decent length and she managed to kick the nail-biting habit. She had beautiful nails for her special day, and I had another happy and loyal client. You never need to turn anyone away from your salon. There is always something you can do to help.

Benefits of offering the service for the nail technician

- Word of mouth and good for salon reputation
- Increases profit and sales
- Will improve technician's speed and techniques
- Builds a good relationship/rapport with client
- Provides an opportunity to give aftercare advice
- Promotes personal and professional development
- Develops communication skills
- Adds experience to your CV and makes you more employable
- Makes technician more valuable to the salon
- Builds a good name for the industry

Benefits of the treatment for the client

- Makes client more comfortable with technician
- Improves overall look of client's hands
- Improves client's confidence
- Promotes the client's feel-good factor
- Relaxing and therapeutic experience
- Will not need to do much to nails in between visits
- Enjoys a professional service
- Something to tell friends about

Ask the experts

Q What is acrylic masque powder?

A This is a pink powder that allows you to create a false nail bed to which you can apply tips or sculpt nails.

Q How long will it take me to create a set of false nail beds?

A Approximately 30 minutes.

Q Will acrylic nail enhancements be suitable for a holiday in a warm country?

A Yes of course, you can do everything you normally would in your day-to-day life.

Top Tip

Never turn a client away – there is always something you can do to help and in return your client will be loyal to you and your salon.

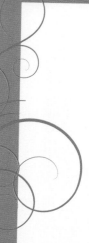

A client with long, natural nails that have a tendency to break will be an excellent candidate for a natural nail overlay. The choice of colour could be the reason that UV gel is chosen over wraps. If, on the other hand, the client finds that their nails split, chip and break, the technician may recommend that wraps are applied as the fabric — silk or fibreglass — will securely keep the nail from splitting further. A client with bitten nails or irregular nail shapes should be recommended liquid and powder as a system. It is the strongest product and has the ability to correct irregular nail shapes and cover imperfections. UV gel should be recommended to clients who wish to have an element of flexibility and a more natural-looking finish.

Occupation and lifestyle

The client's occupation and lifestyle will influence the service chosen. You will need to use questioning techniques to understand this information. Clients who work with their hands a lot should be recommended acrylic, as it is the strongest system. People who work in the medical industry may be limited to the length and colour applied, so you might recommend an overlay to add strength rather than tips adding length. As UV gel is a non-porous product, it is excellent for clients who constantly have their hands in water or for those clients having nail enhancements applied for a special occasion such as a beach holiday. UV gel does not allow water to penetrate like the other systems, so will not lift as easily. A younger client whose nails are still developing should be recommended a product such as wraps, as this system will be much kinder to the natural nail.

Budget and time constraints

The client's budget and time constraints must be taken into account when recommending a service. You will need to discuss the salon's pricing structure, as well as homecare and future recommended services, as this will enable the client to decide whether or not to maintain the enhancements.

The chemical process involved in the nail enhancement system

All nail enhancement products are based on the same chemical family — acrylic. Acrylic has been used for extending nails for many years. It can be used to sculpt nails or for overlaying a tip. There are three main systems, which are described below.

Liquid and powder system

The liquid part of the liquid and powder system is referred to as **monomer**, although there are other complex elements that make up the liquid part. The powder part of the system is a mixture of **polymers** and **copolymers**. It contains the **initiator** and colourants. The powders are available in an array of colours, which makes the system extremely versatile.

Nail enhancement products also require **accelerators**, initiators, **catalysts** and **energy** in order to work properly.

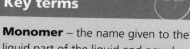

Key terms

Monomer – the name given to the liquid part of the liquid and powder system. Mono means 'one' and mer means 'unit', so a monomer is one part or a single unit of a polymer.

Polymer – a long chain of monomers (poly means 'many'). Polymers can be liquids, but in the nail industry they are usually in solid (powder) form.

Copolymer – polymer made up of two or more types of monomer.

Accelerator – the ingredient that speeds up the setting time of the resin.

Initiator – the ingredient that sets off the reaction, present within the polymer.

Catalyst – chemical that speeds up or slows down a chemical reaction.

Energy – produced in the form of heat, it helps to set the resin.

Polymerisation

Polymerisation is the setting that takes place in all nail enhancement systems, for example when a monomer liquid and polymer powder are mixed together. To start this reaction an initiator is needed and to control the reaction a catalyst is required.

A selection of products for acrylic nails

Primers

Primers are used in many ways. Wood primers prepare wood for the application of paint.
Natural nail primers are used to promote adhesion of nail enhancement services. They act as anchors, similar to double-sided sticky tape. The primer works by creating two bonds: one with the keratin in the natural nail and another that develops through a chemical bond, known as a covalent bond, which links the primer to the nail enhancement.

> **Top tip**
>
> Use primer with caution and avoid contact with the skin, as some primers are very corrosive to the skin and may cause burns.

Brushes

The brush is the most important tool a technician uses. Each nail technician will have a personal preference for the size and shape of the brush they use. The brush is divided into three sections:

- tip — used to pick up the powder and liquid
- barrel or belly — the firmest part of the brush, with a reservoir that holds and dispenses the liquid
- ferrule — the strongest part of the brush, which can withstand firm pressure.

Brushes come in many different shapes and sizes. The smaller the belly, the less liquid it will pick up and so it will only allow you to create smaller beads of acrylic. Avoid handling the bristles of the brush with your fingers and always use a tissue. Never pluck the stray hairs from your brush. Use scissors and cut hairs at the base to avoid the brush falling apart.

> **Top tip**
>
> Store your brush in its original tube to keep the bristles in shape and prevent them becoming damaged. Lie it flat in a drawer to avoid liquid collecting in the area that glues the brush bristles.

> **Key term**
>
> **Oligomer** – short, pre-formed chain of individual monomers. They make the gel harden under UV light.

UV gel system

UV gel is easy to apply and is low in odour compared with other nail systems. Gels are part of the acrylic family and have the same properties as the liquid and powder system. UV gel is semi-liquid and is known as an **oligomer**.

There are different types of gel available, with the main two differences being the viscosity (thickness) and colour of the gel. Low-viscosity gels are used in many thin layers to create strength to a natural nail overlay or over a nail tip. The more viscous gels can be applied using fewer layers. Different brands offer different viscosities, depending on how the product company wishes the application to be carried out.

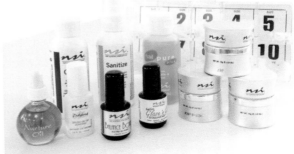

A selection of products for gel nails

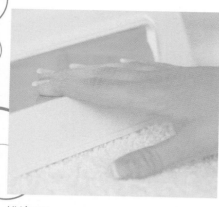

UV lamp

Provide and maintain nail enhancement

Key term

Wattage – a measure of power.

Top tip

Follow the manufacturer's instructions to maintain and prolong the life of your brush.

Top tip

Avoid handling the fabric, as the natural oil on your fingers will prevent the fabric from adhering to the nail plate.

Oligomers

An oligomer is a short, pre-formed chain of individual monomers — because of this it takes less time for the gel enhancement to reach full cure time. When the UV gel is exposed to the energy of ultraviolet (UV) light the polymerisation process begins immediately. The oligomers rush around at great speed linking up with each other. This causes an exothermic reaction, which is a chemical reaction that gives off heat. Gels need UV energy to cure or set the product. UV gels can only be 99 per cent cured; the remaining 1 per cent is left as a sticky residue which must be wiped off at the end of the treatment.

UV lamp

Not all UV lamps are the same. Gel products are formulated to work with the UV lamp for that system or brand. They each require a particular **wattage** to allow the curing process to fully develop. UV lamps must be maintained to a high standard and bulbs replaced every 4–6 months.

Brush

Like liquid and powder, the gel is applied using a brush. There are many types of brush on the market for the application of gel. These tend to be much flatter than acrylic brushes and are mainly made from synthetic products rather than real hair.

Wraps (fibreglass and silk) system

Fabric mesh is used to provide a cross-linked structure and to give the overlay strength and reinforcement. There are two types of fabric:

- fibreglass
- silk.

The one you use is a matter of personal preference. The mesh is supplied either as strips that are cut using special scissors (stork scissors) to the width of the nail or in pre-cut fingers. Some have an adhesive backing, which makes them easier to apply.

Fibreglass

This is fibre with high glass content. It is the stronger of the two meshes, as the glass remains untouched by the resin as a linked structure but can be more difficult to wet than silk.

China silk

This is a very fine mesh of natural silk fibres. It reinforces the structure — the resin soaks into the fibres and the silk becomes an integral part of the resin. It is easier to wet than fibreglass.

Resin

Ethyl cyanoacrylate is the resin or liquid adhesive used in all wrap systems. The liquid encases the fabric and has little strength without it. It is used to wet the fibre so that it cannot be seen and then is built up to an overlay. Also available in brush-on.

Resin activator

Resin activators are used to cure or dry the resin quickly and are available either as a spray or brush-on activator.

Without an activator, the resin will take about 15 minutes to dry. The result will be pliable, peel off easily and not give a good finish. Therefore, an activator must be used to produce a strong overlay. The spray activator must be used at least 15–25 centimetres from the nail. Good ventilation must be available to ensure that the activator does not get into the air.

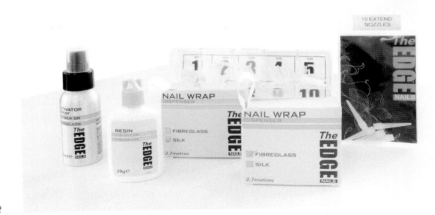

Products for fibreglass/silk nails

Nail and skin analysis and conditions

To learn more about:

● the importance of nail and skin analysis

● nail and skin conditions

● diseases and disorders of the nail and skin

see the unit on Skin analysis on page 147.

Contra-indications preventing or restricting nail enhancement treatments

Contra-indications are divided into two categories: those which contra-indicate or prevent the service and those that restrict the service. During the consultation, you will need to question the client in order to establish if any contra-indications are present, as this will impact on whether the service can be carried out. To learn how to identify contra-indications, see Skin analysis, page 150.

If a contra-indication that prevents treatment is present, it may be necessary to refuse the client the nail enhancement service and refer them to their GP. If possible, offer the client a suitable alternative. It is vital that the safest service possible is offered that also meets the client's needs. It is important also to identify any allergies at this stage so that you know which products to avoid.

It may be that you can adapt or modify the service, which will allow the client to receive the treatment if a contra-indication that restricts is present. The client must be consulted and agree on the service plan prior to the service application.

> **Key term**
>
> **Contra-indication** – reason why a treatment may or may not be carried out, with or without modification of treatment.

> **Top tip**
>
> Avoid nail enhancement treatments where the client has onycholysis, or nail separation, as this could make the condition worse.

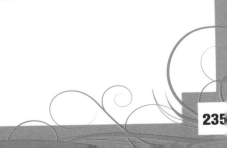

Bitten nails

Severely bitten nails are regularly presented to nail technicians. They are very short nail plates with the free edge bitten away and left with uneven edges. Due to the free edge having been bitten and removed, the skin at the fingertips will have become bulbous without the pressure of the nail plate pushing it down. The nails will look neglected with dry, rough, torn and overgrown cuticles present. The fingertips can be very red and angry-looking, and may be very painful. If this is the case, it may be advisable to recommend to the client that they have a series of manicure treatments prior to nail enhancements being applied.

Where nails are badly bitten, nail enhancements may not last as long as there may not be enough surface area present for the nail tip to stick to and it is difficult to achieve a balanced structure. Allowing the nail to grow a little prior to treatment will ensure that the nail can have a little length without it being too top-heavy on the free edge and falling off. It may also be recommended that the nails are sculpted using acrylic rather than applying tips, as they may be difficult to attach and blend. Once the nail enhancements have been applied, recommend to the client that they return for a maintenance treatment after one week to check for lifting of the product, as this can be an issue for nail-biters. Subsequent maintenance treatments should be carried out every two to three weeks.

Provide nail enhancement services

Now that you have an understanding of the chemical processes involved in nail enhancement systems and the products, tools and equipment available, you are ready to carry out nail treatment techniques. This includes knowing how to maintain and remove nail enhancements.

To learn about the structure and functions of the nail and skin, see Anatomy and physiology, page 121.

How to communicate and behave in a professional manner

To learn more about the importance of communication and professional ethical conduct, see Client care and communication, page 35.

Health and safety working practices

Disposal of waste

Non-contaminated waste should be placed in a sealed or tied bag and placed outside the waste disposal container at the collection point at the end of the working day.

Think about it

To ensure that you maintain high standards while working, obtain a copy of the Code of Practice for Nail Services, which is produced by Habia, the body that sets the standards for the UK nail industry. The guidelines are designed to protect both the nail technician and client during and after treatment.

Cleaning up as you work

Nail technology can be very dusty work and this dust must be cleaned and removed during the service. This will ensure that products do not become contaminated and a hygienic treatment is delivered to the client.

Place lids back on any bottles of product used straight away. This will minimise any release of chemical vapours into the atmosphere and reactions with the air. Caring for products in this way will maintain their effectiveness for longer and prevent them from drying out. Clean up any spillages that occur during treatment to maintain health and safety. This will reduce the potential for harm to you and those around you.

Leaving the work area and equipment in a condition suitable for further nail services

Once the nail enhancement service is complete, the work area must be left in a suitable condition for further nail services. The nail technician must tidy the area as they go. Once they have finished using a product, the area must be cleaned and the product stored away, following manufacturer's instructions. In this way the area will be ready for the next service, so it can be carried out with clean, sterilised products and equipment and delays in the treatment rooms can be avoided. It will minimise the risk of cross-infection and present a professional image.

Ensuring the service is cost-effective

The commercially acceptable service time for an artificail nail enhancement service is two hours. It is important that you can work competently within this time limit, creating balanced, beautiful artifical nails. If you cannot carry out the service in a commercially acceptable service time, it could cause problems in the salon, delaying the changeover of treatment rooms and equipment. This could cause the other nail technicians to fall behind on their appointments, resulting in clients having to wait. A salon cannot run smoothly if the treatments are running behind. Clients expect a salon to keep to the appointment slots made and accommodate their needs. If a salon is known for running late and making clients wait, it cannot create or maintain a professional image. This will have an impact on the salon's ablity to maximise profits.

The importance of positioning yourself and the client correctly

As a nail technician, you may sit at a nail station for long hours at a time, carrying out treatment after treatment. This can cause major problems if your posture is incorrect. The nail station should be wide enough for the treatment to be carried out comfortably, with the client's and nail technician's hands meeting in the middle of the station without the need to stretch arms.

A nail technician's chair should be on wheels, with the facility to raise or lower its height. You should be able to sit comfortably with your hands/arms level with the nail station. If your position is too high or too low, you will experience back pain, which will become progressively worse over a period of time. You should face the client and not sit at an angle. Many technicians find that the nails they

Top tip

If you intend on working as a mobile nail technician, invest in a good mobile, fold-away nail table. This will make you look professional and mean that you won't have to work at uncomfortable or awkward angles at client's tables.

produce are cut at an odd angle, causing them to reshape them at the end of the service, adding extra time to the treatment.

To learn more about the importance of correctly positioning yourself and the client, see Follow health and safety practice in the salon, page 19, and Provide manicure and pedicure treatments, page 165.

Nail treatment techniques

It is impossible to produce good-quality, long-lasting nails with improper preparation.

Many nail technicians blame adhesion problems on particular product systems – the reality is that 99 per cent of the time they are the result of incorrect nail preparation. No matter what nail service you are performing or which product you are using, correct preparation of the nails is vital to ensure that artificial nails do not lift and to maximise the product's benefits.

Natural nail preparation is one of the most important stages of the artificial nail application. Preparation must not be rushed and a thorough job should be carried out. Without sufficient nail preparation, the nail technician will experience lifting of the overlay and possible infection of the cuticle and natural nail.

Lifting of the overlay occurs when a layer of cuticle is left adhered to the nail between the natural nail and the overlay of product including liquid and powder, UV gel and wraps. The cuticle acts as a barrier between the product and nail plate, causing the product to separate from the nail. This usually occurs at the base of the nail. However, over time the lifting can work its way up the nail plate, separating more of the artificial nail. Lifted products can prove to be too tempting for some clients to leave, and results in clients picking off the lifted product in between treatments and damaging the natural nail beneath. The natural nail plate becomes thin and sore, as it can be unknowingly removed alongside the lifted product. The artificial nail becomes unsightly and catches on things, causing the client pain. This can cause a breakdown of the service and the client may not return for further treatment.

Removing this lifted product can be carried out during the maintenance treatment and the artificial nails restored to their original state. However, the process of removing this lifted product is time-consuming and, if not carried out correctly, can cause many problems. Lifting of the product can be eliminated if perfect preparation is carried out.

Pushing back the cuticle

Preparation ensures that the natural nail is free of any cuticle and skin **debris**, leaving the area neat and undamaged. The same preparation is carried out regardless of the artificial nail system that is used. It may be necessary, if the client has bitten nails with very overgrown cuticles, to recommend that a manicure be carried out prior to the artificial nail application, at a separate time. This enables the nail technician to soften the cuticle, push it back and remove the built-up layers of skin and membrane from the nail plate.

Key term

Debris – loose material such as bits of glue, nail filings and waste left over from a treatment.

Preparation will differ depending on the artificial nail brand used to apply the overlay. It involves pushing back the eponychium to expose the natural nail. This can be carried out using a cuticle remover if this is stated in the manufacturer's instructions. Use of products to soften the cuticle is not recommended at this stage. It is absorbed by the nail and can create a barrier between the nail plate and the overlay, which is difficult to remove.

A metal cuticle pusher is used to push back and remove any adhered cuticle and skin membrane from the nail plate. At this stage, it may be necessary to trim any untidy cuticle or hangnail using cuticle nippers, as they can be damaged through use of the files later in the application. There are many cuticle removers available. Most of them have a pusher at one end and a knife/blade at the other.

The technique of pushing back the cuticle and removing the skin from the nail plate must be carried out very carefully; if it is carried out incorrectly it can cause damage, by cutting the skin or digging into/scratching the nail plate. The implement must be used at a flat angle to the nail. The cuticle at the base of the nail must be pushed back, as well as the skin around the side walls. This area can be reached by pulling down on the skin at the side of the fingernail using the thumb and index finger.

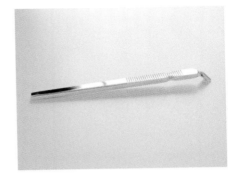

Cuticle remover

Using a file

The nail length must next be removed and the nail shaped to fit the contact area of the tip. The nail, if long, may need to be cut and filed using a natural nail file, to ensure it fits the chosen tips. The file must be used in long, sweeping movements in one direction at a 45° angle to the nail. It must not be used in seesaw movements. This creates heat in the nail and causes the cells to separate, creating splits in the free edge. The free edge must be cleaned of any filed nail debris by bevelling using the file. If this is not done, it will feel very uncomfortable for the client.

Preparing the natural nail

Once the layer or membrane of skin/cuticle is removed and the nail has been shaped, it is then lightly exfoliated or buffed to remove any debris. This is carried out using a 220/240 grit file or block. It is important that this is carried out carefully, avoiding the cuticle and surrounding skin. It is recommended that you move the block in the direction of nail growth, from the cuticle to the free edge, lifting the buffer back to the base of the cuticle each time. The corner of the block should be used to get into the nail grooves and beside the side walls of the nail to remove any excess debris. These movements should never be carried out from side wall to side wall without lifting the block from the nail, as this will cause friction, build heat and thin the nail below.

Once this preparation is complete, any cuticle and dust should be removed using a nail brush. The nail must then be cleaned and sterilised using a lint-free pad and the recommended nail sanitising solution. The nail should be rubbed with this solution and not just wiped, to ensure it is thoroughly cleaned and dehydrated. The nail is now ready for application of any of the artificial nail systems.

Top tips

- When using new files and buffers it is important that they are prepared prior to use. The edges of the files can be very sharp and if you are not careful, the client's nail and surrounding skin can be damaged by the file cutting the skin. The sharp edges of the file must be blunted before they are used. This can be done by using an old file and running it along the edges of the new file. This will remove the sharp corners and avoid the file slicing the client's skin.

- When using a three-way buffer to create a high-gloss shine, it is important that it is used in the direction of the nail growth. This will avoid damage to the nail and will stimulate nail growth.

- Dehydrating the natural nail ensures maximum adhesion of the overlay.

Provide and maintain nail enhancement

Step-by-step natural nail preparation

All steps need to be carried out to fully prepare the natural nail for all the artificial nail systems, including liquid and powder, UV gel and wraps (fibreglass and silk).

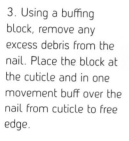

1. Prepare the natural nail for application of artificial nail systems.

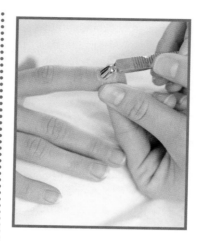

2. Apply cuticle remover to aid cuticle removal and then push back the cuticle using the metal cuticle pusher. Remove the excess skin membrane from the natural nail by holding the tool at a flat angle and pushing at the cuticle and side walls.

3. Using a buffing block, remove any excess debris from the nail. Place the block at the cuticle and in one movement buff over the nail from cuticle to free edge.

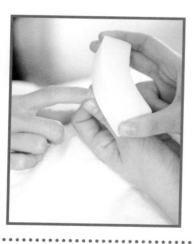

4. Reduce the length by filing the nail using a natural nail file in one direction and shape the free edge to fit the artificial nail tip.

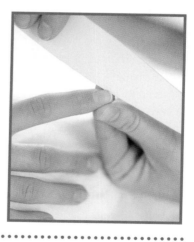

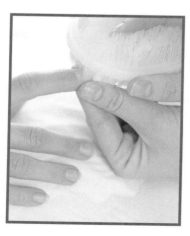

5. Remove any dust and cuticle using a nail brush.

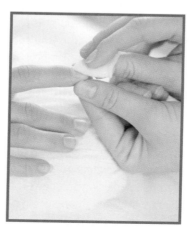

6. Using a lint-free pad and steriliser, clean and dehydrate the natural nail thoroughly by rubbing the nail.

Tip application

Follow the step-by-step process above to prepare the client's natural nails ready for the application of tips.

Nail tips are applied to the natural nail to add extra length and are combined with another nail service overlay. The plastic nail tips come in different shapes and sizes and it is important to select the right tip for the client and technician to work with. The application of the tip is extremely important — a poor application may cause the final result to be vulnerable to breaks and will look untidy. After completing this stage, the tip must look like it is part of the natural nail, as the overlay's job is to add strength, and if there are any mistakes you will not be able to rectify them.

How to choose the correct tip

Try to choose a tip that follows the same curve of the natural nail. Some clients have very flat nails, others may have curved nails. There are many different-shaped tips on the market and, depending on the manufacturer, they have various names, some with large contact areas, which should be **pre-tailored**, and others with smaller contact areas, ready to be applied. Choosing the wrong shape will cause a number of problems such as air bubbles between the tip and nail bed, which will show through the overlay and encourage bacteria or fungi to breed.

It is vital that the tip's contact area covers no more than one-third of the nail plate. The area of the tip that comes into contact on the natural nail is known as the contact area or stress area (see below). The larger the stress area, the more likely it is that the nail enhancement will come under stress and possibly break and fall off. Therefore, the smaller the contact area between the natural nail and nail tip, the more secure the tip will be. Remember that the overlay that is applied over the natural nail and tip provides the strength. The more coverage of product on the natural nail, the stronger the nail will be.

Nail tips come in ten different sizes and, depending on the brand of artificial nail system being used, 1 is usally the biggest and 10 the smallest. When choosing the tip size for each finger you must ensure that it covers the nail plate from side wall to side wall. When sizing a tip, ensure that you hold the tip so that its side runs along the side wall of the natural nail. Press down gently while holding the tip to see how it will look when glued on — this will allow you to check that it is the right size and fits the nail correctly. When it is in position, hold it there and, moving the finger, look at the other side wall of the nail, checking that the tip meets this side wall also.

If you are unsure, you must always try the size above and below to ensure you get the best fit. After application you must not have a gap at the side walls when the skin is pulled back. The tip may need to be pre-tailored prior to application. Pre-tailor the tip before it is adhered to the natural nail. It is always better to size up a tip and then pre-tailor it for a proper fit.

The application of a correct-sized tip is vital for the longevity of the artificial nail. Too small a tip will create a great deal of discomfort for the client. In order to make the tip adhere to the natural nail, you will need to apply pressure,

Top tip

Always begin any nail enhancement procedure by preparing the natural nail. Follow the step-by-step natural nail preparation.

Key term

Pre-tailor – tailoring the tip's contact area before it is glued onto the natural nail.

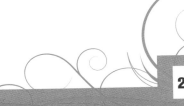

Top tips

- Spend time choosing the correct tip; this can make all the difference to a professional look.

- Always pre-tailor a tip to fit before application, as you cannot change it once it is attached to the natural nail.

flattening the natural curve of the tip. Once the tip is in place, it will try to spring back into its natural curve, pulling the natural nail below with it. This can cause the natural nail to feel tight and pinched, which can be very painful for the client. It will also be too small on the side walls and gaps will appear when the tip starts to grow out. The client will find that this will catch and become strained, causing the nail enhancement to snap off at the tip. A tip applied that is too big will stick and dig into the side walls of the natural nail. This will catch and rip off, damaging the natural nail below.

Features of a tip

Contact (stress) area/well area – This is the area that will fit onto and make contact with the natural nail. The contact area should never cover more than 30 per cent of the natural nail plate. The contact area can be reduced using curved scissors or a file.

Stop point – This is the small ridge on the underside of the contact area that acts as a stop point when the tip is applied to the nail plate. The natural nail free edge should fit snugly into this to create a seal when bonded.

Side walls – Tips either have parallel or tapered side walls to enhance the shape of the natural nail. The sides of the tip at the contact area are reinforced in order to provide maximum strength in this vulnerable area.

Upper arch/lower arch – Just like natural nails, tips have different-shaped upper arches – from flat to very curved. It is important that you select a tip of the correct size and shape when fitting it to the natural nail.

'C' curve – This is the natural curve on the nail from side wall to side wall. Never compromise on the fit of the 'C' curve; the tip should always fit comfortably.

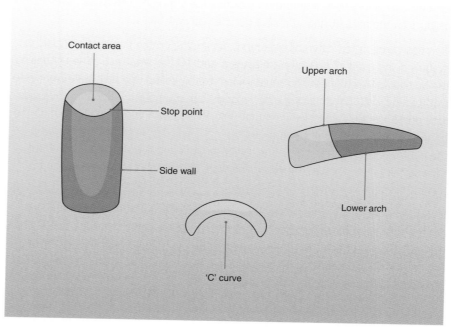

Features of a tip

Step-by-step tip application

Always begin a tip application procedure by preparing the natural nail — see step-by-step natural nail preparation on page 240. All steps are to be carried out for all the artificial nail systems including liquid and powder, UV gel and fibreglass and silk wraps.

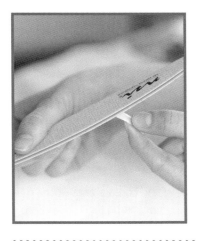

1. Pre-tailor the tip prior to application by holding the tip and using an artificial file at a 45° angle until the tip has been shaped to fit the natural nail. This will make the blending of the tip easier at a later stage.

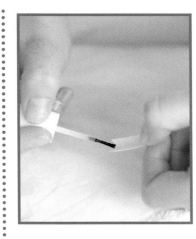

2. Place a small amount of adhesive in the contact area of the tip. Spread the adhesive across the contact area.

3. Pull the tip down until the contact area meets the free edge of the natural nail and bring it to a 45° angle. Once the tip is in place, apply even downward pressure to press out all of the air bubbles from under the tip. Hold for at least 10 seconds to allow a secure and airtight adhesion. Using a lint-free pad, wipe and remove any excess glue from the tip.

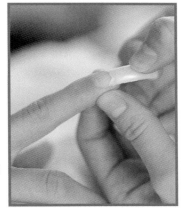

4. Cut the tip to size.

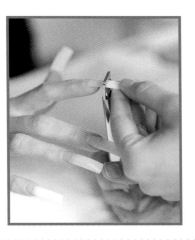

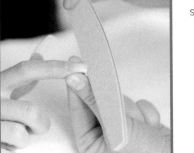

5. File the free edge to shape.

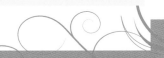

Top tip

Correctly adhere the tip to the natural nail to ensure longevity.

Removing air bubbles

If you see any air bubbles under the applied tips, it is important that you remove and reapply them, as these areas may become a source of bacterial or fungal infection. Air bubbles can also cause the structure to become insecure and may cause the tip to crack and fall off. The positioning of the air bubbles will indicate what the problems with application were:

- If the air bubbles are in the middle of the contact area of the tip, it indicates that when the tip was pushed downwards on the nail, it was not taken from a 45° angle. It was most likely just applied to the nail without squeezing out the air before it was adhered.

- If the air bubbles are positioned on the wings of the contact area, it will indicate that there was not enough glue applied to the contact area and it was not spread over the contact area.

- If the air bubbles are positioned at the furthest end of the contact area, beside the natural nail, it indicates that the tip was not pushed down fully onto the nail plate and so there is an area of tip not in contact with the natural nail.

- If the air bubbles are positioned at the inner side of the contact area at the free edge of the natural nail, it indicates that when the tip was pushed down onto the nail it was pushed too far, it pulled up at a slight angle and has started to come away from the free edge of the natural nail.

Blending the tip

The next step of the application process is to blend the tip to the natural nail. You must be careful when blending the tip seam line. Only ever blend in one direction and use long, sweeping movements with the file to avoid friction to the nail bed, or it will result in the client feeling heat or a burning sensation on the nail plate. Begin at the edge of the tip working down towards the seam. You must ensure that the shiny surface of the tip is removed. Using very light pressure, file over the base of the tip near the seam, avoiding the natural nail. The contact area on the tip will become thinner and thinner, until it cannot be seen.

Blending, if not carried out correctly, can cause an enormous amount of damage to the natural nail, including excessive thinning of the nail plate if the nail is caught by the artificial nail file. Ridges can form at the base of the tip and the natural nail. In the nail industry, this is known as 'red rings of fire'. A nail technician can identify when the artificial nails were applied using the ring of fire as an indicator.

Care must be taken to avoid the natural nail when blending in the tips. If the tip is not blended in sufficiently, it can cause ghost shadowing, known as visible demarcation lines. This is the line of contact area of the tip visible under the overlay. To remove this line, the tip requires further blending. This can cause a beautiful full set of overlays to look amateurish and it can be rectified easily if identified prior to the overlay application. If it is not dealt with at this stage, the full set of nail enhancements may need to be removed and reapplied.

Top tip

New artificial nail files can have very sharp edges. Use your old file to remove these sharp edges by running it along the file edge.

Step-by-step tip blending process

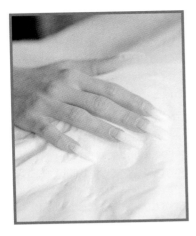

1. The tips are now applied and need to be blended into the natural nail.

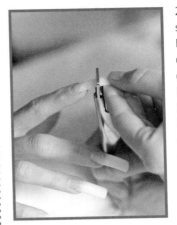

2. Use a tip cutter to gently squeeze and cut the nail tip. Ensure that you are wearing the correct PPE, including safety goggles. If tip cutters are used, the tip will be cut in a straight line and no cracking will result, because the tip cutters act as a guillotine, and there will be no discomfort to the client. However, if the technician tries to cut the plastic tip using nail clippers, this will cause the sides of the tip to bend upwards and possibly crack, which will be uncomfortable for the client. It may also cause the plastic to turn white where it was stressed and this will show through the overlay.

3. Use a 180 grit file to create the desired shape on the tip. If creating a square shape, just remove the sharp edges and corners.

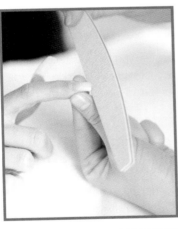

4. Use the file in a flat position on the contact area and length of the tip. Be careful when working near the seam line of the natural nail to avoid removing the shine from the tip and thinning out the tip. (Ensure that you do not burn into the natural nail, as this will cause friction (heat), leave a red mark, thin the client's natural nail and be very painful.)

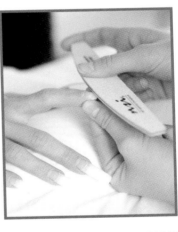

5. Use a white block for the finish.

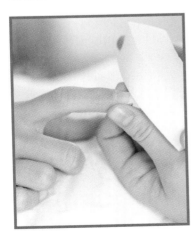

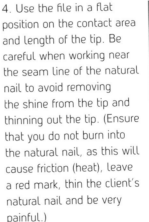

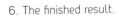

6. The finished result.

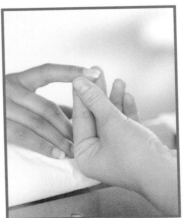

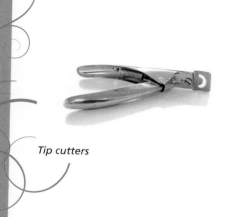

Tip cutters

Provide and maintain nail enhancement

Application of overlay

The application of natural nail overlays has become very popular over the past ten years with some nail product companies specialising in products used for this purpose alone. Natural nail overlays are used to give strength to the natural nail, allowing them to grow at their own pace and gradually giving natural length to the nail. The natural nail below the overlay is protected and so does not split or break as the nail might normally do. It is a way for the client to grow their own natural nails. Many clients who begin with a full set of nail extensions eventually end up with their own nails covered with an overlay.

Natural nail overlays are produced using two of the three artificial nail systems — UV gel and wraps. Liquid and powder is not a product that is commonly associated with this treatment, as it is too thick and bulky on the natural nail. UV gel and wraps flex with the natural nail below and give excellent results. UV gel allows for the use of a variety of colours, creating a permanent varnish effect, including French polish, that lasts longer on the nails. This treatment allows clients to be introduced to artificial nail products with the possibility of it being carried out on both fingernails and toenails.

Always begin an overlay application procedure by preparing the natural nail — see step-by-step natural nail preparation on page 240. Then follow the steps for application of tips on page 243.

Natural nail overlays are applied to the natural nail using either UV gel or wraps, which include fibreglass or silk. It is important when working with these products that you leave a free margin around the cuticle and side wall area of the nail.

This will avoid the product coming into contact with the skin and causing lifting. If the product comes into contact with the skin, it can cause overexposure and allergic reactions to the products used. This is especially common on clients where UV gel is applied.

Top tip

Apply overlay to all nails in the correct sequence following manufacturer's instructions.

How services can be adapted to suit client service needs, nail and skin conditions

Correcting problem nails requires an artistic and creative touch. When working on different shape nails such as flat nails, fan nails, bitten nails, ski-jump nails, crooked nails and hooked nails the application process of the tips will differ. The steps are similar to the basic application procedure; what changes is the way the materials are tailored to correct the problems. It is important to ensure that you follow the natural shape of the nail when applying the structure. However, not all natural nail shapes are perfect and so it is your job to correct the natural imperfections during the tipping stage followed by a planned overlay application to create the desired effect.

Correcting nail shapes

To learn about fingernail shapes, see Provide manicure and pedicure treatments, page 178.

Flat nails

Do not struggle to fit a nail tip onto the natural nail. Go one size up and pre-tailor the tip into a V-shape, avoiding any unnecessary pressure on the tip. This will allow the tip naturally to fit flatter to the nail plate. Apply the artificial nail system and apply more product above the stress area, creating a higher apex arch to give a more pronounced upper arch.

Fan nails

This is where the edge of the nail is wider than the base and the side of the walls. This nail shape is not very elegant if the shape is not corrected. Trim the natural nail as close to the free edge as possible. The correct tip size should be chosen carefully. When shaping the free edge, the side walls need to be narrowed in to compensate for the wide free edge.

Bitten nails

This is probably the biggest challenge for a technician. Size and pre-tailor the tip without regard to the length of the contact area, which must then be trimmed to half the length of the natural nail plate. Remove a small arch from the tip along the side wall line of the tip to relieve the pressure at the puffed skin by the free edge. This will allow the tip to sit securely against the nail plate.

Ski-jump nails

This is where the nail curves upward towards the tip, and is a relatively common shape. If a tip were put on to this nail shape without any correction, the nail would appear to be pointing upwards. Begin by filing the natural nail's free edge as close to the upturned edge as possible. Remove some of the contact area of the tip. When applying the tip, look at the side view to make sure the tip is curving down, even though the nail is curving the other way.

Crooked nails

A crooked nail is corrected by applying the nail tip in alignment with the finger rather than the growth of the natural nail.

Hooked nails

This nail has an exaggerated upper arch and the free edge has a tendency to curve over the end of the finger. The solution for this problem is to remove any free edge on the natural nail. A deep, curved nail tip should be chosen for this nail shape and care must be taken when applying the tip as there should be no gap between the underside of the nail tip and the nail plate.

Liquid and powder

It is always good to practise product control before attempting to create your first overlay. This will allow you to get the correct consistency. Consistency is determined by the amount of polymer powder blended with the monomer liquid.

> **Top tip**
>
> There are many systems of nail extensions available on the market today, and their application methods vary. Always follow the manufacturer's instructions to achieve the most effective and desired results.

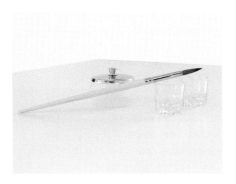

Dappen dish and acrylic brush

When the bead is perfect	When the bead is too wet	When the bead is too dry
• Strength and toughness • Clarity • Prevention of overexposure • Proper set and cure times	• Potential lifting and weakness • Bubbles • Overexposure • Lengthened set and cure times • Shrinkage	• Lifting • Weakness • Bubbles

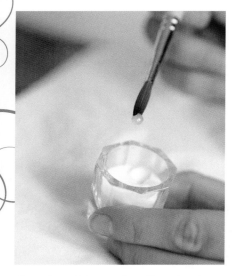

Correct consistency of acrylic on brush

It is important to get the liquid to powder consistency right. This can be achieved by the correct mix ratio:

- Wet consistency – 2 parts monomer to 1 part polymer: this creates good adhesion but can lead to cracking, lifting and peeling.

- Dry consistency – 1 part monomer to 1 part polymer: offers a strong enhancement but has little adhesion.

- Medium/wet consistency – 1.5 part monomer to 1 part polymer: combines the above, creating a strong and flexible enhancement with good adhesion.

If the product is too wet, the bead will fall off the brush; if the product is too dry, the bead will look uneven and have dry powder visible. A bead that is smooth and shiny in appearance and does not fall off the brush is the correct mix.

Make sure the brush is free from debris and then dip it into the liquid. Practise pressing and wiping the brush on the side of the Dappen dish to check how much liquid the brush will hold. Create a bead by using only the flat tip of the brush, gently drag and press into the powder. When a bead is on the brush it should have a slightly dimply look, not too shiny and not too firm.

Top tip

Train and trust your eye to determine the correct mix ratio and bead size.

Key term

Smile line – a curve on the nail that is created naturally by the hyponychium or a coloured artificial overlay or nail varnish.

Top tip

Check the shape of the nail from both sides and down the barrel to ensure a balanced and even structure as you apply product to each section of the nail.

At the end of the treatment, clean the brush in the monomer and wipe off any excess product. If using brush cleaner, take care to remove all brush cleaner before using the brush again, as this will contaminate the new monomer being used.

Top tip

When a smaller bead is required, extract more liquid from the brush by wiping it along the edges of the Dappen dish. Then dip it into the powder. Similarly, if you require a larger bead, do not wipe as much liquid out of the brush prior to dipping it into the powder.

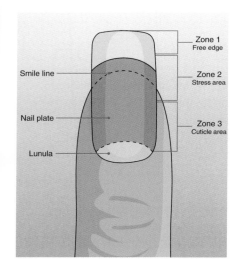

Zones of the nail

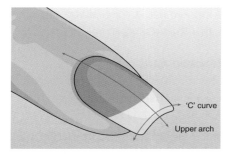

Apex arch

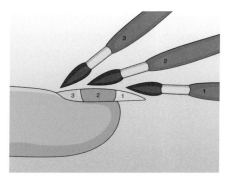

Three positions for applying acrylic beads

Step-by-step clear liquid and powder overlay application process

1. Prepare the natural nail as described in the step-by-step on page 240. Tip and blend the natural nails and tips as described on page 245. Remove dust with a dust brush. Sanitise and dehydrate the nail using a lint-free wipe and steriliser. Apply primer to the natural nail, avoiding contact with the soft skin tissue and the plastic tip.

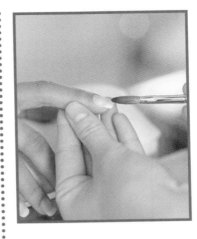

2. Using clear acrylic powder to pick up your first medium bead, place the bead in the middle of the free edge (zone 1). Using the end of the brush, press the bead down.

3. Keep the brush at an angle that allows the product to remain at its thickest point at the smile line. Push the product evenly across the nail, pressing and pushing the product over the tip (zone 1).

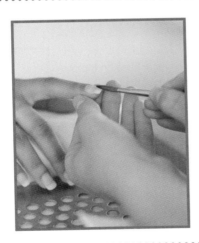

4. Using clear acrylic powder, pick up the second large bead. Place it onto the middle of the nail just above the stress area (zone 2) to create the apex arch. Press the product out towards the side walls, keeping most of the product in the middle of the nail. Draw the brush down over the product to smooth the surface.

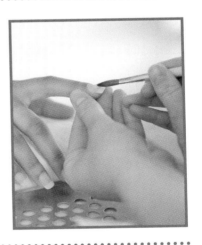

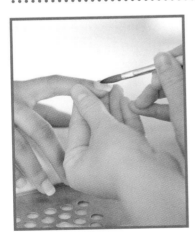

5. Pick up the third small bead and place in the middle of the nail (zone 3). Angle your brush to avoid 'flooding' the cuticle area. Press and push the bead towards the cuticle. Draw the brush down over the product to avoid a ridge at the cuticle area and to smooth the application. Repeat steps 2–5 on all nails.

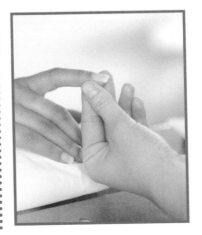

6. The finished result.

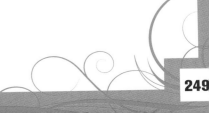

UV gel

In the UV gel system, the gels are mixed for you and so all of the problems related to improper mix ratio with liquid and powder do not exist. Remember to keep your tools clean. Brushes must be thoroughly cleaned using a lint-free pad and a gel wipe-off solution. When you have finished the treatment, replace the lids on all pots and dispose of rubbish correctly.

Step-by-step clear UV gel overlay application process

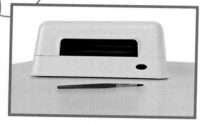

1. The key tools and equipment for gel nails

2. Prepare the natural nail as described in the step-by-step on page 240. Tip and blend the natural nails and tips as described on page 245. Remove dust with a dust brush. Sanitise and dehydrate the nail using a lint-free wipe and steriliser. Apply primer to the natural nail, avoiding contact with the soft skin tissue and the plastic tip.

3. Using the clear UV gel, pick up a very small bead of gel and apply a base coat of thin gel over each nail, placing both hands under the UV lamp to cure, following manufacturer's instructions.

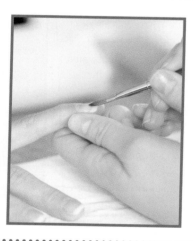

4. Using clear UV gel, pick up a large bead on the end of the brush and place it in zone 2. Work the gel into zone 3, with small circular motions. Leave a margin around the cuticle and side walls to ensure product does not touch surrounding soft tissue. To create the apex arch, work the gel into zone 1, ensuring the bulk of the gel stays in zone 2.

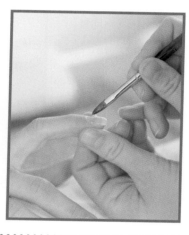

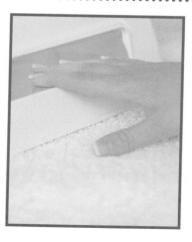

5. Check the structure of the nail from all angles, to ensure it is even. Keep the client's hands level and place under UV lamp. Cure for the recommended time as per manufacturer's instructions. Repeat procedure on two nails at a time, leaving thumbnails until the end. Continue applying gel until all fingers are complete, then carry out the same process on both thumbs.

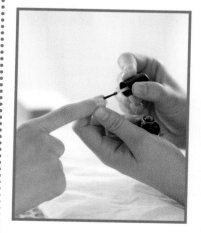

6. Once all nails are cured, remove sticky residue using a lint-free pad and gel wipe-off solution. File, buff and blend the nail, then apply a thin layer of UV gel top coat. If required by manufacturer's instructions, cure in UV lamp. Check the shape of the nail from both sides and down the barrel to ensure an even structure. Apply more gel if required.

Wraps (fibreglass and silk)

Step-by-step fibreglass and silk wraps application process

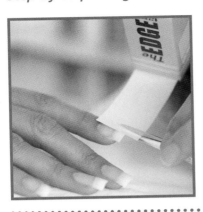

1. Prepare the natural nail (see page 240). Apply tips and blend into the natural nail (page 245). Remove dust, sanitise and dehydrate the nail. Using a pair of stork scissors, measure and cut the fibreglass or silk to fit the width of the nail to be worked on.

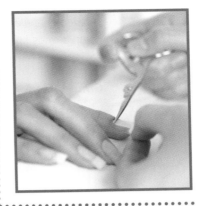

2. Remove sticky backing paper. Do not touch the wrap — oils/bacteria from your hands could prevent the resin from sticking or cause infection. Using tweezers or scissors, apply the wrap to the nail. Make sure it covers the nail but leave a margin. Use the backing paper to press onto the nail.

3. Trim the length of the wrap to slightly shorter than the nail tip. This will allow the resin to seal the tip and prevent lifting.

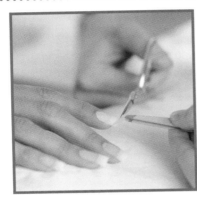

4. Measure and cut the fibreglass or silk, creating a small strip to reinforce the apex arch.

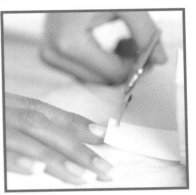

5. To reinforce and add strength to the apex arch, apply the small strip of wrap across the stress area of the nail.

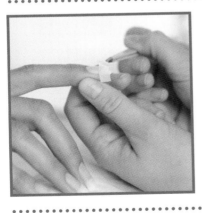

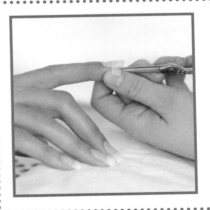

6. Cut the excess wrap from the sides of the stress strip.

7. Apply a small amount of resin down the centre of the nail, from cuticle to free edge, creating a line in the middle of the nail. Using a nozzle, push the resin into the wrap and across each side of the nail, encouraging the wrap to become sheer.

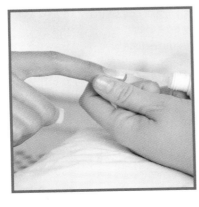

8. Hold a spray activator 15–25cm from the nail and spray once to cure the resin. Repeat steps 7 to 8 on each finger until three layers have been applied to create the apex arch. Check the shape of the nail to ensure it is even. Apply more resin and activator if required.

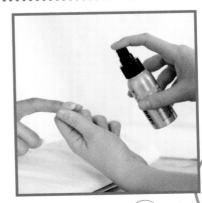

Finish filing

Using buffing and filing techniques will allow you to create a balanced nail with an even shape and length and a smooth, even surface. This process is often referred to as finish filing or buffing. The process is carried out to complete all nail enhancement systems.

Guidelines for filing

- Use a 180 grit file or higher to start off the process.
- Use a new file on each client or have a client file that is stored with their client record card and reused each visit.
- Have a firm hold of the client's finger. This will allow you to control where the file comes into contact.
- Avoid filing too much in the one area, as this will cause heat friction to the fingernail and will be very uncomfortable.
- Roll the finger from side to side to keep the file moving evenly along the surface.

> **Top tip**
>
> When applying wraps, ensure you have applied the resin evenly over the fibre or silk so that no fabric is uncovered. When you buff the product smooth at the end it will show the mesh pattern through the nail wherever the product was too thin or not there at all.

Step-by-step finish file process

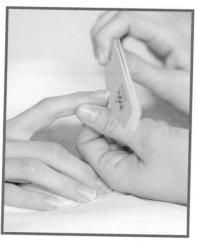
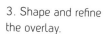

1. Create the shape of the artificial nail to meet the client's needs by using the file at the free edge and along the side walls, ensuring that the nail is not creating a fan shape.

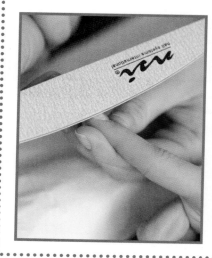

2. Turn the hand to the side, hold the file at a flat angle and buff the side walls, tapering the product from the sides to create a gradual thickness to the middle of the nail. Turn the hand to the other side and repeat. Once complete, the barrel of the nail should look even on both sides.

3. Shape and refine the overlay.

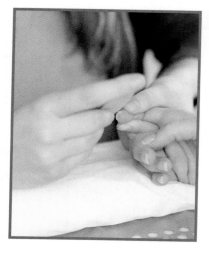

4. Working at the cuticle line with the file at a 30° angle, blend the product line so that the overlay is flush with the natural nail. Be careful not to file over the natural nail at the base of the cuticle. There should be no ridge at the join from natural nail to overlay.

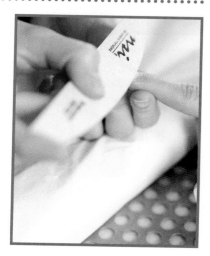

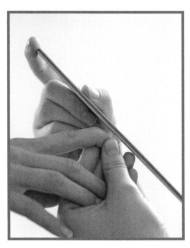

5. Look down the barrel of the nail. Use the file at a flat vertical angle in sweeping movements away from you, to buff and blend away bumps. Ensure you are left with an even layer of product that thins at the side walls. Buff the apex arch, to smooth and remove the bulk of product. Be careful not to remove too much. The apex arch area should be the thickest part of the artificial nail.

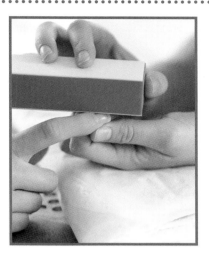

6. Bevel the nail and check the shape at the side walls. The side of the tip should continue in a line from the side walls. When working with both liquid and powder and wraps, use the three-way buffer to create a surface shine. Finish by applying a layer of oil to the nail.

How to maintain nail enhancements

Most clients start out as full-set clients. Subsequently, they become a maintenance client or a natural nail client. Skilfull maintenance is as important as application and will keep clients returning regularly.

Like hair, nails are continually growing and what was put on to a nail near to the nail fold will be in a different place in two weeks' time. There will be a gap at the base of the nail and the small area of the exposed nail plate will have cuticle attached to it. This regrowth can be very obvious.

There may also be some lifting of the overlay that is not very obvious, or at times there may even be a slight reaction to the products. After a period of natural nail growth, the structure that was created during application with the two curves meeting at the apex or stress area of the nail to create the strongest nail possible will have moved further away from the nail bed and could be on the free edge. This will unbalance the nail and make it susceptible to breakages. During maintenance, these problems are rectified and the nail enhancements returned to their original state.

Maintenance treatments include a treatment that allows the nail technician to check for any problems and infill the small area of regrowth, removing the ridge at the base of the cuticle by applying new product to this area. If required, the apex that has moved to the wrong place may need to be removed and repositioned into the correct place. Maintenance treatments vary in application depending on the rate of natural nail growth. An artificial nail that has severe lifting of the overlay must be removed correctly and reapplied. If 50 per cent of the artificial nail is missing, it must be removed and reapplied.

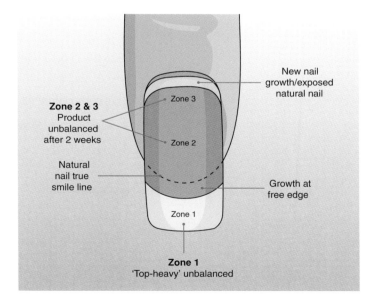

New nail growth/exposed natural nail

Zone 2 & 3 Product unbalanced after 2 weeks

Zone 3

Zone 2

Natural nail true smile line

Growth at free edge

Zone 1

Zone 1 'Top-heavy' unbalanced

Maintaining a nail enhancement by redoing the tip or reapplying product

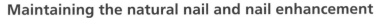

Maintaining the natural nail and nail enhancement

Before nail enhancements can be maintained, you must carry out a full consultation, identifying and recording any problems or changes that have occurred. As part of this, a service plan will be created, detailing any remedial work that is required to return the artificial nails to their original state.

Nail preparation takes up to 90 per cent of the time during a maintenance treatment:

1 Assess the nail – check for cracks, identify the length and check the side walls for curling away of product.

2 Refine the nail enhancement by reshaping and refining the side walls.

3 In zone 3, prepare the cuticles by pushing them back. Use light filing movements over any lifted product to thin it down and allow it to crack away and dissolve under the file. Thin the infill line at the cuticle and remove the shine from the new natural nail.

4 In zones 1 and 2, check for any cracks and splits. In zone 1, if length has been removed, the barrel will be very thick as you will be in the centre of the old apex arch. This must be thinned down and the bulk removed. In zone 2, the side walls may need to be tapered in and any further lifting in this area removed.

5 The nail must be sterilised in preparation for the overlay product.

Using nail maintenance techniques to restore the nail enhancement

Liquid and powder

1 Apply the nail primer to the exposed natural nail only.

2 In zone 1, apply a small bead of clear acrylic and press and push the product to the cuticle line, ensuring that a margin is left around the nail.

3 If required, reapply acrylic to zone 2 at the apex arch, drawing the brush down over the entire nail.

4 Repeat on all nails.

5 Finish file the nail and apply oil to the finished nails.

UV gel

1 Apply the nail primer to the exposed natural nail only.

2 Apply a thin layer of base coat gel and cure under the UV lamp.

3 Pick up a small bead of clear gel and apply it to zone 3. Work it out to the edge of the nail by the cuticle, ensuring that a margin is left around the nail. Reapply gel to the apex arch if required.

4 Cure under UV lamp for 2 minutes or according to the manufacturer's instructions.

5 Repeat on all nails.

6 Finish file the nail and apply oil to the finished nails.

Wraps

If the client is returning for a maintenance treatment for the first time, they may not require the wrap to be applied as the growth area will be minimal. Only reapply the wrap if there is significant lifting, a large regrowth area or it is the second maintenance treatment.

1 If required, cut a small amount of wrap to fit in the regrowth line and apply using the backing paper.

2 Apply a small amount of resin to the regrowth area of the nail and blend it up on to the rest of the nail.

3 Apply the activator as previously directed.

4 Reapply the resin and activator until the desired thickness is achieved.

5 Repeat on all nails.

6 Finish filing the nail and apply oil to the finished nails.

Natural nail repair

The natural nail can be repaired using a wrap overlay. This is the only system that can be used to complete this technique. The vulnerable area will be reinforced by applying the fabric including silk or fibreglass over the split and overlayed using resin and activator.

Use buffing and filing techniques to leave the nail balanced with a smooth, even surface shine and to the required shape and length.

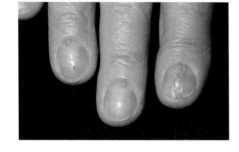

A badly split nail

How to remove nail enhancements

If artificial nails are removed incorrectly, this may cause:

- thinning of the natural nail plate

- increased risk of infection

- damage to the surrounding skin

- damage to the nail plate

- loss of business

- client dissatisfaction.

When carrying out a buff-off removal it is possible to over-buff, causing excessive thinning of the natural nail. This can be extremely painful and cause sensitivity when applying pressure to the fingertips or soaking them in warm water.

If the nail is not prepared prior to a soak-off removal with the application of a barrier cream or oil, the artificial tip remover or acetone will dry out the nail and surrounding skin. When carrying out a soak-off removal some nail technicians can get a little impatient; if the tip remover is not left to work and dissolve the overlay effectively, the product is then scraped off. This can cause damage to the natural nail below by scratching or gouging the nail plate.

Removal of UV gel – buff-off

Most of the UV gel on the market is non-porous, so the removal will require buffing off. When carrying out a buff-off removal, care must be taken not to damage the natural nail beneath by overfiling and thinning the nail, which will create sensitivity.

1 Reduce the length of the free edge using tip cutters and files.

2 Begin by buffing down the gel overlay. Ensure that friction is not created by vigorous filing, as this can be very uncomfortable for the client. The product should never be forcefully removed by picking or scraping. This will cause damage to the nail below.

3 Repeat on both hands until the product has been completely removed.

4 Continue with the natural nail preparation before reapplying the new nails or perform a natural nail manicure if the client no longer wishes to wear nail extensions.

Removal of liquid and powder and wraps

Soak-off method

Liquid and powder and wraps are both porous products, which means that they allow products such as acetone to penetrate them. The acetone or tip remover works by breaking down the structure of the nail enhancement. This is the soak-off method. This method can be approached in many ways, depending on the tools and equipment available. Acetone must be used in glass or ceramic bowls as it has the ability to melt products and could cause damage to plastic bowls.

1 Pour approximately 2—3 centimetres of acetone into two glass bowls and place the bowls into two larger bowls containing hot water. (Warming the acetone will accelerate the soak-off of the product.)

2 Prepare the area for treatment by applying oil or a barrier cream to the skin prior to immersing the nails in the acetone.

3 Place the fingertips in the acetone and cover the bowl with a towel. This helps to keep the acetone warm and prevent acetone fumes from being released into the air.

4 Leave the fingers soaking for approximately 20 minutes.

5 Remove the first hand from the acetone and begin to tease the product off using an orange stick. Do not use force to remove the product as it will damage the natural nail plate.

6 Repeat on both hands until the product has been removed. Submerge the nails if required in the acetone once more.

7 Dispose of the acetone by soaking it up with couch roll and placing it in the bin.

Top tip

When using acetone always use a glass or ceramic bowls. Acetone will dissolve a plastic bowl.

Top tip

Never pour acetone down the sink as it can damage the pipes.

Foil method

1 Soak a cotton wool pad in acetone and wrap it around the nail.

2 Cut a square of foil and wrap it around the nail and finger.

3 Repeat this step for all nails that need to be soaked off.

4 After 10 minutes, unwrap one nail and gently ease the product off using an orange stick.

5 Continue the process until all the product is removed.

6 Ask the client to wash their hands.

7 Gently buff smooth each nail with a white block.

8 Offer the client a manicure.

Contra-actions that may occur during and following service and how to respond

Contra-actions can occur during the service, for example the technician may cut the client's skin or burn into the nail plate with excessive filing, or after the treatment, if the client develops an allergy to the products used.

It is important that you respond to any contra-actions that occur during the treatment and it is your responsibility to educate the client on what to do if they encounter any further contra-actions when they get home. The table below identifies the main contra-actions, how they are caused and what actions should be taken.

Key term

Contra-action – an allergic reaction to any aspect of the treatment. The skin may appear red, swollen and itchy.

Contra-action	Causes	Solution
Cracking of product	Incorrect mix ratio Trauma to the applied product	Remove product and reassess the mix ratio used Remove the product and reapply, ensuring no further trauma is created
Bacterial/fungal infection of nail	Improper preparation Contaminated tools Lifting of the overlay	Remove product, sterilise nail and equipment thoroughly and advise client to contact GP. Once infection has cleared up, ensure effective nail preparation is carried out
Irritation or allergic reaction	Chemical overexposure Inefficient consultation	Remove product and advise client to contact GP. Try another artificial nail system once the symptoms have cleared up. Carry out a full consultation, recording all information and gaining client's signature
Yellowing of product	UV light destruction Staining of varnish used	Buff any visible yellowing using a white block and advise the client to use a base coat and a top coat
Breakage of artificial nail	Not following aftercare advice Incorrect tipping Unbalanced apex arch	Client to return to the salon and have the remaining product removed from the nail and reapplied, ensuring the correct size tip is selected and the apex arch is sufficiently thick
Lifting of product	Product applied too thinly Incorrect nail preparation	Client to return to the salon and have any remaining lifted product removed and reapplied, ensuring the product is not too thin at the cuticle and nail preparation is carried out effectively

Contra-actions – causes and solutions

Top tip

Always ask the client to pay before painting their nails to avoid smudging nail varnish. They could also put on their coat.

Top tip

At the end of the treatment, remember to record the results of the service. To learn more about record cards, see Client care and communication in beauty-related industries, page 42.

Top tip

Always provide the client with an informative aftercare advice leaflet. This will ensure they have all the information to hand on how to look after their nails. It will also ensure they have your contact details. Giving good aftercare advice ensures no complaints can be made.

Contra-actions also cover things that the client should avoid doing after treatment. For example:

- ensure that the client has paid for the treatment, put on their coat and removed anything needed from their pocket or handbag to avoid smudging the varnish
- wear rubber gloves when hands are in water or when using chemicals
- do not use nails as tools
- do not pick any lifting material
- treat nails in the same way as you would the natural nail.

The importance of completing the service to the satisfaction of the client

To learn more the importance of client feedback, see Client care and communication in beauty-related industries, page 47.

Provide aftercare advice

Aftercare advice should be given to clients to give them the necessary understanding and skills to maintain and protect their nails at home. This will result in the nail enhancements lasting longer and being more durable. It avoids the possibility of contra-actions occurring and should result in client satisfaction with the service and advice that they have received. Regular maintenance services should be recommended to the client. The frequency of maintenance treatments will vary depending on the rate of natural nail growth but is usually every two to three weeks. However, the client must be advised to return to the salon if they accidently damage their nail enhancements and not try to fix them at home as this can result in contra-actions such as infection.

Homecare advice

Advise the client to:

- apply cuticle oil daily — this will protect the natural nail below and also stimulates circulation to the area, bringing nutrients to the natural nails
- regularly use a quality hand and nail cream
- use a protective base coat to prevent staining of the artificial nails
- use a protective top coat
- use a non-acetone varnish remover
- wear gloves when carrying out household chores.

Future treatment needs

Advise the client to:

- have regular salon maintenance treatments every two to three weeks

- return to the salon if any lifting or breaks occur

- return to the salon if they want to remove the nails so that they can be correctly soaked or buffed off

- avoid activities which may cause contra-actions.

You could also recommend other appropriate salon treatments such as nail art.

Check your knowledge

1. What are the three main artificial nail systems available?

2. What is polymerisation?

3. What zone is the free edge?

4. What are tip cutters used for?

5. What solvent is used to remove nail enhancements?

6. What damage can nail enhancement products do to the natural nail plate?
   a) Thinning and softening
   b) Thickening and hardening
   c) Thinning and hardening
   d) Softening and thickening

7. At what angle should you hold your file when filing?
   a) 90°
   b) 45°

8. Why is it important to provide good aftercare advice? (Note: you can choose more than one answer.)
   a) To make the salon manager happy
   b) To appear professional
   c) So the client can look after her nails at home
   d) To make extra work for everyone

9. What is a contra-indication?

10. How often should you advise your client to return for maintenance?
    a) Every five weeks
    b) Every two to three weeks
    c) When the client feels like it
    d) Once a month

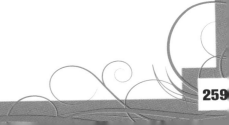

Getting ready for assessment

City & Guilds	VTCT
	VRQ
Evidence requirements: • To achieve this unit you must practically demonstrate in your everyday work that you have met the standards for extending, maintaining and repairing nails • The standards cover things you must do (performance criteria), things you must cover (range) and things you must know Knowledge and understanding criteria will be assessed by: • practical tasks • written and oral questioning • knowledge and understanding tasks(s) in an assignment • or an online test	Service times: • Nail enhancements (full set) – 120mins • Nail enhancement maintenance (1 colour) – 90mins • Nail enhancement removal – 60mins • Natural nail overlays – 75mins Evidence: • It is strongly recommended that the evidence for this unit be gathered in a realistic working environment • Simulation should be avoided where possible • You must practically demonstrate that you have met the required standard for this unit • All outcomes, assessment criteria and range statements must be achieved • Knowledge and understanding in this unit will be assessed by a mandatory written question paper. These questions are set by VTCT Knowledge and understanding will be assessed by: • a mandatory written question paper • oral questioning • a portfolio of evidence

Create an image based on a theme within the hair and beauty sector

What you will learn

■ Plan an image

■ Create an image

Introduction

Nail services is a very creative, **visual** industry. Artistic beauty therapists are drawn to it because it allows them to express themselves in their designs. This unit looks at the planning and research that goes into creating an image based on a theme, from first ideas to the final product, and all the work that takes place in between. This process will help you to develop your career, not only on the practical side but also by providing you with the skills required to communicate with others in the industry.

You will need to demonstrate a variety of skills in the planning stage, including independent research skills using media and whatever interests you. From here, you can find something that you are passionate about that will come across in your image. Without this passion, it will be hard to grab the attention and imagination of your target audience.

Throughout the unit, you will need to demonstrate that you can work safely, following your training establishment's and the manufacturers' guidelines to create the image. It is easy to get carried away with ideas and forget the simple health and safety procedures that must be adhered to.

Mood boards will help you to plan and coordinate the creations and theme that you put together during your research. They should be exciting and filled with ideas, colours, textures and techniques that you want to express in your image. Mood boards are a very visual tool, used in many industries, which may help to sell your idea to your audience as they get drawn into your artistic creation.

When going through the process from planning to creation of the image, **self-evaluation** is the key to further personal development. You should be constantly assessing your plan and ideas until the final image has been created. The whole process should then be evaluated to see if the image fitted its purpose and followed the ideas laid out in the planning stage. This will help with future projects and refining your skills when creating an image.

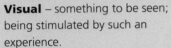

Key terms

Visual – something to be seen; being stimulated by such an experience.

Self-evaluation – appraisal of one's work, involving an evaluation of the process.

Plan an image

How to identify media images to create a theme

Media can play an important part when deciding on the theme for your image. We are influenced more than we think by what we see in magazines, adverts, TV and on the Internet. When researching, it is a good idea to collect images that attract your eye and fit with your theme. You can get inspiration from a wide range of media.

Many people base their image around **media styling**, sometimes combining different aspects to create one overall look. **Cultural and ethnic influences** might inspire you too. To be even more creative you may decide to follow a fantasy theme where anything goes, and you could draw on many different influences to create something unique.

Key terms

Media styling – styles that would be influenced by celebrities, films, television and music.

Cultural and ethnic influences – influences from various cultures from all over the world and various religions.

The target audience

You need to decide who your target audience is — who you want your image to appeal to. You can then select the forms of media that are appropriate for the age range. Younger audiences will be influenced by television adverts, the Internet, magazines and current music, while an older audience may be more interested in television documentaries and newspapers. There is a variety of radio and television programmes to suit all ages; some will be more appropriate than others.

Recording initial ideas

The beginning of the process, when you start your search for a theme, can be very daunting, as sometimes too many ideas come at once or you may have no ideas at all. When asked to put together an idea it is not uncommon at first to have a mental block.

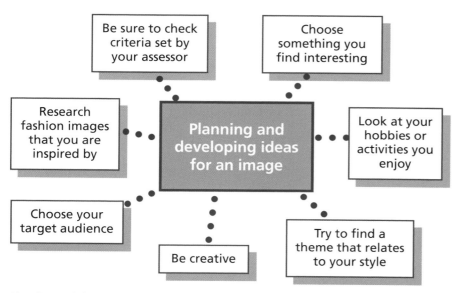

Planning and developing ideas

Normally, we can become creative and imaginative with a theme or topic that interests us. Without the interest, you will find it hard to sell your image to the target audience. The final image should be a reflection of your personality, so first take a look at your own lifestyle and sense of style.

Mind maps are an excellent tool to start jotting down initial ideas. All ideas that you think of should be recorded, even if they are very different. Once you have recorded some initial ideas, it is a good idea to leave the project for a while and come back to it later. This will give you time to think and you may find you are drawn back to one particular idea. The break allows you to work through the **concepts** and develop them further. If you have too many ideas, continually trying to develop them all into a theme may mean that the concept is lost.

At this stage you may find it better to work with other members of your group as you can bounce ideas off one another. Sometimes it only takes one person to plant a seed and the ideas then come rushing through and take the concept to another level.

> ### Key term
>
> **Concept** – the initial idea for the theme of your image.

Every person likes to work in different ways. The table below looks at the advantages and disadvantages of working within a team or on your own. Your salon may dictate how you work for this unit, so check with them before you start.

Top tip

The work you produce in the planning stage does not have to be neat, but you should have evidence of it to place in your portfolio to show how your initial ideas developed into the final image.

Individual planning	Group planning
<ul><li>You can explore more personal themes that interest you</li><li>It may be more challenging to develop your original ideas further</li><li>You can work at your own pace</li><li>It may be harder to stay motivated</li><li>The reward is greater when the final image is created</li><li>All responsibility lies with yourself</li></ul>	<ul><li>You may have to settle on a theme you are not enthusiastic about</li><li>You can bounce ideas off each other to take the concept to the next stage</li><li>One person may influence the group too much</li><li>The rate at which you work may be quicker as each person can have a different job role</li><li>The buzz of working in a group can keep you motivated</li></ul>

The purpose of a mood board

A mood board is a visual tool to present your ideas. It should be bright, colourful and attract the eye and show the journey you have taken to reach your final theme. It will aid the planning process for your image and will tie together themes and concepts in the early stages.

Creating the mood board

Collecting resources

When creating your mood board you will need to have a wide range of resources to hand. There is no right or wrong way of making a mood board — it should just consist of your ideas and inspirations. A3 paper is a good size to use, as anything smaller will not have the same impact. It is also advisable to lay out the materials to show how they work together. Anyone looking at the mood board should immediately be able to identify what your theme is going to be.

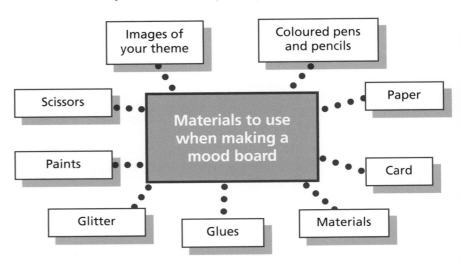

During your research, try to collect examples of everything that has influenced your theme. These will need to be evidenced on your mood board, but try to avoid putting too many different ideas on to the mood board, as they may confuse both you and the target audience of your overall theme.

Following health and safety guidelines

Protecting yourself and your working area is important at this stage — it can get very messy! Be careful where you work, as certain pens and paints may stain. Any spillages should be cleaned up immediately — you will risk spoiling your work if an accident were to happen. Keep the area organised so you can find the materials you need. There may be other people working in the same area, so avoid spreading your materials all around as they may be a trip hazard.

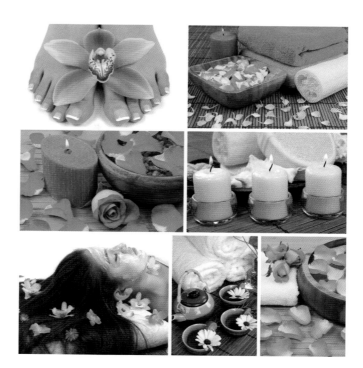

Example of a mood board

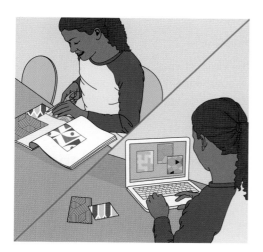

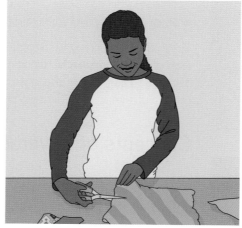

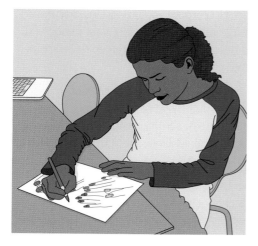

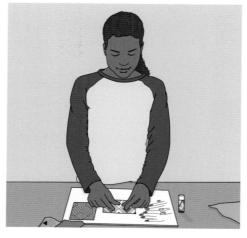

Creating a mood board

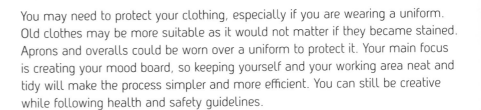

You may need to protect your clothing, especially if you are wearing a uniform. Old clothes may be more suitable as it would not matter if they became stained. Aprons and overalls could be worn over a uniform to protect it. Your main focus is creating your mood board, so keeping yourself and your working area neat and tidy will make the process simpler and more efficient. You can still be creative while following health and safety guidelines.

Evaluating the mood board

Although you will evaluate your final theme, it is also important to evaluate throughout the process. You may find ideas you placed on the mood board do not work as well as you first thought. This is the whole idea of the process – you can constantly change and update your theme. It will not be perfect at the first attempt.

Ask yourself these questions:

- Does the mood board fully express the concept of the theme?
- Does it identify colour schemes and materials you will use?
- Does it have a range of images relating to the theme?
- Is there a wide range of resources used on the mood board?
- Do the materials and colour schemes complement each other?
- Have you explained your choice of resources?

At this stage, you may wish to gather the views of your target audience in the form of **market research**. Handing out a **questionnaire** to the target audience will help you to gather their thoughts and ideas. It can help with decision making if you are unsure of any elements of your image.

Concepts of advertising to a target audience

Advertisements have a greater effect on us than we imagine, partly because the effect can often be subconscious. This section looks at how you can use advertising to promote your image to the target audience.

The mood board will be your main advertising tool. However, there are many other resources that you may wish to use to promote your image. As discussed earlier, your advertising tools must clearly outline the theme of your image and how it relates to the industry. Once you have decided on the target audience for your image, you can then choose suitable promotional tools.

Without advertising, companies would not be able to generate sales of their products, and audiences would be ill informed of the choices available. When promoting your image you will need to be able to communicate to your audience – they should be intrigued by your design – and convince them to give positive feedback.

- Positive advertising: this form of advertising will promote sales of a product and have the desired effect on the target audience. Examples of positive advertising include clients recommending the salon to friends and family, an

Key terms

Market research – gathering of information and data before introducing new products or concepts.

Questionnaire – set of questions given out for people to complete. Helps to gather information and opinions on a variety of topics.

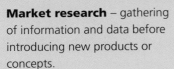

Check it out

Provide evidence when you make changes, so your assessor can see you have continually assessed and evaluated your theme. This could be in the form of a written paragraph identifying and explaining the changes you are going to make.

Top tip

Even though the image you create may not be promoting a product for sale, you are promoting your creativity and passion for the nail services industry.

Create an image based on a theme within the hair and beauty sector advertising campaign that increases sales, professional working relationships with other professional organisations, and advertisements in trade magazines.

- Negative advertising: inappropriate advertising methods may fail to have the effect you had planned and not allow you to connect with the target audience, which can lead to poor or negative feedback. Unfortunately, if your method of advertising does not appeal to the target audience, they may be left uninterested and unlikely to be inspired by your theme. Examples of negative advertising include an advertising campaign that fails to increase sales or even reduces business.

Nowadays anything can be used to advertise, and we are constantly bombarded with images wherever we go — from traditional methods, such as television adverts, to modern techniques such as mobile phone apps. The diagram below suggests ways to promote your image.

Check it out

You will need to present your image to your peers. Even if they are not your target audience you must demonstrate how you would adapt your presentation to appeal to them. Your assessor and peers may then ask questions about your image and how it came about.

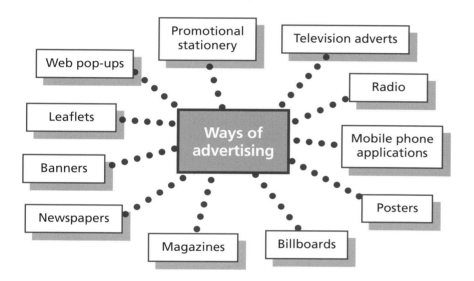

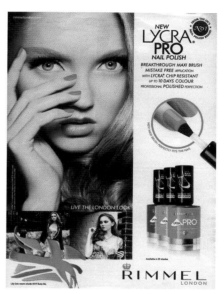

Sample advertisement

How to present a mood board to others

Once you have designed your image and carried out your research, you are ready to promote it to the target audience. For your qualification, you may be asked to carry out role play to create a realistic environment to carry out your promotion. Usually in the form of a presentation to your peers, it is your chance to communicate with the audience and take them on the journey of how your image was created. Along with the mood board, you may find it helpful to produce a chart showing each stage in your planning. Your chart will need to cover the following:

- Areas of interest and inspiration
- Initial ideas jotted down
- Shortlist of ideas
- Why you selected your theme
- What factors influenced your choice

Think about it

Can you think of any other advertising methods to add to the list above? Highlight the ones that you find particularly effective.

Check it out

Produce a chart showing your planning stages, using the areas suggested above. You may wish to include more details and other areas as appropriate.

- Who the theme is aimed at — target audience
- What textiles/colours/tools will help create the image
- How you will create the image — what skills are needed
- Creation of the mood board.

From the many methods of advertising available to you, it is advisable to select only a few of them to use in your promotion. Too many different methods may mean your message is lost and your target audience confused about what you want to achieve.

Presentation skills

Many people find the thought of having to do a presentation daunting — it can make them feel anxious and under pressure. If you are unsure about your topic, you may feel even more anxious. Having good knowledge and understanding of what you are going to talk about can increase your confidence levels. The positive aspect of presenting your image is that it is your chosen topic and one you feel passionately about.

Setting up the presentation

When setting up your presentation consider the following:

- Location — ensure there are no distractions or anything that may create too much background noise, for example radios, that the working area is well lit and there is plenty of room for people to sit comfortably.

- Preparation — ensure you have everything you need before commencing. Having to stop halfway because you have forgotten something is not professional.

- Display — check that your mood board and any other props you will be using can be seen clearly by your audience.

If your preparation is thorough it will make you feel more confident before the presentation begins. Remember your audience wants to hear about your ideas and inspirations, and they want to feel inspired too. Lack of preparation will make you feel tense and anxious, which will come across in your presentation.

Making the presentation

When making your presentation follow the suggested guidelines below.

- Speech — talk clearly and loudly enough for everyone to hear. Do not rush as your audience may not be able to understand you.

- Time — rehearse so you know roughly how long your presentation will take. Your training establishment may define how long it should take. Too long and your audience may start to switch off; too short and you may not have given them all the necessary information.

- Feedback — invite the audience to ask questions at the end. There may be areas of your image they want explained further. This shows they are interested in your image and not that they weren't listening properly.

- **Body language** – it is advisable to stand up during the presentation, as this looks professional. Sitting down inhibits the projection of your voice and it may appear that you are uninterested.

- Posture – stand up straight and use arms/hands as you talk, as this emphasises the points you are making.

Key term

Body language – communicating using, for example, gestures, expression and posture.

The salon's requirements for preparing the client, yourself and the work area

After the research and planning, you are now nearly ready to start creating your image. This will take place within a professional area of your training establishment and often with other learners around. You may all be participating and creating your image at once.

Your professional environment may become a buzz of excitement as you prepare your tools and equipment. It is not uncommon for people to become overexcited and this can have a detrimental effect on the whole atmosphere. This is out of your control, so just keep focused on the task in hand to avoid being distracted.

Remember that you will be under assessment during your preparation, not just when you are actually creating your image. Stay professional and calm and listen carefully to your assessor, who will be giving you instructions of their expectations and how to meet the assessment criteria. When receiving these instructions you should briefly stop your preparations so that you can pay full attention and not risk missing important points.

As you will be working closely alongside your peers, teamwork is still vital. Help each other in your set-up and respect other learners' working areas and equipment. Do not borrow items that are not yours unless you have asked permission.

During your preparation it is a good idea to write down a step-by-step guide as to how you will create your image on the day. This will ensure you carry out the steps in the correct order.

Choosing your model

Your model, who will act as the client, will play an important role in helping present your image and bring all your research and planning to life.

Here are some points to remember when selecting your model:

- Can they commit to the day and any rehearsal days?

- Select someone who fits the theme of your image.

- As the image will be photographed, good skin, bone structure, healthy hands and nails are essential.

- Check the condition of the skin on the body if this is going to play a part in creating your image.

- Ensure they help to prepare themselves for the day – skin, hair, nails etc.

Top tip

It is a good idea to get together with your model to discuss the concept of your image and then have a run-through. Even if you do not have access to all the equipment at home, you can still practise elements of your image. This will also give your model a chance to see what will be expected of them on the day and ensure they feel comfortable about how they will be presented.

- Choose someone who is enthusiastic about the theme, as this will help to convey it.

On the day, give your model clear guidelines on what they need to wear while the image is being created. It may be advisable to protect their clothing in case products come into contact with it. Advise them not to wear any of their own jewellery unless it will form part of the image. This means you do not have to worry about the security of these items while you are working.

Preparation of your working area

In all the excitement of preparation of the working area, it is easy to forget about health and safety and general organisation. Remember, you will be continually assessed throughout the process, so good preparation will ensure that the creation of your image will go as smoothly as possible. Not having the correct tools and equipment on hand may prevent you from being able to create a part of your image.

On the day, remember to have with you:

- plans of your image
- rough step-by-step procedure
- products
- clean equipment
- mood board
- clothing, if applicable
- consumables — tissues, cotton wool etc.

It may take you some time to create your image, so your working area should be comfortable for both you and the model. Only have the tools you need to create your image — store anything else in a separate area. There is also a risk that clothing could get products on it, which could spoil it. The less cluttered your working area is at the start, the easier it will be to maintain it during the process.

There may be other members of your team in the professional environment and your untidy area could be a hazard to them. Your assessor will also need to walk around watching the images being created, so it must be safe for them also.

It is essential that the preparation of your area is carried out in a suitable amount of time. Your training establishment may insist that all learners start creating their image at the same time, so it would be unfair to hold other people up while you continue your set-up. Be logical when preparing your equipment and products — this will help you to avoid visiting the dispensary several times to get a selection of products. Keep focused on the task in hand and don't be distracted by the other people in your area.

Due to the types of products used in nail enhancement, you must demonstrate that you can set them up safely and in accordance with the relevant legislation. Your working area will be busy and full of a variety of products. These must be stored in suitable containers that follow your training establishment's requirements. It may not be possible to have out all the products that you wish,

Top tip

Remember to carry out **patch tests** on your model before the day of the presentation, as you will be using a variety of products on them. You must ensure they are all suitable for application on your model.

Key term

Patch test – testing of products (for example body paints or hair colour) to ensure client is not allergic to any of the ingredients. Should be carried out 24–48 hours before treatment and recorded on the client's record card.

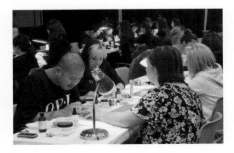

Have only the necessary tools and equipment for creating your image

due to their nature — check where would be the most suitable place to keep them until they are required. Your assessor may decide to retain certain products which learners can access when required. Apart from any health and safety issues, this will help to ensure that learners do not keep products to themselves and that everyone has access to them.

To learn more about health and safety guidelines, see Follow health and safety practice in the salon, page 1.

Preparing yourself

Finally, do not forget to prepare yourself for the activity ahead.

- Ensure you are in correct uniform, including suitable shoes.

- Secure your hair up and away from your face — this not only looks professional but will ensure your hair does not contaminate products or spoil your image.

- Protect your clothing with aprons and, if applicable, wear gloves to protect your hands, as some of the products you use may stain.

Create an image

How to communicate in a salon environment

During the activity, you will need to show that you can use the following methods to communicate:

- Speaking — to your assessor, model (client), peers and audience.

- Listening carefully to any instructions you are given and any questions asked by the audience at the end of the presentation.

- Body language — promoting yourself as a professional nail technician.

- Reading — following assessment criteria, manufacturers' instructions and relevant health and safety guidelines.

- Recording — showing your mood board and chart of planning stages.

- Following instructions — from your assessor and from manufacturers.

- Using a range of related terminology — showing your professionalism and your knowledge of the subject.

Technical skills required for creating a theme-based image

When creating your image you will be using a wide variety of beauty skills, not just from the nail services industry. All aspects of your model will come together to represent your theme, so you will need to be creative in all areas: fashion, hair, make-up and nail art/enhancements.

> **Top tip**
>
> As you will be carrying out practical treatments, you will still need to complete a detailed consultation plan to ensure your client (model) has no contra-indications that may prevent or restrict the treatment.

Fashion

From your research you will have selected fabric and materials that represent your theme. It does not necessarily mean you have to completely dress your model, but having clothes to match the theme will strengthen your image. It could be dressing of the hands and hair, if these are going to be the main aspects of your image.

Hair

You are not expected to be a hairdresser. However, if you are creating a complete look, the hair will need to be dressed in a way that complements the theme. It is your chance to be creative and experiment with styles that match your theme. In your rehearsal ensure your model's hair is suitable for the style you want. Keep it to a style that is straightforward to create on the day and make sure you allow enough time.

Make-up

Once again, you can be creative and experimental with products and application methods. There is a wide range of products available on the market to suit all themes, from high-street brands to more specialised theatrical brands. Patch testing will highlight if any of the products are not suitable for your model. During the rehearsal, plan a step-by-step guide as to how make-up will be applied and in what order — use a picture from your research to help guide you.

Nail art and enhancements

You alone will know what your skill level is like for this area. Some people have a real flare for nail art while others can struggle with the application methods. Work within your own abilities, to ensure you feel confident in the application methods. Stretching yourself will add extra pressure on the day and may make you feel anxious as you create your image. Being comfortable in what you are creating will keep you relaxed and focused on the task in hand.

For your image you may wish to use all, one or a variety of the skills highlighted above. Whichever you choose, ensure they complement each other and when viewed together express the same theme. If you decide to make one area your key feature, keep others subtle so they do not distract from the main image.

Safe and hygienic working practices

During the creation of your image, you must demonstrate that you can work safely and adhere to your training establishment's health and safety guidelines. If you fail to do this, you could be putting yourself, your model (client) and any other people in your working area at risk.

Here are some important points to remember:

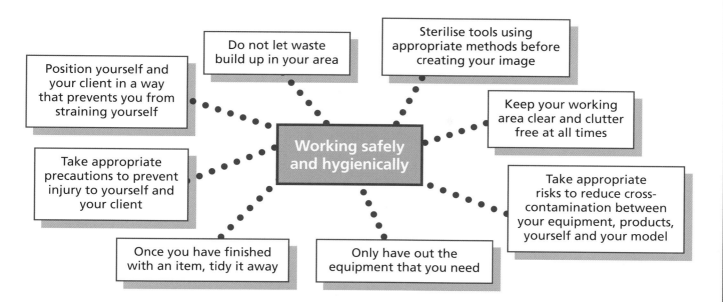

Methods of sterilisation

All tools and equipment need to be sterilised before you begin. Throughout the presentation, ensure they are kept sterile wherever possible. Avoid dropping them on the floor — if this happens, re-sterilise them. Have a sterilising solution such as Barbicide in your working area if appropriate.

Use disposable consumables and brushes where appropriate.

Disposal of waste

Waste left in your working area will increase the risk of contamination. Place all disposable materials in a waste bin and empty if it becomes full — do not let it overflow.

If you have left-over products, follow your training establishment's policies for disposal. For example, do not pour acetone down the sink. If there is any contaminated waste, ensure it is placed in the yellow bins so it can be disposed of appropriately.

COSHH

Particularly when you are creating images for nails you will need to adhere to COSHH regulations and store products appropriately. The working area must be kept well ventilated to avoid a build-up of fumes, and fans should be turned on if appropriate. Ensure all products are returned to their appropriate storage place when you have finished with them.

Personal protective equipment (PPE)

Protect yourself and your model throughout the session by wearing appropriate PPE. Your establishment will expect you to be in uniform and your client's clothes to be protected. When working with nail enhancement materials, wear a mask to prevent inhalation of dust and goggles to prevent products coming into contact with your eyes.

Salon life

My story

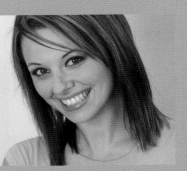

My name is Jenny and I have just finished my qualification in nail technology. As part of our course we had to create an image based on a theme. During the process we had to make presentations and create a mood board of ideas before creating the final look.

I found this experience quite daunting, as it seemed such a large project and I did not know where to start. There were so many areas to think about and all my other peers seemed to be racing ahead of me. My first hurdle was choosing a theme. I had so many in my head that I was not sure what direction to go in. After sitting down and discussing the project with my lecturer I began to start whittling down my choices. We started to look at my hobbies and interests and a common theme appeared, which was dance. I had always been a keen dancer and took classes from when I was little until a teenager. Ballet had always been my main passion, so I started to explore famous productions. Eventually I came up with the concept of Swan Lake.

After deciding on my theme I still felt quite daunted about the work ahead of me, so my lecturer helped me come up with a series of steps to work through. This really helped me break down the project into smaller, more manageable tasks. As I worked my way through each one I gathered ideas and evidence to place on my mood board. Before I knew it, it was full up. I was really proud of my mood board and I couldn't have been more excited to create my final image. My feedback from my lecturer was very positive, as she could see how much passion I had put into the project. From feeling quite overwhelmed at the beginning I turned it completely around by using my own background to guide me.

Ask the expert

Q Hairstyling is not one of my strengths. Will this have a detrimental effect on my image?

A No – everyone has strengths and weaknesses. Ensure your final image shows off areas that you have greater skills in. Opt for a hairstyle that is fairly simple to achieve but still complements your theme. If you choose something too adventurous, there is a greater risk of it going wrong.

Top Tip

Do not worry if you find the process daunting; just be sure to ask for help. It can sometimes be hard admitting that you need help when the rest of your peers are progressing well. Remember that everyone learns and develops their skills at different rates.

Finalising your image

All the hard work in your preparation will pay off when the final image is created. When you have carried out the necessary application take time to check your image for any improvements before it is presented. Small errors such as excess product left on the skin or uneven application could have a detrimental effect on your assessment. It is also a good idea to check that you have not forgotten to apply anything to your model that will complete the entire image.

Tidy up your working area so that when your image is viewed it shows a clean and hygienic place – untidiness could detract from your image.

Methods of evaluating the effectiveness of the creation of a theme-based image

During the planning stages, you constantly evaluated your image, developing new ideas and changing your concept until the final image was created. Many people do not even realise they are evaluating their work. They believe they are just changing their mind, but this is evaluation.

Verbal feedback

This can come from many different people in your working environment. Your model will comment on how well the process has gone and give their opinion of the final image. Your peers may also express opinions of your work — remember that your image and concept will not appeal to everyone. You have created an image that is based on your creativity and everyone has their own personal taste. Your assessor will give you verbal feedback on your final image and what you have achieved from an assessment aspect. Take the time to listen to everyone's comments, as it will help towards personal development.

Written feedback

This may take the form of a questionnaire that you hand out (see the example below), asking for feedback from your peers and any other people viewing your image. When completing the project this process may help you to assess how successful it has been and which areas could have been improved. Your assessor will give you written feedback to form part of your portfolio. This will show how you have covered the assessment criteria and in some cases which areas need more work. You should take time to read through the comments and ask questions if there is anything you do not understand or are unsure of.

Date:	
What are your favourite aspects of the created image?	
What are your least favourite aspects of the image?	
Does the image clearly represent its theme?	
If not, what could be changed?	

Example of a feedback questionnaire

Photographic evidence

For your portfolio you will need to have photographic evidence of your final image. It will need to clearly translate the creativity and work that has gone into the whole process. The diagram below shows some tips on taking photographs of your work.

Check it out

Your completed questionnaires can be kept as portfolio evidence. They should be anonymous, that is they should not ask for the names of people who fill them in.

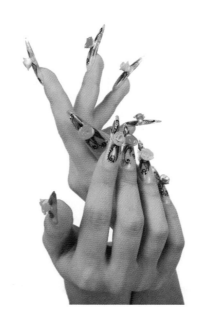
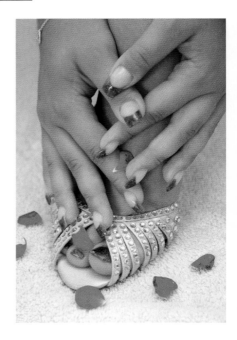

Photographs of final images

Create an image based on a theme within the hair and beauty sector

Top tip

Take care when taking your photographs, as this will be the only evidence of your image once everything is removed from your model. Ensure photos are saved onto a computer so they can be printed for your portfolio.

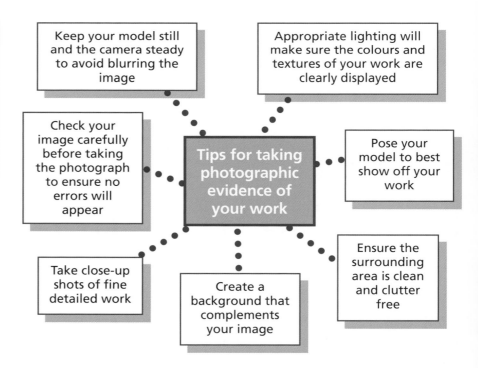

Keep your model still and the camera steady to avoid blurring the image

Appropriate lighting will make sure the colours and textures of your work are clearly displayed

Check your image carefully before taking the photograph to ensure no errors will appear

Tips for taking photographic evidence of your work

Pose your model to best show off your work

Take close-up shots of fine detailed work

Create a background that complements your image

Ensure the surrounding area is clean and clutter free

Your training establishment may wish to use your photographs to form a presentation of their learners' work, so make sure they are stored appropriately. This is an excellent way to show new and potential learners the exciting work they can be part off.

Self-evaluation

Your training establishment will encourage you to give your thoughts and opinions on your final image based on a theme. They may provide you with an evaluation form or you could create one yourself for your portfolio (see example below). You need to look at the whole process from start to finish and perform a **critical analysis** of each step. Some people find it hard to evaluate their own work, so perhaps take a step back and look at it as if it were someone else's piece of work. You will find there will be elements of the image you love and some you are not so keen on. Actually creating the image and using your technical skills will highlight what you found difficult and what areas you felt you excelled in. Given another chance, would there be anything you would do differently or change about your final image? This way of thinking shows self-evaluation, as you are identifying potential improvements to your work.

Why evaluation is so important

The process of evaluation may seem insignificant after the final image has been created, but it is important to highlight what you have gained from the whole experience. The experience you have in your training establishment will help form your future career and the areas you wish to specialise in.

The evaluation process should include negative areas as well as positive. What would we learn if we were always told there was no need to improve? There would be nothing for you to work towards and achieve. You need to be able to deal with positive and negative feedback whether it comes from yourself or someone else.

Positive feedback

This will give you a rush of confidence and make you feel proud of what you have created. It gives the whole process a purpose and makes you feel that all the hard work and frustrating times were worth it. It will highlight what your strengths are and ascertain your skill level in the nail services industry. Listen carefully to the feedback given, as it is easy to be carried away with the rush of excitement that praise gives.

Negative feedback

This is always harder to deal with and accept than positive feedback but is equally important. Without negative feedback we would have no determination to improve and achieve more in our careers. If you find negative feedback hard to accept, it is best to review it at a later date when you have more of an open mind. Have the feedback written down and read through it later when you can take on board what the other person is saying. Never take the feedback as being a personal attack — it is purely about the work that has been created. Constructive criticism should help you to

> **Key term**
>
> **Critical analysis** – objective analysis of your work and performance.

Date:	Theme of image:
Was your preparation sufficient for creating the image?	
Was your final image exactly as planned?	
If not, what was different?	
What did you find challenging about the process?	
What was your favourite part of the process?	
If you were to create this image again, would you do anything differently?	
Learner's signature:	Tutor's signature:

Example of a self-evaluation form

Check it out

Give more examples of how the Plan, Do, Review, Improve model is used in your training.

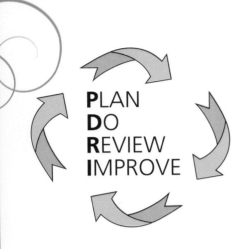

PLAN
DO
REVIEW
IMPROVE

1. Plan your client's treatment

2. Carry out your client's treatment

3. Evaluate the treatment and how the procedure went; seek feedback from your client

4. Improve your skills – the more you do something, the better you will become at it and the more chance you will have of achieving a high-standard result

Plan, Do, Review, Improve model and personal development flow chart

improve your skills and give advice on ways to improve your work. It should help you progress further in your training and give you something to work towards.

Personal development

The nail services industry is competitive and nail technicians are always trying to find new and creative ways to show off their skills and artistic side. This unit should help you to show your passion for the industry and the many different elements of your talent.

The evaluation of others and your self-evaluation will help determine the next stages of your career. Positive comments will highlight where your strengths are and what areas you could specialise in. This works well if your positive feedback matches the areas that you are interested in. When you do not feel passionately about something it is difficult to see yourself using the skill in the future, but the evaluation process should open your eyes and mind to areas of the industry you may not have considered before.

Similarly, negative feedback can highlight areas that need to be improved, which could be worked on in your training establishment, or push you to develop your skills further by attending external training courses. It can give you the motivation to improve on your weaknesses, showing you are well driven – and that is a personality trait employers will want to see. Throughout your training and career you may find some tasks too challenging, but then, through sheer determination, you can succeed, and use your determination as a strength.

The diagram below shows how a continual cycle of evaluation will keep you on a path of improving your skills. This can be applied in all areas of your training and education, even when carrying out nail services on your client.

Frequently asked questions

Q   What material should I create my mood board on?

A   You will need a large piece of strong card. Too small and you will not be able to fit much on. You will need to be able to transport it, so the card will have to be durable.

Q   If my model does not completely fit my theme will it matter?

A   A model that will complement your theme is best, otherwise you will have more work to do when creating your image. You will have to use more styling techniques to change the model's appearance, which could take up more of your valuable time.

Check your knowledge

1. What is the purpose of a mood board?

2. List five different media images that could be used to create your image.

3. What advertising methods would most appeal to a younger audience?

4. Compare the benefits and downfalls of working individually or within a group.

5. What legislation is linked to creating your image?

6. Why is positive body language important when making a presentation?

7. What may happen if you have not fully prepared for creating your image?

8. What combination of skills can you use to create your image?

9. List three methods of evaluating your image.

10. Why is evaluation so important for your personal development?

Getting ready for assessment

VRQs
City & Guilds
Service times: Not applicable to this unit

Evidence:
• Practical tasks to demonstrate you can plan and create an image

Knowledge and understanding will be assessed by an:
• assignment or online test |

Index